MEDICATED INTRAUTERINE DEVICES

DEVELOPMENTS IN OBSTETRICS AND GYNECOLOGY

VOLUME 5

1. J.E. Jirásek, Human fetal endocrines, 1980. ISBN 90-247-2325-6.
2. P.M. Motta, E.S.E. Hafez, eds., Biology of the ovary, 1980. ISBN 90-247-2316-7.
3. J. Horský, J. Presl, eds., Ovarian function and its disorders, 1980. ISBN 90-247-2326-4.
4. D.W. Richardson, D. Joyce, E.M. Symonds, eds., Frozen Human Semen, 1980. ISBN 90-247-2370-1.

Series ISBN 90-247-2334-5

MEDICATED INTRAUTERINE DEVICES

PHYSIOLOGICAL AND CLINICAL ASPECTS

edited by

E.S.E. HAFEZ
Detroit, Michigan, USA

and

W.A.A. VAN OS
Haarlem, The Netherlands

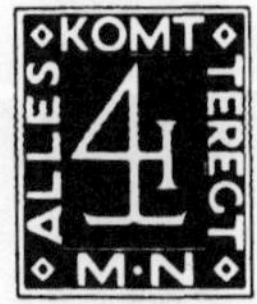

1980

MARTINUS NIJHOFF PUBLISHERS
THE HAGUE / BOSTON / LONDON

Distributors:

for the United States and Canada

Kluwer Boston, Inc.
190 Old Derby Street
Hingham, MA 02043
USA

for all other countries

Kluwer Academic Publishers Group
Distribution Center
P.O. Box 322
3300 AH Dordrecht
The Netherlands

Library of Congress Cataloging in Publication Data CIP

Main entry under title:

Medicated intrauterine devices.

(Developments in obstetrics and gynecology; v. 5)
Contributions from an international symposium held June 27-30, 1979 in Amsterdam.
Includes index.
1. Intrauterine contraceptives. Medicated – Congresses. 2. Intrauterine contraceptives – Congresses.
I. Hafez E.S.E., 1922- II. Os, W.A.A. van. III. Series.
RG137.3.M42 613.9'435 80-14373

ISBN-13: 978-94-009-8874-3 e-ISBN-13: 978-94-009-8872-9
DOI: 10.1007/978-94-009-8872-9

TABLE OF CONTENTS

II. CLINICAL ASPECTS

III. FUTURE DEVELOPMENT

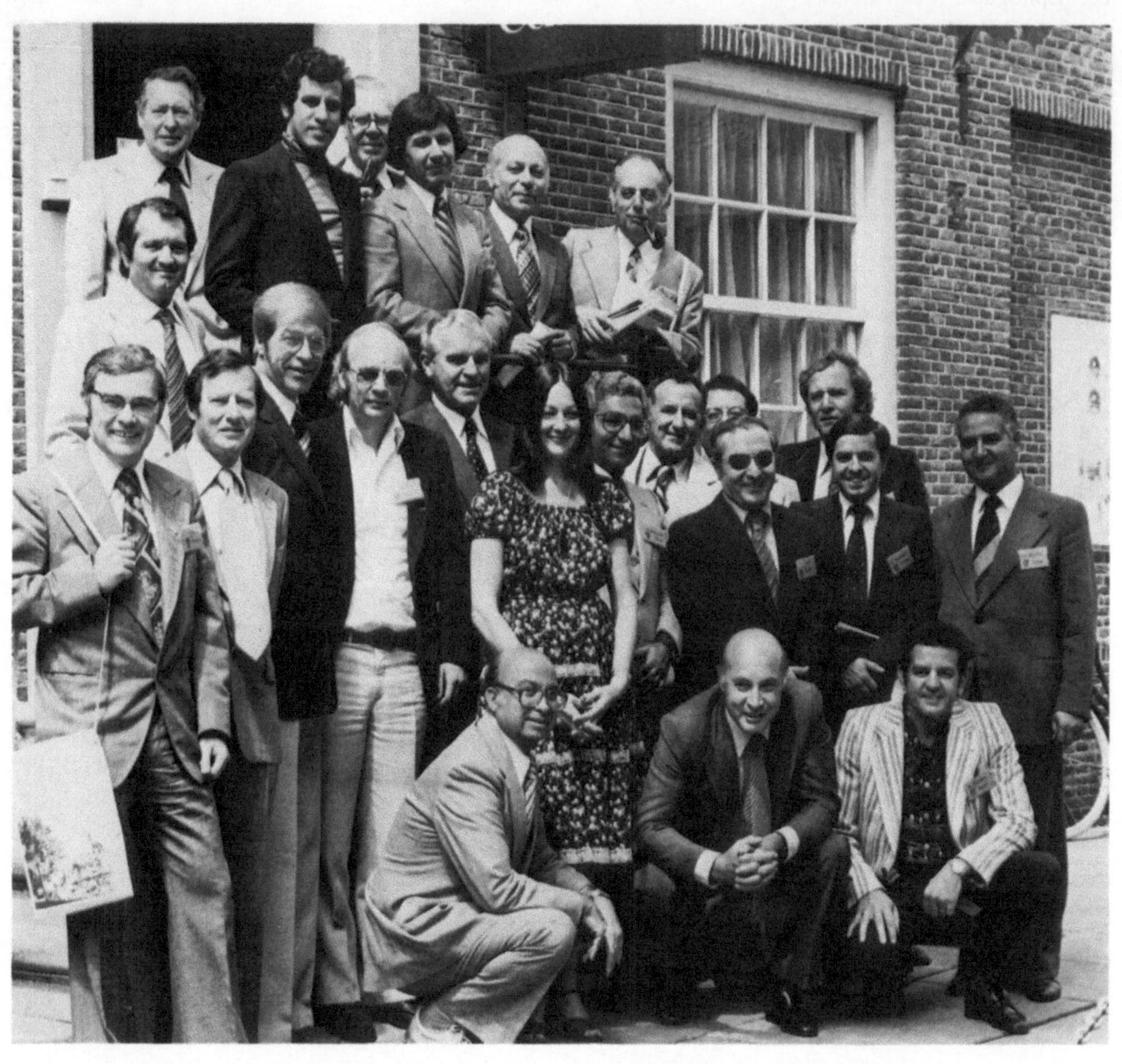

Medicated IUDs and Polymeric Delivery Systems International Symposium, June 27-30, 1979, Amsterdam, The Netherlands.

CONTRIBUTORS

ABDALLA, M.I.: Reproductive Endocrinology Research Unit, Department of Obstetrics and Gynecology, Faculty of Medicine, Cairo University, Cairo, Egypt

AMIRIKIA, H.: Department of Gynecology and Obstetrics, Wayne State University School of Medicine and Hutzel Hospital, 4707 St. Antoine, Detroit, Michigan 48201, USA

ANDOLŠEK, L.: University Gynecological Clinic of Ljubljana, 61000 Ljubljana, Slajmerjeva 3, Yugoslavia

BARWIN, B.N.: Hôspital général d'Ottawa, 43 Bruyère, Ottawa, Ontario K1N 5C8, Canada

BATÁR, I.: Department of Obstetrics and Gynecology, Medical University, Noi Klinika, Debrecen, Hungary

BAYAD, M.A.: Reproductive Endocrinology Research Unit, Department of Obstetrics and Gynecology, Faculty of Medicine, Cairo University, Cairo, Egypt

BELLER, F.K.: Frauenklinik, Abteilung Geburtshilfe und Gynäkologie der Westfälischen Wilhelms-Universität, Westring 11, D-4400 Münster, Federal Republic of Germany

BERGSTEIN, N.A.M.: Department of Obstetrics and Gynecology, Ziekenhuis Zevenaar, The Netherlands

BUCKINGHAM, M.S.: University of Southampton, Southampton General Hospital, Tremona Road, Southampton SO0 4XY 772, United Kingdom

CHANTLER, E.: University Hospital of South Manchester, Withington Hospital, Nell Lane, West Didsbury, Manchester M20 8LR, United Kingdom

COOPER, M.T.: Bureau of Medical Devices, Health Protection Branch, Health and Welfare Canada, Tunney's Pasture, Ottawa, Ontario K1A 0L2, Canada

EL-BADRAWI, H.H.: Department of Gynecology and Obstetrics, C.S. Mott Center for Human Growth and Development, Wayne State University School of Medicine, Detroit, Michigan 48201, USA and Faculty of Medicine, Cairo University, Cairo, Egypt

ELSTEIN, M.: University Hospital of South Manchester, Withington Hospital, Nell Lane, West Didsbury, Manchester M20 8LR, United Kingdom

GIBOR, Y.: Alza Corporation, Palo Alto, California, USA

GIESSEN, R.H.M. van der: Department of Obstetrics and Gynecology, Ziekenhuis Zevenaar, the Netherlands

HAFEZ, E.S.E.: Department of Gynecology and Obstetrics, and Department of Physiology, Wayne State University School of Medicine, Medical Research Building, 550 East Canfield, Detroit, Michigan 48201, USA

HASSON, H.M.: Department of Obstetrics and Gynecology, Grant Hospital of Chicago, Northwestern University School of Medicine, 2424 North Clark Street, Chicago, Illinois 60614, USA

IBRAHIM, I.: Reproductive Endocrinology Research Unit, Department of Obstetrics and Gynecology, Faculty of Medicine, Cairo University, Cairo, Egypt

KOSONEN, A.: Copper and Copper Alloy Division, Outokumpu Oy, PO Box 60, SF-28101, Pori 10, Finland

LUDWIG, K.S.: Anatomisches Institut der Universität, Pestalozzistrasse 20, CH-4056 Basel, Switzerland

LUUKKAINEN, T.: Steroid Research Laboratory, Department of Medical Chemistry, University of Helsinki, Siltavuorenpenger 10A, SF-00170 Helsinki 17, Finland

MALL-HAEFELI, M.: Sozialmedizinischer Dienst der Universitätsfrauenklinik, CH-4056 Basel, Switzerland

NOOYER, C.C.A. de: St. Elisabeth's of Groote Gasthuis, Department of Obstetrics and Gynecology, Boerhaavelaan 22, PO Box 417, 2000 AK Haarlem, The Netherlands

OS, W.A.A. van: Department of Obstetrics and Gynecology, St. Elisabeth's of Groote Gasthuis, Boerhaavelaan 22, PO Box 417, 2000 AK Haarlem, The Netherlands

OSMAN, I.: Reproductive Endocrinology Research Unit, Department of Obstetrics and Gynecology, Faculty of Medicine, Cairo University, Cairo, Egypt

PERCIVAL SMITH, R.: Student Health Service, University of British Columbia, Room 114, Wesbrook Place, Vancouver, British Columbia V6T IW5, Canada

RHEMREV, P.E.R.: Department of Obstetrics and Gynecology, St. Elisabeth's of Groote Gasthuis, PO Box 417, 2000 AK Haarlem, The Netherlands

SCHMIDT, E.H.: Frauenklinik, Abteilung Geburtshilfe und Gynäkologie der Westfälischen Wilhelms-Universität, Westring 11, D-4400 Münster, Federal Republic of Germany

SCIARRA, J.J.: Department of Obstetrics and Gynecology, Northwestern University Medical School, 333 East Superior Street, Room 490, Chicago, Illinois 60611, USA

SPORNITZ, U.M.: Anatomisches Institut der Universität, Pestalozzistrasse 20, CH-4056 Basel, Switzerland

STRYKER, J.C.: Department of Gynecology and Obstetrics, Wayne State University School of Medicine: Hutzel Hospital Pregnancy Drug Addiction Program, Hutzel Hospital Annex, 4707 St. Antoine, Detroit, Michigan 48201, USA

THIERY, M.: Division of Obstetrics, University Hospital, De Pintelaan 135, B-9000 Ghent, Belgium

THOMSEN, R.J.: Department of Obstetrics and Gynecology, 97th OBN OGA Hospital, Postfach 28, 6000 Frankfurt/Main, Federal Republic of Germany

TOPPOZADA, M.: Department of Obstetrics and Gynecology, University of Alexandria School of Medicine, Shatby Maternity Hospital, Alexandria, Egypt

UETTWILLER, A.: Laboratorien des Kantonsspitals Bruderholz, CH-4101 Bruderholz, Switzerland

VOSSENAAR, T.: Organon International BV, PO Box 20, 5340 BH Oss, The Netherlands

WERNER-ZODROW, J.: Sozialmedizinischer Dienst der Universitäts-frauenklinik, CH-4056 Basel, Switzerland

WHEELER, R.G.: International Fertility Research Program, Research Triangle Park, North Carolina 27709, USA

ZATUCHNI, G.I.: Program for Applied Research for Fertility Regulation, Northwestern University, 1040 Passavant Pavilion, 303 East Superior Street, Chicago, Illinois 60611, USA

PREFACE

Extensive basic research and clinical trials have been conducted on inert and medicated intrauterine devices. In the last decade, substantial progress has been made in understanding the modes of action and the physiological mechanisms of IUDs – progress resulting from modern techniques and instrumentation in microanatomy, immunology, pathology, endocrinology, biochemistry and biophysics. Such studies, however, are scattered in such a wide spectrum of journals that the clinician and family planner can hardly keep up to date with the advances.

An attempt is made in this volume to coordinate physiological and clinical parameters. Little is known about the possible role of diet, diseases and environmental factors.

The contributors, from a wide selection of professional groups, each have considerable experience in some aspect of reproductive physiology, gynecology, or family planning. There is in this volume an attempt to provide a total coverage of current progress in medicated intrauterine devices. The volume is intended for a broad readership, including physicians, medical workers, medical personnel, and administrators in family planning. It is hoped that this volume will serve as a stimulus to basic scientists and clinicians concerned with intrauterine devices to intensify their research toward better contraceptive techniques.

September 1980

E.S.E. Hafez
Detroit, Michigan
USA

ACKNOWLEDGEMENTS

Basic research, clinical trials, preparations of manuscripts, scanning electron microscopy, editorial assistance and presentation of results have been generously supported by the following institutions and organizations:

Alza Corporation, Palo Alto, California, USA
Battelle, Pacific Northwest Laboratories, Richland, Washington, USA
C.S. Mott Center for Human Growth and Development, Wayne State University, Detroit, Michigan, USA
Frauenklinik der Westfälischen Wilhelms-Universität, Universität Frauenklinik, Münster, Federal Republic of Germany
Freie Universität Berlin, Berlin, Federal Republic of Germany
Hutzel Hospital, Detroit, Michigan, USA
International Fertility Research Program (IFRP), Research Triangle Park, North Carolina, USA
International Planned Parenthood Federation, London, United Kingdom
Kensington, Chelsea and Westminster Area Health Authority (NE District) of the National Health Service, United Kingdom
Ministry of Foreign Affairs, Directorate-General for International Cooperation, The Hague, The Netherlands
Multilan SA, Fribourg, Switzerland
Outokumpu Oy, Finland
Program for Applied Research for Fertility Regulation (PARFR), Northwestern University, Chicago, Illinois, USA
Pathfinder Foundation, Chestnut Hill, Massachusetts. USA
St. Elizabeths of Groote Gasthuis, Haarlem, The Netherlands
Wayne State University School of Medicine, Detroit, Michigan, USA

Thanks and appreciation are due to the contributors who prepared their chapters meticulously; to Ms. Lori Rust for editorial skills; to Ms. Elma van Ekeris, Ms. Penny Stoops and Ms. Jackie Smieska for editorial assistance; and to Mr. Jeffrey Smith of Martinus Nijhoff for his cooperation during the publication of this volume.

E.S.E. H.
W.A.A. v. O.

FOREWORD

The role of the physician in improving the quality of life for the individual, and in family and community health, necessitates his familiarity with the benefits and risks of fertility regulation methods. The direction of the physician's activities – whether he provides care for the individual or within the framework of health programs – will further determine his need to be informed about social, political, religious and economic factors that influence population changes. It should be recognized that population change can never be examined as an isolated phenomenon. A uniform approach on a worldwide basis is not possible when evaluating regulation of population changes. The variations existing in different communities, regarding demographic characteristics, understanding of population issues, and the acceptability of the available contraceptive methods, preclude uniformity.

There is a relationship between state of health and fertility. Notwithstanding other factors that may be involved, fertility regulation for health reasons is universally accepted. The social and economic consequences of population growth have induced many countries to set up national programs for fertility regulation, but it is ultimately up to the individual physican to apply his knowledge and expertise of existing methods in the most responsible way.

Developments in the field of fertility regulation in recent years may not have been revolutionary, but advances have been made. In the area of oral contraceptives, the doses administered have lessened without the apparent sacrifice of contraceptive reliability. Epidemiological investigations have made major contributions to the identification of risk factors, allowing for a better selection of women with regard to the choice of contraceptive method. Among these methods, the intrauterine device (IUD) presently occupies a predominant position.

The first publications regarding a practical IUD date from the beginning of this century, but the widespread application of such devices did not occur until about 1960, since then the devices in existence have improved. Research efforts have been geared toward making IUDs as effective as possible while at the same time minimizing the number of side effects. The results indicate that acceptability no longer poses significant problems.

As with all other methods of contraception, it is essential for the physician to put the benefit-risk ratio of the IUD in a proper perspective. Therefore, he must have thorough knowledge, not only of the practical results obtained with certain devices but also of the objective scientific data accumulated in the process of development.

This book deals mainly with one intrauterine contraceptive device. Different aspects of research that have led to the profiling of this device are described. The positive, favorable clinical results obtained over a number of years have justly made the IUD widely acceptable.

It is hoped that the reader of this book will gain an insight not only into the present and possible future methodologies in IUD development, but also into the possibilities and limitations of practical application of this particular device which, according to the reported clinical results, has definite advantages.

T. Vossenaar

This volume is dedicated to

WALTER H. SEEGERS

Chairman of the Department of Physiology
upon his retirement from Wayne State University

MEDICATED INTRAUTERINE DEVICES

PHYSIOLOGICAL AND CLINICAL ASPECTS

1. HISTORICAL: ERNST GRÄFENBERG AND THE GOLDEN YEAR OF THE SILVER RING

R.J. THOMSEN

On a windy, cold winter night some months ago I sat in a small room in an ancient castle near Münster, in northern Germany. Not far away was the village where my grandfather was born and raised and then lured by the exciting appeal of nineteenth-century America. And it was in that timeless castle, an ideal setting for such a narrative, that to me was unfolded in detail the saga of Dr. Ernst Gräfenberg and the intrauterine ring contraceptive device which bears his name. Nearby on my right sat Dr. Jack Lippes, the father of the Lippes loop, another classic IUD. He, too was largely a listener that night, for across the room, handling an assortment of antique contraceptive devices as if to pull from them hidden details and legends, was Dr. Hans Lehfeldt, who regaled Dr. Lippes and myself with anecdotes about the life of Dr. Gräfenberg and the days when only the farsighted and brave sought effective contraceptive technology for women under their care. Regarded from the exponential view of eternity, fifty years is a mere speck, but it can be a long time nonetheless, as we mortals chart our endeavours. The year 1979 marked one such epoch, half a century of progress in medicine important to humanity, and of German-American history in which this progress became intricately woven.

The year 1979 – irrespective of the history of the IUD – was certainly a year of introspection for both Germany and America. The traumas our two great countries face are manifest in a world apparently beyond their control in its unbridled passions and unforgiving in its recall of past wrongs. In the context of today it does not seem inappropriate to allude to the reality of the past fifty years – five of history's most turbulent decades. For in the history of intrauterine contraception political and medical developments have often interacted. Turning, then, to Dr Gräfenberg and his time, I first spotlight the year 1929. The location was London, where Gräfenberg spoke before the International Sexual Reform Congress, backed by the years of contraception research he had been quietly performing. He had first publicly discussed his ring intrauterine contraceptive device in 1928 at the Berlin postgraduate course chaired by Dr. Margaret Sanger. Also participating in this course was Dr. Lehfeldt, already a junior colleague and admirer of Dr Gräfenberg. But it was from the platform of the September 1929 congress in London that Dr. Gräfenberg first propounded intrauterine contraception and from which its golden anniversary should be dated. His third presentation of the subject, at the Seventh International Birth Control Conference in Zurich in September 1930, added but inadequately to the acceptance needed to ensure the method's survival.

Tainted by preantibiotic disasters rightfully attributed to the cervico-uterine pessaries foisted upon women about the turn of the century, the Gräfenberg's Ring was hardly received with enthusiasm by the leading lights of German gynecology – their reaction was soon to come. However, before detailing the rise and fall of the Gräfenberg Ring, a summary of the highlights of Dr. Gräfenberg's busy early life must be attempted. Ernst Gräfenberg was born in 1881 at Adelebsen, a small community in the green hills some fourteen kilometres from the old university town of Göttingen. The family name was taken from a nearby hill, Gräfenberg (Count's Hill), when nineteenth-century German Jews were permitted to bear family names. Leaving school in 1900, Gräfenberg went on into medicine, studying at the universities in Göttingen and Munich. His doctoral thesis, 'Die Entwicklung der Knochen, Muskeln und Nerven der Hand' [The development of the bones, muscles and nerves of the hand], was lauded and reputably published. His studies first led him to practice ophthalmology, working in that department at the University of Würzburg. As though to give encouragement to those of us who find it difficult to choose among the many interests and rewards life presents, Gräfenberg then acutely changed his professional interests. Gynecology thereafter became his work; he studied under Dr. Richard Werth and Dr. J. Pfannenstiel at the University of Kiel, where his training was completed in 1910. Thereafter, for the next three decades, the multiple facets of Dr. Gräfenberg's professional pursuits effused from Berlin. There he maintained a private practice of obstetrics and gynecology in addition to being the chief of gynecology at a city hospital. From observation and investigation of those patients Gräfenberg produced medical publications on a widely varied spectrum of subjects, including serological tests for pregnancy and venereal disease, pelvic anatomy, tuberculosis, dysmenorrhea, syphilis and associated congenital anomalies, and obstetric anesthesia. He was the pioneer in elucidating the cyclical variation of vaginal secretory acidity as related to ovulation. Dr. Lehfeldt's extensive review of Gräfenberg's contributions attests to wide clinical interests in addition to his classic, founding contribution to intrauterine contraception.

Gräfenberg's writings and clinical interests manifest themselves as an extension of his early and growing concern for the medical emancipation of women. Abortion, birth control, sexual realization – each claimed an considerable amount of his thought and professional effort. Typically relevant were the thoughts he expressed during the 1929 London presentation of the ring IUD: 'A satisfactory contraceptive method is most important in dealing with psychosexual disturbances in women. By removing fear and the necessity for objectionable preparations, many physical and mental inhibitions are removed'. Lest we forget, the sexual and medical rights of women in this century's first third were only cosmetically different than those under which their sisters of the Middle Ages suffered, slaved, or died. Still in the world's preantibiotic history and with but redimentary anesthesia and surgical support from our modern perspective, women in the 1920s could often anticipate infective morbidity or death as a consequence of sex and childbirth. Hemorrhage added to the grim toll. From this perspective is Gräfenberg's work best appreciated. Whether in the charity ward or among the socialites of his practice on Berlin's fashionable Kurfürstendamm, Gräfenberg keenly perceived the plight of women and sought to alleviate it. Of additional credit to Dr. Gräfenberg's pioneering contribution to intrauterine contraception is that it was done in the face of the inherent opposition of German medicine to both change and invasion of the uterus.

The bias of gynecology against intrauterine devices was not irrational in that preantibiotic, patent medicine milieu. From late in the nineteenth century a plethora of various cervico-uterine pessaries had been espoused for everything from hysteria and dysmenorrhea to abortion and even contraception. Typical of the devices in Gräfenberg's Germany was the wishbone spring pessary patented in 1902 by Dr. Carl Hollweg. A possible slight improvement of the 1920s was the device of Dr. Karl Pust. His cervico-uterine pessary made of silkworm gut attached to a cervical glass button was eventually distributed for use in over twenty thousand women. In a 1923 issue of *Deutsche Medizinische Wochenschrift*, Pust claimed that there were no pregnancies among the 453 women in whom he had inserted his silkworm pessary. Candidly titled, 'Ein brauchbarer Frauenschutz' [A useful protection for women], Pust's report further made the somewhat improbable claim that there were no serious complications for the method. Unconvinced, other gynecologists denounced the Pust device.

Tangentially, intrauterine silkworm gut was first reported for use as an intrauterine contraceptive by Dr. Richard Richter, a German doctor in the small town of Waldenburg (Walbrzych), near Breslau (Wroclaw). Richter plainly titled his report, 'Ein Mittel zur Verhütung der Konzeption' [A means of preventing conception]; this was frankly audacious at a time when it was illegal to prescribe birth control. Aware of both the valid objections to intrauterine tampering and the earlier use of silkworm, Gräfenberg's first efforts utilized silkworm gut in a star shape. This gave way to a silkworm gut ring which was further refined and made visible on X-ray by wrapping it with a wire of German silver. Finally evolved as the device called the Gräfenberg Ring, the circle of tightly wound German silver has been analytically studied in modern times and found to contain nickel, zinc, and 26 percent copper. Ten years of systematic evaluation involving hundreds of insertions predated Gräfenberg's 1929 report of the ring IUD. Shortly thereafter, a scattering of other European physicians added statistics verifying both the increased clinical use of the ring and the mounting number of damaging reports of pelvic infections associated with its use. The demise of the Gräfenberg's Ring swiftly followed his original optimistic reports. His fourth and last public presentation of the subject was in 1931 at the German Congress of Gynecology meeting in Frankfurt. Composed of but seventeen printed lines, the report was denounced by virtually all of the attending leading lights of German gynecology including Dr. Ludwig Fraenkel, professor and chairman of gynecology at Breslau, and Dr. S. Aschheim. So damning was the denouncement and so authoritative the denouncers that for all practical purposes the Gräfenberg ring was banished. The nearly concurrent Nazi ban on contraception in promotion of national fertility soon assured the total disappearance of intrauterine contraception from German medical practice.

Despite the ignoble treatment the ring was afforded in its demise, the attribution to Dr. Gräfenberg of the origination of the intrauterine contraceptive device is based not on first use of the method, but on the scientific thoroughness with which he investigated and reported the use of the ring. In elucidating its effectiveness, complications, physiological impact on the uterus, and safe insertion and removal techniques, Gräfenberg contributed a scientifically valid foundation upon which the method could be resurrected under the changed atmosphere of medical practice and population problems facing the world as it approached the sixth decade of the twentieth century. The unfinished character of the ring's story was akin to many aspects of Dr. Gräfenberg's life subsequent to the 1931 Frankfurt confrontation. The cloud of national socialism fell ever more darkly on Germany's Jews as the uncertainties of the early thirties turned into terrible realities. Many Jewish doctors fled Germany, including some who would become prominent in supporting IUD usage in the 1960s. Dr. Hans Lehfeldt left in 1934, encouraging a similar course for his friend Gräfenberg. Seemingly insulated by his position as gynecologist to the wives of the rich and of high-placed Nazi politicians and diplomats, Gräfenberg was misled about his safety and stayed in Berlin. Possibly augmenting his hopeful presumption of safety was his patriotic credential of having served in the First World War as a medical officer on the Russian front. Nevertheless, in 1937 he was imprisoned near Berlin. Surviving, as Dr. Lehfeldt conjectures, because the warden's wife was his patient, Gräfenberg languished in prison until his release was ransomed by Dr. Margaret Sanger for a large sum in American dollars in 1940. Gräfenberg arrived in New York in 1941 by a circuitous route through Siberia and Japan, with a short professional stop in Chicago. He assumed a busy life of obstetrical and gynecological practice, his continued interest in contraception being manifest in his work at the Margaret Sanger Research Bureau. Furthermore he helped Dr. Herbert Hall in the development of a stainless steel ring IUD eventually marketed as the Inhiband. Texts tracing IUD history state that warnings given Dr. Gräfenberg against attempting the use of his ring were so effective as to preclude his ever again utilizing the method. This is not correct. Dr. Hans Lehfeldt asserts as 'irrefutable' his personal knowledge that his friend Gräfenberg used modified ring IUDs amid the strict confidentiality of his private New York practice.

Scant public notice and no professional accolades marked the death of Dr. Gräfenberg on 28 October 1957, after a prolonged, debilitating struggle against Parkinsonism. An unfortunate irony of human existence is the frequency with which deserved recognition for a person's noteworthy accomplishments is withheld until after his death. Dr. Gräfenberg's death predated by but two years the modern rebirth of intrauterine contraceptive research, use, and general acceptance. In 1959, Dr. Alan Guttmacher, having adamantly opposed IUDs during Gräfenberg's life, condoned the experimental use of handmade IUDs at Mount Sinai Medical Center by Dr. Lazar Margulies. Dr. Gräfenberg had himself practiced at Mount Sinai for a fifteen years. Guttmacher's change of mind was precipitated by his alarm over the world's burgeoning population and reinforced by the 1959 publications from Israel and Japan of studies documenting Gräfenberg and Ota ring IUD insertions in thousands of women. By 1960, Margulies was marketing his plastic spiral, the Gynekoil, through the Ortho Pharmaceutical Company. It was the first of the deluge of devices which flooded gynecological practices in the 1960s. The rapidity of the acceptance of intrauterine contraception can only be compared to the precipitous decline of the Gräfenberg Ring after its condemnation in 1931 at Frankfurt.

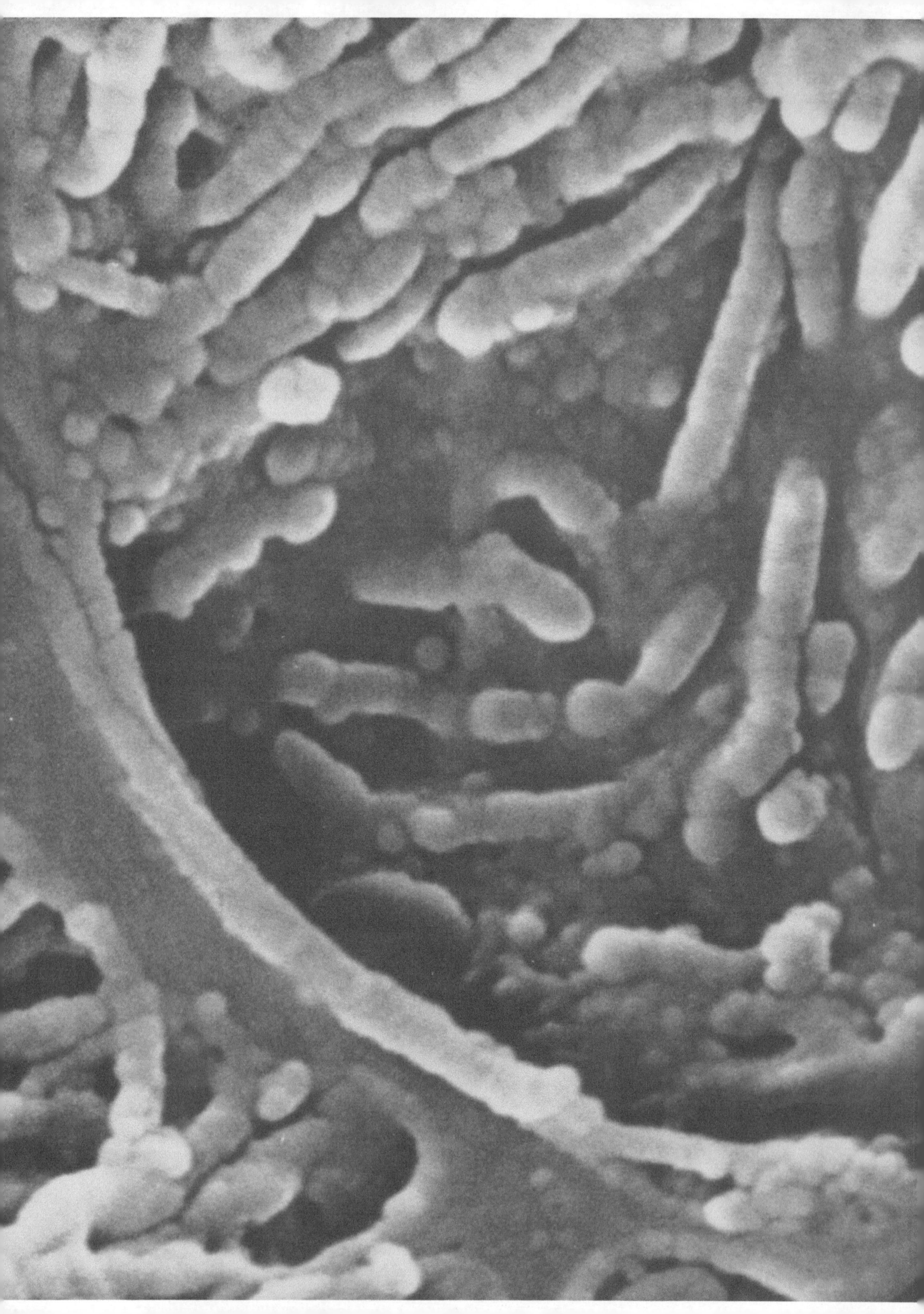

I. PHYSIOLOGICAL ASPECTS

2. UTERINE GEOMETRY AND IUD PERFORMANCE

H.M. Hasson

Individual variations in the size and shape of the human uterus are probably greater than variations in the size and shape of the human foot. It is, therefore, unfortunate that, whereas individual fitting of shoes is an accepted custom, selective fitting of IUDs is not. Furthermore, the current method of selecting IUD size, on the basis of bimanual pelvic examination and sounding of the uterus for total axial dimension, is grossly inadequate. Estimating external uterine size does not give an indication of the internal dimensions of the endometrial cavity (Wittman and Chow 1976; Tejuja and Malkani 1969), and measuring total uterine length is not useful in identifying endometrial cavity length (Hasson 1976; Wittman and Chow 1976). As IUDs are normally placed in the endometrial cavity exclusive of the cervical canal, knowledge of cervical length is essential for the proper placement of an IUD above the cervix; knowledge of endometrial cavity dimensions is necessary for proper fitting of the device.

I. UTERINE GEOMETRY

I.A. Geometric parameters of the endometrial cavity

The endometrial cavity is generally triangular in configuration. It possesses an axial dimension and various transverse and anterior-posterior diameters. It is a space that is capable of being distended. Numerous studies have shown considerable variations in the shape, size and potential capacity of individual endometrial cavities (Hasson et al. 1976; Püroinen and Kaihola 1975; Adel et al. 1971; Kamal et al. 1971; Lewis and Zuspan 1970; Tejuja and Malkani 1969; Burnhill and Birnberg 1966; Shubeck 1965; David and Israel 1964; Mann 1962). These uterine parameters cannot be estimated by bimanual pelvic examinations (Wittman and Chow 1976; Tejuja and Malkani 1969) or by sounding the uterus for the total dimension (Hasson et al. 1976; Wittman and Chow 1976). The length of the cervical canal and the length of the endometrial cavity can be determined easily with the use of a Wing Sound (Hasson 1974), but the development of a practical instrument to gauge uterine transverse dimensions is still under way. With the use of conventional graphic technique, the shape of the endometrial cavity can be determined if the axial dimension and two or more transverse dimensions are identified. The assessment of uterine potential capacity, defined as degree of distensibility, is more difficult. This uterine parameter has been evaluated with the use of an intrauterine balloon (Hasson 1975; Mann 1962) and with special hysterographic techniques (Rozin et al. 1967). However, it is difficult to translate degrees of intrauterine balloon distention or amounts of injected contrast material into actual anterior-posterior dimensions of the endometrial cavity.

I.B. Functional cyclic changes

Dynamic cyclic changes in uterine shape and size normally occur in women during different phases of the menstrual cycle (Püroinen and Kaihola 1975; Mann 1962). The variations in uterine shape are based on a cyclic alternating inverse tonal relationship between the uterine fundal and isthmic segments (Mann 1962). During menstruation the isthmic segment is wide, short and hypotonic. Following ovulation, it becomes increasingly narrow, long and hypertonic (Johnstone et al. 1974; Mann 1962; Mann et al. 1961; Youssef 1958). Changes in the uterine fundal segment occur in reverse order. Myometrial activity is most prominent during menses (Behrman and Burchfield 1968), at which time rhythmic contraction waves arise in the fundus and spread to the cervix (Behrman et al. 1969). Changes in uterine shape and activity that occur during representative phases of the menstrual cycle are shown in Figure 1.

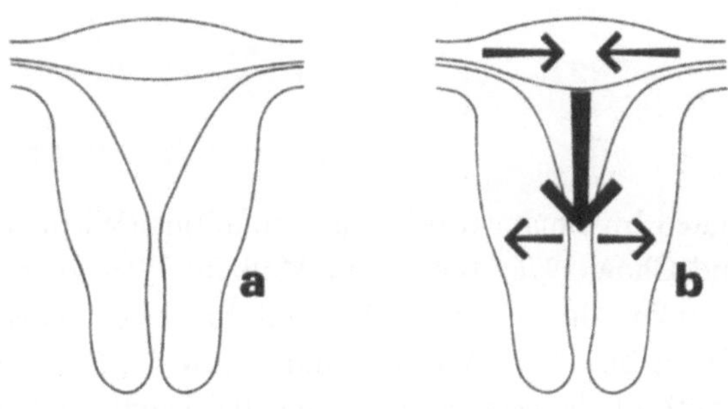

Figure 1. Changes in uterine shape, dimensions, and contractility pattern during menses. (a) Specific uterus on cycle day 18. (b) Anatomic and functional changes occurring in the same uterus on cycle day 1: (1) contracted fundus with reduced transverse diameter; (2) relaxed isthmus with increased transverse diameter; (3) definite fundus-to-cervix muscle propagation waves.

I.C. *Abnormalities*

Abnormal variations in uterine topography may be congenital or acquired. During embryonic life the müllerian duct system initially develops as a pair of ducts, one on each side. Subsequently, the lower portions of the ducts fuse to form the vagina and uterus, while the upper portions become a pair of fallopian tubes. Failure of fusion or improper fusion of the müllerian ducts results in a wide variety of developmental uterine anomalies, the extent of which depends on the degree of the fusion defect (Crosby and Hill 1962). The incidence of congenital uterine anomalies in patients utilizing IUDs was four percent in two hysterographic studies (Adel et al. 1971; Kamal et al. 1971) and nine percent in another study (Mazher et al. 1968). Leiomyomas are the most notable examples of acquired lesions that distort the shape of the endometrial cavity and reduce the uterine area accessible to an IUD.

II. THE SIGNIFICANCE OF UTERINE GEOMETRY TO IUD PERFORMANCE

II.A. *Endometrial cavity length*

The geometric relationships of a properly inserted IUD with a specific fairly rigid length to endometrial cavities with various inappropriate axial dimensions are indicated in Table 1 and illustrated in Figure 2. The optimum geometric relation is one in which the IUD is shorter than the endometrial length by 1.25 to 1.75 cm (Hasson et al. 1976). This distance probably represents the narrow lower uterine segment and/or isthmus. Placing the IUD entirely above the isthmus and fitting it properly in the upper uterine segment can be expected to produce favourable results. In fact, correctly fitted IUDs placed in this optimum position, regardless of their shapes, have been associated with better performance records than IUDs that did not fit the

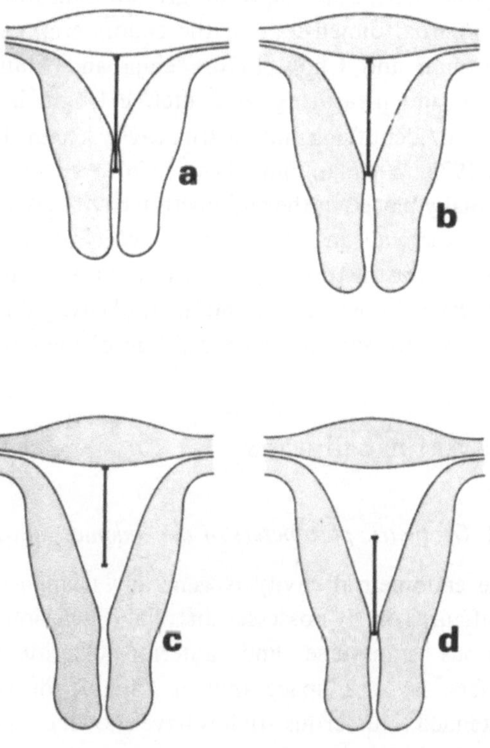

Figure 2. Geometric relation of a properly-inserted IUD with a specific fairly rigid length to endometrial cavities with various inappropriate axial dimension. (a) ECL < DL. (b) ECL = DL. (c) ECL > DL by 2 cm; initial IUD position. (d) ECL > DL by 2 cm; possible subsequent IUD position. ECL: endometrial cavity length; DL: device length.

Table 1. Relation between uterine geometry and IUD performance.

Geometric variable	*Possible mechanical result*	*Possible clinical outcome*
ECL = DL	IUD in the isthmus	expulsion, pain?
ECL < DL	IUD in the cervix endometrial injury myometrial distension	expulsion, pregnancy, infection, pain? bleeding, infection, pain? expulsion, pain
ECL > DL by 2 or more cm	IUD in the isthmus	expulsion, pregnancy*, pain?
FTD significantly smaller than DGTD**	endometrial injury myometrial distension	bleeding, infection, perforation, pain? expulsion, pain
FTD significantly greater than DGTD**	IUD in the isthmus	expulsion, pregnancy*, pain?
IUD thickness significantly greater than uterine capacity**	endometrial injury myometrial distension	bleeding, infection, pain? expulsion, pain
IUD thickness, surface area, or volume significantly smaller than uterine capacity, surface area or volume**	geometric factors, not related to device position, resulting in an inadequate contraceptive effect*	pregnancy*
Reduced available uterine space	IUD in cervix and/or isthmus myometrial distension	expulsion, infection, pregnancy, pain? expulsion, pain

ECL : endometrial cavity length
DL : device length
FTD : Fundal transverse dimension
DGTD : device's greatest transverse dimension
* : only if IUD is inert
** : the specific degree of disproportion has not been identified.

upper segment and those that were partially placed in the isthmus or cervix (Hasson et al. 1976; Sakurabayashi et al. 1969).

When the length of the IUD is equal to that of the endometrial cavity, the lower portion of the device comes to rest in the uterine isthmus, which is characteristically more irritable and ejective than the upper uterine segment (Mann 1962). Irritation of the uterine isthmus triggers myometrial contractions that promote expulsion. Distortion or distension of the lower uterine segment may also induce painful sensations that are independent of uterine contractions. Other investigators have reported findings that clearly support this important concept. Mazher et al. (1968) observed that for most asymptomatic patients wearing the loop IUD the length of the device did not exceed 75 percent of the length of the endometrial cavity. These investigators also noted that the lowermost portion of the loop was always above the uterine isthmus in all asymptomatic wearers.

Both Shubeck (1965) and Margolis (1975) attempted to optimize IUD performance by filling the uterine cavity with resilient nontraumatic devices. Schubeck experimented with a rapidly-polymerizing silicone device; Margolis used a fluid-filled balloon. The length of both devices was equal to the endometrial length, by virtue of design. The clinical outcome was revealing. Shubeck experienced an expulsion rate of thirty percent; Margolis reported slightly better results.

If the IUD is longer than the endometrial cavity, a portion of the device may protrude into the cervical canal. Devices partially contained within the cervix are more prone to expulsion. Partial presence of a bioactive IUD in the cervix decreases the device's contraceptive capability. If the amount of the bioactive agent remaining within the endometrial cavity is insufficient to prevent conception, pregnancy may occur. Retrograde penetration of the cervical barrier by an IUD increases the possibility of transcervical bacterial migration into the endometrial cavity and pelvic infections.

If IUD length is greater than endometrial cavity length and the device does not slide into the cervical canal by virtue of design or circumstance, the large device becomes impacted in the endometrial cavity. Such a device, depending on its shape, causes generalized myometrial distension or localized tenting distortion and diffuse endometrial compression or focal penetration injuries. These conditions are manifested clinically as pain, bleeding, expulsion, infection, or even perforation.

The clinical data accumulated with the use of various IUDs confirm these observations. For instance, pregnancies in the presence of bioactive IUDs have been recorded frequently when the devices were partially displaced into the cervix (Pharriss 1978; Tatum 1977; Zador et al. 1976; Newton et al. 1975; Sivanesaratnam et al. 1975; Scommegna et al. 1974; Shaila et al. 1974; Landeman et al. 1973). Partial presence of an IUD in the cervix (Tatum 1977), embedding of an IUD in the uterine wall (Bernstine et al. 1975; Schiffer et al. 1975; Taylor et al. 1975), and traumatic endometrial erosion or excessive compression caused by an IUD (Lomax et al. 1976; Bernstine et al. 1975; Schiffer et al. 1975) have been implicated as predisposing factors in pelvic infection. A definite relationship was reported between expulsion, bleeding and pain and the presence of Dalkon Shield, Lippes Loop, Cu-T and Cu-7 IUDs in the cervix (Wittman and Chow 1976; Ostergard 1975; Adel et al. 1971).

We have found that insertions of loop A in nulliparous women were associated with an unacceptably high event rate, although most of the devices were completely contained within the endometrial cavity (Hasson et al. 1976). Other authors have also stated that loop IUDs are unsuitable for use in nulliparous women (Howard 1972; Shirley 1975). The explanation is related in part to a length disparity between the IUD and the cavity. The endometrial length of many nulliparous women is less than in standard preinsertion length (28 mm) of loop IUDs (Hasson 1974). The loop is capable of changing its length following insertion (Dass et al. 1971). When the IUD is placed in a small endometrial cavity, its length decreases as the device is compressed within the confines of the cavity. However, such axial compression of the loop also increases the centrifugal force distributed by the device to the uterine wall.

When IUD length is significantly smaller than endometrial cavity length, the IUD may gravitate downward until its greatest transverse dimension abuts the uterine wall. In certain cases, the IUD becomes partially or totally lodged within the lower uterine isthmic segment, triggering uterine activity that may promote expulsion and give rise to painful sensations. Furthermore, inert IUDs that do not cover the fundus may not prevent pregnancy. Hysteroscopic studies have demonstrated the occurrence of pregnancy in the upper uterine segment when small IUDs were lodged in the lower uterine segment (Sakurabayashi, et al. 1969). The unsatisfactory performance of small IUDs in large endometrial cavities has also been documented by hysterography (Mazher et al. 1968). We have identified in our studies the significance value of the relative disproportion between the length of the endometrial cavity and that of the IUD. When endometrial length was greater than IUD length by 2 cm or more, event rates increased significantly (Hasson et al. 1976).

II.B. Transverse uterine dimensions

The geometric relationships of a properly inserted IUD with a specific fairly rigid greatest transverse dimension to endometrial cavities with various inappropriate fundal transverse dimensions are shown in Table 1 and diagrammed in Figure 3. The optimum geometric relationship is one in which the greatest transverse dimension of the IUD is equal to or slightly in excess of the fundal transverse dimension or one of the immediately receding transverse dimensions that follow in the direction of the cervix. In order to distribute pressure evenly to the endometrium, the transverse IUD member that comes in contact with the uterine wall should be resilient and atraumatic. The device can then abut the

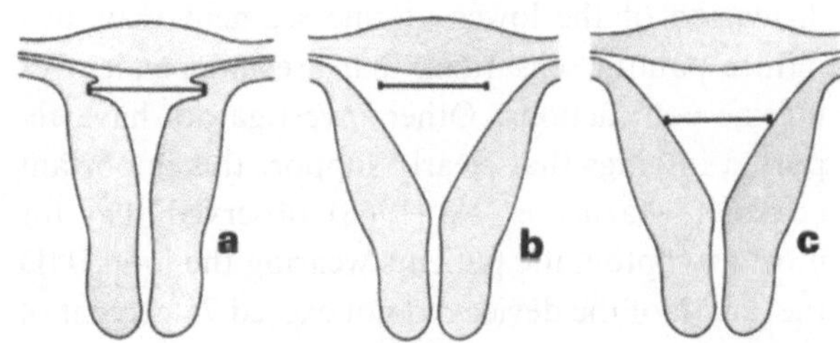

Figure 3. Geometric relation of a properly-inserted IUD with a specific fairly rigid greatest transverse dimension to endometrial cavities with various inappropriate fundal transverse dimensions. (a) FTD significantly smaller than DGTD. (b) FTD significantly greater than DGTD; initial position of IUD member with greatest transverse dimension. (c) FTD significantly greater than DGTD; possible subsequent position of IUD member with the greatest transverse dimension. FTD: fundal transverse dimension; DGTD: device's greatest transverse dimension.

uterine wall without creating excessive compression or focal injury. These geometric relationships and physical properties promote IUD retention and stability while minimizing endometrial trauma (Hasson, 1978b; Kamal et al. 1971). On the other hand, IUDs with fairly rigid and fixed transverse dimensions that are significantly greater or smaller than the fundal transverse diameter have unfavourable geometric relationships with the endometrial cavity.

Unfortunately, the specific degree of disproportion that causes adverse mechanical effects and clinical events has not yet been identified. If the fundal transverse diameter (FTD) is significantly smaller than the device's greatest transverse dimension (DGTD), the device compresses or embeds in the uterine wall at the point or points of contact. Traumatic injury to the endometrial lining follows, and bleeding results from physical damage to the endometrial blood vessels. Uterine perforation may occur in localized areas of impingement by embedded tips of the device. Relatively anaerobic conditions that favour the growth of facultative anaerobes arise as a result of traumatic erosion of the endometrium and embedment of the device in the uterine wall, so the natural resistance of affected tissues is reduced. The patient is thus made more vulnerable to pelvic infections. The tenting distortion of the uterine cavity produced by an excessively wide IUD distends the myometrium, thereby stimulating uterine contractions which produce painful sensations and increased probability of expulsion of the device.

Guidoin et al. (1976), Shaw and Moyer (1974), and Kar and Chandra (1965) report that endometrial bleeding is caused by physical damage to the endometrium in areas of IUD contact. In a hysterographic study of 48 randomly selected women wearing Cu-T IUDs, Khatamee and Lehfeldt (1975) found that partial embedment or complete perforation of the uterine walls by the transverse arms of the device had occurred in 65 percent of the patients. Other investigators (Strecker and Kraus 1976; Landeman et al. 1973) also documented uterine wall perforations by the horizontal bar of the Cu-T. The significance of endometrial ulceration or embedment of the device in the uterine wall in the occurrence of pelvic infections has been discussed by several authors (Scott 1978; Lomax et al. 1976; Bernstine et al. 1975; Schiffer et al. 1975; Taylor et al. 1975). The relationship between excessive myometrial distension and the clinical problems of pain, bleeding and expulsion is well established (Kamal et al. 1971; Sakurabayashi et al. 1969; Tejuja and Malkani 1969; Mazher et al. 1968).

On the other hand, if the fundal transverse diameter is significantly greater than the device's greatest transverse dimension, the IUD gravitates downward into the endometrial cavity until the device meets resistance (Kamal et al. 1975). The level at which surface resistance occurs is where the transverse diameter of the device becomes greater than the transverse diameter of the uterine cavity (Hasson 1978b). In certain instances downward movement of the IUD continues until the device is partially or completely impacted in the lower uterine segment and isthmus. The effect of such an unfavourable IUD-uterine relationship on clinical outcome has already been discussed.

II.C. Anteroposterior uterine dimensions

The geometric relationship of an IUD with inappropriate thickness to an endometrial cavity with a specific anteroposterior dimension is presented in Table 1 and illustrated in Figure 4. It is not yet

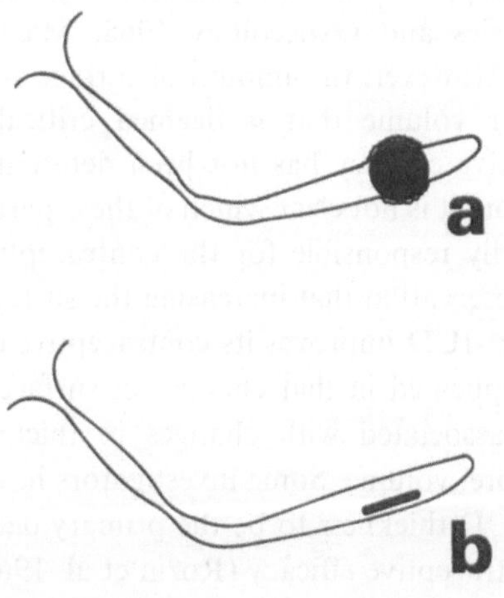

Figure 4. Geometric relation of IUDs with inappropriate thickness to an endometrial cavity with a specific capacity. (a) IUD thickness significantly greater than the anteroposterior dimension of the endometrial cavity. (b) IUD thickness significantly smaller than the anteroposterior dimension of the endometrial cavity.

possible to estimate the anteroposterior dimensions of the endometrial cavity, so it is impossible to fit an endometrial cavity precisely with an IUD or to quantitate the degree of disproportion that may exist between device thickness and uterine potential capacity. Rozin et al. (1967) reported that extreme distension of the endometrial cavity was associated with loss of uterine contractility. However, more convincing evidence was subsequently developed to indicate that excessive myometrial distension predictably results in augmented uterine contractions (Joelsson et al. 1976) and the occurrence of the clinical problems of pain, bleeding and expulsion (Kamal et al. 1971; Sakurabayashi et al. 1969; Tejuja and Malkani 1969; Mazher et al. 1968). Furthermore, significant compression of the endometrium by a disproportionately thick device is more likely to provoke undesirable injury. At any rate, the need to consider IUD thickness as a factor of performance has been largely eliminated because of the availability of bioactive contraceptive agents: contraceptive efficacy is independent of the thickness of the bioactive device.

It is generally accepted that inert IUDs whose surface area, thickness or volume is considerably smaller than the uterine surface area, capacity or volume are associated with higher pregnancy rates (Bernstine et al. 1975; Wheeler et al. 1974; Tietze 1970; Zipper et al. 1969; Advisory Committee on Obstetrics and Gynecology 1968; Mazher et al. 1968). However, the amount of surface area, thickness or volume that is deemed critical to contraceptive efficacy has not been determined. Furthermore it is not clear which of these parameters is primarily responsible for the contraceptive effect. The observation that increasing the surface area of an inert IUD improves its contraceptive capability is complicated in that changes in surface area are often associated with changes in thickness and, therefore, volume. Some investigators have considered IUD thickness to be the primary determinant of contraceptive efficacy (Rozin et al. 1967). These geometric parameters do not affect the contraceptive ability of bioactive IUDs, which is derived primarily from the added medication.

II.D. Functional cyclic uterine changes

The dynamic changes that take place in uterine shape and dimensions during different phases of the menstrual cycle modulate the relationship between the IUD and the host endometrial cavity. Conditions operative during menstruation produce a generally negative effect on IUD-uterine relations, as illustrated in Figure 5. The combined effects of increased fundal activity and isthmic hypotonia tend to compress, distort, displace and expel the IUD. Powerful uterine forces cause the IUD to move within the uterine cavity following insertion. While the significance of this important phenomenon has been recognized by some investigators (Dass et al. 1971; Phatak 1969; Mazher et al. 1968), it is not generally appreciated. These dynamic cyclic uterine changes necessitate accommodative adjustments in the design of IUDs and reevaluation of the concept of IUD fitting. For instance, the lower end of the IUD must be sufficiently expanded to resist downward movement of the device into the isthmus and cervix. Furthermore, because uterine dimensions are neither static nor fixed, the dimensions of the IUD should be capable of adaptive change. It is also clear that fitting of IUDs does not require exact and precise measurements of uterine dimensions but rather more approximate assessments of these changing parameters.

II.E. Abnormal variations in uterine topography (anatomy)

Congenital malformations and acquired lesions of the uterus affect IUD performance to the extent

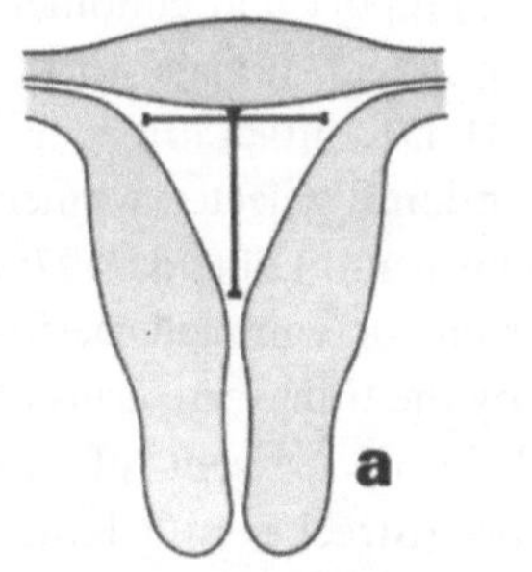

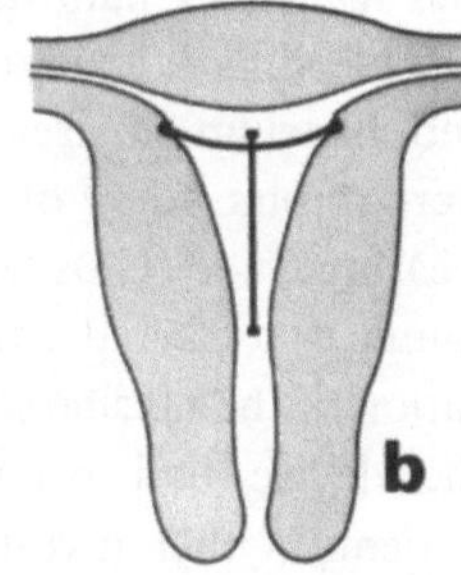

Figure 5. Effect of menses on IUD-uterine relations. (a) Position of an IUD with specific axial and greatest transverse dimensions in a specific uterus on cycle day 18. (b) Changes in geometric relation of the same IUD and uterus occurring on cycle day 1, provided that the diameter of the lower end of the device is not enlarged sufficiently to resist downward gravitation and the IUD member possessing the greatest transverse dimension is fairly rigid.

that they reduce the uterine space available for IUD deployment. In the case of a congenital fundal septum (Figure 6), the IUD could be placed entirely below the tip of the septum if the device lacked adaptive features allowing it to utilize uterine areas above that level (Hasson 1978b). The uterine septum may force the IUD to become displaced into the uterine isthmus or even into the cervix (Kamal et al. 1975; Adel et al. 1971; Mazher et al. 1968). The device thus becomes impacted in the narrow lower confines of the endometrial cavity, which distend it and distort its shape; the uterine fundus is left uncovered. The likelihood of expulsion, bleeding, pain and infection is increased (Table 1), while contraceptive efficacy is decreased. Pregnancies in unprotected areas of bicornuate uteri have been reported (Sakurabayashi et al. 1969; Mazher et al. 1968). The mechanical and clinical effects of a uterine leiomyoma depend on the size and position of the tumor.

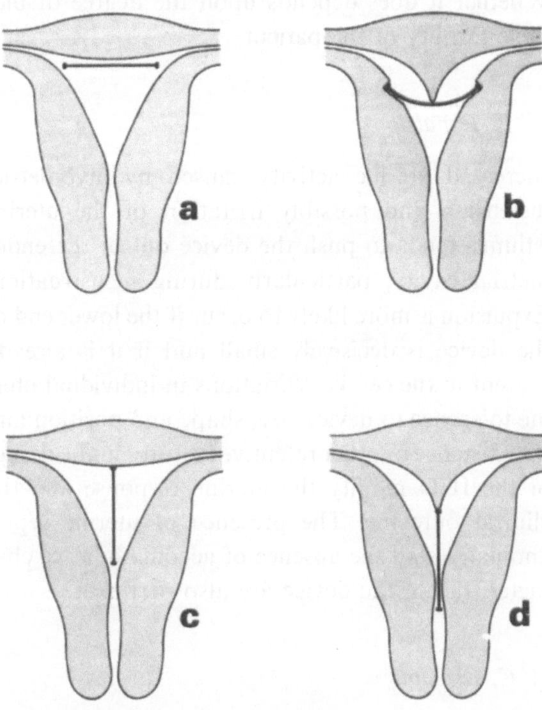

Figure 6. Effect of a congenital uterine fundal septum on IUD-uterine relations. (a) Transverse IUD-uterine relation of an IUD with a specific greatest transverse dimension placed in a normal uterus. (b) Transverse IUD-uterine relation of the same IUD placed in a uterus with a fundal septum. (c) Axial IUD-uterine relation of an IUD with a specific length placed in a normal uterus. (d) Axial IUD-uterine relation of the same IUD placed in a uterus with a fundal septum. The circumstances of (b) and (d) occur provided that design of the IUD does not allow it to utilize uterine space above the lower end of the septum.

III. GEOMETRIC FOUNDATIONS OF IUD COMPLICATIONS

Certain design qualities of an IUD appear to influence its performance regardless of associated uterine characteristics (Table 2). Devices possessing small lower-end diameters tend to descend into the uterine isthmus or cervix during menstruation, particularly if downward IUD movement is not restrained at a higher level. Progressive endometrial injury terminating in uterine perforation may result from the use of IUDs possessing a dependent vertical arm (Hasson 1978a, 1978b; Tatum 1977; Wei 1975; Nygren and Johansson 1974; Tacchi 1968). Should the vertical arm become displaced downward in response to uterine contractions, it may slide smoothly into the cervical canal. However, if the vertical arm is in an oblique position it may impinge upon the isthmic or cervical mucosa. Eventually, it may penetrate the uterine wall because of continued downward pressure generated by additional uterine contractions (Tatum 1977; Wei 1975).

Devices possessing spicular projections or sharp edges provoke injuries that may result in uterine bleeding or perforation as well as pelvic infections. Pointed IUD projections commonly become embedded in the uterine wall. The endometrial areas into which IUD projections have anchored show tissue proliferation and serious damage. During uterine contractions that cause a reduction in endometrial cavity size the spicular projections could not only compress and penetrate the endometrium but also distend and penetrate the myometrium. Myometrial injury and distension may cause painful contractions and eventually perforation (Guidoin et al. 1976). Uterine perforations caused by pointed tips of IUD transverse arms have been observed (Strecker and Kraus 1976; Landeman et al. 1973) and documented by hysterography (Khatamee and Lehfeldt 1975).

The mechanical effects and clinical results of using an IUD with pointed members are best illustrated by the Majzlin Spring experience. This device is made of a 0.4 mm-gauge stainless steel wire

Table 2. Effect of pertinent device characteristics on IUD performance.

Geometric variable	*Possible mechanical result*	*Possible clinical outcome*
IUD with a small lower-end diameter	IUD in cervix and/or isthmus.	Expulsion, pregnancy, infection, pain?
IUD with a dependent vertical arm with a pointed tip	IUD in the cervix and/or isthmus Endometrial injury	expulsion, pregnancy, infection, pain? bleeding, infection, perforation, pain?
IUD with sharp edges or other pointed tips	endometrial injury	bleeding, infection, perforation, pain?

that is formed with 12 elbowlike projections. When it was used as an IUD, the metallic projections penetrated the endometrium, became embedded in the myometrium and occasionally perforated the uterine wall, as was demonstrated by hysterography and examination of the surgical specimens (Taylor et al. 1973). These mechanical effects were associated with an unacceptably high rate of severe bleeding, pain and infection. Of the wearers, one percent developed extensive pelvic infections characterized by intense cellulitis. The findings suggested that spring embedment in the uterine wall created a portal of entry for the bacteria (Taylor et al. 1973).

The adverse clinical effects of unfavourable relationships between the geometric parameters of the IUD and those of the endometrial cavity, as well as effects that result from independent uterine or device characteristics, are mediated through the mechanical determinants outlined in Table 3.

IV. GEOMETRIC FACTORS ASSOCIATED WITH INDIVIDUAL EVENTS

IV.A. Pregnancy

For inert IUDs there appears to be a positive correlation between the amount of device surface area and thickness or volume and the contraceptive efficiency. Even though the critical values of pertinent device parameters have not been identified, it is generally accepted that devices whose surface area, thickness or volume are significantly smaller than corresponding uterine parameters do not provide an adequate contraceptive effect. Partial presence of an inert IUD in the cervix serves to diminish the device's contraceptive effect to the extent that the device is not present in the endometrial cavity. In the case of bioactive IUDs, contraceptive efficacy is essentially related to the amount of active agent located within the endometrial cavity. If the amount of active agent contained in the cavity is reduced as a result of improper placement or downward displacement of the device into the cervix, conception may occur. Whether it does depends upon the degree of biologic fertility of the patient.

IV.B. Expulsion

Increased uterine activity caused by myometrial distension and possibly irritation of the uterine isthmus tends to push the device out of the endometrial cavity, particularly during menstruation. Expulsion is more likely to occur if the lower end of the device is decisively small and if it is already present in the cervix. Variations in individual uterine tolerance to device size, shape and position and the existence of other retentive features in the design of the IUD modify the uterine response and the clinical outcome. The presence of uterine septal anomalies and the absence of accommodative characteristics in the device are also pertinent.

IV.C. Bleeding

The mechanical effect of IUDs on endometrial cells is one of pressure (Hafez et al. 1975). Compression of endometrial tissues in areas of IUD contact may be sufficient to produce superficial ulcerations. Endometrial bleeding arises as a result of the kinetic surface changes as well as of other biological alterations. The severity of bleeding is generally related to the degree of tissue damage. Thus, it appears that, with present technology, a certain

Table 3. Geometric foundations of IUD complications.

Unfavourable mechanical determinant	*Geometric basis***	*Associated clinical problems*
Low device position:		
IUD in the isthmus	1.1., 1.2, 1.3^+, 1.5^+, 2^+, 3.1, 3.2.	expulsion, pregnancy*, pain?
IUD in the cervix	1.1, 2^+, 3.1, 3.2.	expulsion, pregnancy, infection, pain?
Geometric factors, not related to device position, that result in an inadequate contraceptive effect	1.7.	pregnancy*.
Endometrial/myometrial injury due to device penetration and/or compression	1.1^+, 1.4, 1.6, 2^+, 3.2, 3.3.	bleeding, infection, perforation, pain?
Myometrial distension sufficient to cause increased uterine activity	1.1^+, 1.4, 1.6, 2^+.	expulsion, pain?

* only if IUD is inert
** numbers in this column refer to the following adverse geometric factors:
1. *Unfavourable IUD-uterine relations:*
1. DL > ECL
2. DL = ECL
3. DL < ECL by 2 or more cm
4. DGTD $\gg$FTD^{++}
5. DGTD $\ll$FTD^{++}
6. IUD thickness $\gg$uterine capacity
7. IUD thickness, surface area or volume $\ll$ uterine capacity, surface area or volume^{++}

2. *Reduced uterine space*
due to a congenital fundal anomaly or a space-occupying lesion

3. *Unfavourable IUD features:*
1. Small lower-end diameter
2. Dependent vertical arm with a pointed tip
3. Sharp edges or other pointed tips

$^+$ the design of the IUD is a factor in determining whether the problem occurs
$^{++}$ the specific degree of disproportion has not been identified
DL: device length
ECL: endometrial cavity length
DGTD: device's greatest transverse dimension
FTD: fundal transverse dimension.

amount of abnormal uterine bleeding is unavoidable with IUD use, at least in some patients. The utilization of IUDs with sharp edges or pointed tips causes localized penetration injuries of the endometrium. More extensive injuries may take place if the length, width or thickness of the device, regardless of shape, is significantly greater than the corresponding endometrial cavity parameter.

IV.D. Pain

The relationship between excessive myometrial distension and painful sensations is well documented. However, it is not clear whether pain also arises from endometrial injury or isthmic irritation unaccompanied by uterine distension. The expression of pain may be modified by psychological, cultural and social factors.

IV.E. Infection

Presence of the IUD in the cervix and endometrial/myometrial injury are the two mechanical factors implicated in pelvic infections associated with IUD use. The underlying cause is interference with the cervical and the tissue resistance barriers. Relatively anaerobic conditions favouring facultative anaerobes exist within pockets of the uterine wall in which pointed IUD tips are embedded. The risk of an IUD wearer developing a pelvic infection under these conditions is increased for the following reasons:

1. Breaks in the natural surface of the endometrium provide an entry site for the bacteria;
2. The anaerobic environment found within the pockets of device embedment facilitates the growth and multiplication of facultative and obligatory anaerobes;
3. The damaged cells found in the affected areas offer little resistance to the invading organisms and may actually serve to increase their virulence by acting as a culture medium.

The occurrence of a pelvic infection also depends on the degree of device contamination at the time of insertion; whether the device has an appendage formed with multiple filaments; the presence of preexisting pelvic inflammatory disease; and the exposure to sexually transmitted organisms.

IV.F. Perforations

Uterine perforations inflicted at the time of IUD insertion result from faulty technique. Perforations that occur later are caused by impingement of one or more device tips on the uterine wall. Lateral uterine wall perforations are made by devices with pointed transverse arms. Devices with a dependent vertical arm that has a pointed tip cause retrograde penetration.

In summary, it appears that, with few exceptions, the performance record of a IUD is basically determined by its geometric relationship to the host endometrial cavity.

REFERENCES

Adel SK, Ghoneim MA, Sobrero AJ: Hysterography study of long-term effects of intrauterine contraceptive devices. Fertil Steril 22: 651, 1971.

Advisory Committee on Obstetrics and Gynecology: Report on intrauterine contraceptive devices, Washington DC, Food and Drug Administration, 1968.

Behrman SJ, Burchfield W: The intrauterine contraceptive device and myometrial activity. Am J Obstet Gynecol 100: 194, 1968.

Behrman SJ, Archie JT, O'Brien OP: Myometrial activity and the IUCD II: propagation waves. Am J Obstet Gynecol 104: 123, 1969.

Bernstine RL, Davidson AR, Duncan GW, et al.: Review and analysis of the scientific and clinical data on the safety, efficacy, adverse reactions, biological action, utilization, and design of intrauterine devices, Springfield, Va, US Department of Commerce, National Technical Information Service, PB-249-614, 1975.

Burnhill MS, Birnberg CH: The size and shape of the uterine cavity determined by hysterography with an intrauterine contraceptive device as a marker. Int J Fertil 11: 187, 1966.

Crosby WM, Hill EC: Embryology of the Müllerian duct system: review of present-day theory. Obstet Gynecol 20: 507, 1962.

Dass A, Bhagat S, Bhargava K. et al.: Hysterography and the Lippes Loop. Int J Gynaecol Obstet 9: 232, 1971.

Davis HJ, Israel R: Uterine cavity measurements in relation to design of intra-uterine contraceptive devices. In: Intra-uterine contraception, Segal SJ, Southan AL (eds), Amsterdam, Excerpta Medica International Congress, Series 86, 1964, p 135-141.

Guidoin R, Courtney JM, Brault R, et al.: Intra-uterine devices: a SEM study on the Dalkon Shield. Biomater Med Devices Artif Organs 4: 81, 1976.

Hafez ESE, Barnhart MI, Ludwig H, et al.: Scanning electron microscopy of human reproductive physiology. Acta Obstet Gynecol Scand [Suppl] 40: 8, 1975.

Hasson HM: Differential uterine measurements recorded in vivo. Obstet Gynecol 43: 400, 1974.

Hasson HM: Ballooned uterine elevator cannula. Am J Obstet Gynecol 123: 658, 1975.

Hasson HM: Copper IUDs. J Reprod Med 20: 139, 1978a.

Hasson HM: Factors that affect IUD performance: a review and recommendations. J Reprod Med 21: 137, 1978b.

Hasson HM, Berger GS, Edelman DA: Factors affecting IUD performance I: endometrial cavity length. Am J Obstet Gynecol 126: 973, 1976.

Howard G: Use of intrauterine devices in nulliparous women, Lancet 2: 1339, 1972.

Joelsson I, Gidlund L, Anzen B, et al.: In vivo determination of the stress-strain relation of the human myometrium. Acta Obstet Gynecol Scand 55: 325, 1976.

Johnstone FD, Boyd IE, McArthy TG, et al.: The diameter of the uterine isthmus during the menstrual cycle, pregnancy and the puerperium. J Obst Gyn Br Comm 81: 558, 1974.

Kamal I, Hefnawi F, Ghoneim M, et al.: Dimensional and architectural disproportion between the intrauterine device and the uterine cavity: a cause of bleeding. Fertil Steril 22: 514, 1971.

Kamal I, Ghoneim M, Talaat M, et al.: Retention and expulsion of IUDs. In: Analysis of intrauterine contraception, Hefnawi F, Segal SJ (eds), Amsterdam, North-Holland Publishing, 1975, p 359-366.

Kar AB, Chandra H: Uterine bleeding in rhesus monkeys after insertion of an intrauterine device. Indian J Exp Biol 3: 269, 1965.

Khatamee MA, Lehfeldt H: Hysterographic studies in women wearing copper T devices. Adv Planned Parenthood 10: 90, 1975.

Landeman R, Kay R, Wilson K: A two man experience with the Copper T intrauterine device. Contraception 7: 477, 1973.

Lewis RG, Zuspan FP: A method for determining contour volume of the uterine cavity. Contraception 2: 249, 1970.

Lomax CW, Harbert GM, Thornton WN: Actinomycosis of the female genital tract. Obstet Gynecol 48: 341, 1976.

Mann EC: Cineradiographic observations on intra-uterine contraceptive devices. In: Intra-uterine contraceptive devices, Tietze C, Lewit S (eds), Amsterdam, Excerpta Medica international congress series 54, 1962, p 91-96.

Mann EC, McLarn WD, Hayt DB: The physiology and clinical significance of the uterine isthmus I: the two-stage intrauterine balloon in the diagnosis and treatment of cervical incompetence. Am J Obstet Gynecol 81: 209, 1961.

Margolis AJ: A fluid-filled intrauterine device: initial clinical trials. Am J Obstet Gynecol 122: 470, 1975.

Mazher K, Kamal I, Hefnawi F, et al.: A simple technic of hysterography for evaluating side effects and mode of action of intrauterine devices. Fertil Steril 18: 353, 1968.

Newton J, Elias J, McEwan J, et al.: Evaluation of the Copper 7 in England. In: Analysis of intrauterine contraception, Hefnawi F, Segal S (eds), Amsterdam, North-Holland Publishing, 1975, p 291-302.

Nygren KG, Johansson EDB: Retrograde cervical perforation by the Copper T device. Acta Obstet Gynecol Scand 53: 383, 1974.

Ostergard DR: The Dalkon Shield intrauterine device: a review of current status. J Reprod Med 14: 64, 1975.

Pharriss BB: Clinical experience with the intrauterine progesterone contraceptive system. J Reprod Med 20: 155, 1978.

Phatak LV: Intrauterine distortion and displacement of an IUD. Indian J Med Res 57: 89, 1969.

Püroinen O, Kaihola HL: Uterine size measured by ultrasound during the menstrual cycle. Acta Obstet Gynecol Scand 54: 247, 1975.

Rozin S, Schwartz A, Shenker JC: Studies of the mode of action of intrauterine contraceptive device. Obstet Gynecol 30: 855, 1967.

Sakurabayashi M, Mohri T, Ono T, et al.: Studies on intrauterine contraceptive devices IV: the position of IUD in the cavity of uterus and nidation of fertilized ova. Acta Obst Gyn Jpn 16: 275, 1969.

Schiffer MA, Elguezabal A, Sultana M, et al.: Actinomycosis infections associated with intrauterine contraceptive devices. Obstet Gynecol 45: 67, 1975.

Scommegna A, Avila T, Luna M, et al.: Fertility control by intrauterine release of progesterone. Obstet Gynecol 43: 769, 1974.

Scott WC: Pelvic abscess in association with intrauterine contraceptive device. Am J Obstet Gynecol 131: 149, 1978.

Shaila NG, Lane ME, Sobrero AJ: A comparative randomized double-blind study of the Copper-T 200 and Copper-7 intrauterine contraceptive devices with modified insertion techniques. Am J Obstet Gynecol 120: 110, 1974.

Shaw ST, Moyer DL: Problem bleeding with IUDs In: Intrauterine devices: development, evaluation and program implementation, Wheeler RG, Duncan GW, Speidel JJ (eds), New York, Academic Press, 1974, p 99-103.

Shirley RL: The Dalkon Shield in private practice: a disappointment. Am J Obstet Gynecol 121: 564, 1975.

Shubeck F: Use of polymerizing plastics in pregnancy prevention: preliminary report. Obstet Gynecol 25: 724, 1965.

Sivanesaratnam VV, Puvan IS, Sinnathuray TA: Evaluation of Copper 7 intrauterine device in Malaysian Women. Med J Aust 2: 298, 1975.

Strecker JR, Kraus H: Unusual uterine perforation by the Copper T intrauterine device and removal by laparoscopy. Contraception 13: 47, 1976.

Tacchi D: Uterine perforation by a Saf-T-Coil intrauterine contraceptive device. J Obst Gyn Br Comm 75: 1176, 1968.

Tatum HG: Clinical aspects of intrauterine contraception: circumspection 1976. Fertil Steril 28: 3, 1977.

Taylor ES, McMillan JH, Greer BE, et al: The intrauterine device and tubo-ovarian abscess. Am J Obstet Gynecol 123: 338, 1975.

Taylor WW, Martin FG, Pritchard SA, et al.: Complications from Majzlin spring intrauterine device. Obstet Gynecol 41: 404, 1973.

Tejuja S, Malkani PK: Clinical significance of correlation between size of uterine cavity and IUD: a study by planimeter-hysterogram technique. Am J Obstet Gynecol 105: 620, 1969.

Tietze C: Evaluation of intrauterine devices: ninth progress report: cooperating statistical program. Stud Fam Plann 55: 1, 1970.

Wei PY: Downward displacement of IUDs and related problems of accidental pregnancy and cervical penetration. In: Analysis of intrauterine contraception, Hefnawi F, Segal SJ (eds), Amsterdam, North-Holland Publishing, 1975, p 367-371.

Wheeler RG, Buschbom RL, Marshall RK: A rational basis for IUD design and development. In: Intrauterine devices: development, evaluation and program implementation, Wheeler RG, Duncan GW, Speidel JJ (eds), New York, Academic Press, 1974, p 163-190.

Wittman BK, Chow TTS: Diagnostic ultrasound in the management of patients using intrauterine contraceptive devices. Br J Obstet Gynaecol 83: 802, 1976.

Youssef AF: The uterine isthmus and its sphincteric mechanism, a radiographic study I: the uterine isthmus under normal conditions. Am J Obstet Gynecol 75: 1305, 1958.

Zador G, Nilsson BA, Nilsson B, et al.: Clinical experience with the uterine progesterone system (Progestasert). Contraception 13: 559, 1976.

Zipper JA, Tatum JH, Pastene L, et al.: Metallic copper as an intrauterine contraceptive adjunct to the T device. Am J Obstet Gynecol 105: 1274, 1969.

3. CORROSION OF COPPER IN UTERO

A. Kosonen

The improved antifertility effect of a copper-bearing IUD is based on the continuous release of copper, this being essential to maintain the antifertility effect of the IUD. This release is a result of the reaction between the copper and the uterine secretions; the copper corrodes in utero. The behaviour of the corrosion as presented here has been gathered from observations of approximately 100 copper-releasing IUDs, primarily CU-T200s which have been removed after 3-72 months of use. These observations are compared further with those of other investigators. The corrosion damaging the copper limits the life of the IUD, so the elimination of this disadvantage would prolong the effective lifetime of the device.

I. THE DISSOLUTION MECHANISM

In the dissolution process, it is not possible for copper atoms to leave their neighbouring atoms without first reacting with the oxidizing agents present in the solvent. This reaction causes compounds to form on the surface of the metal. These in turn dissociate in solution, forming cupric ions, CU^{++} (Leidheiser 1971). The dissolution mechanism of copper in uterine secretions has been accurately described (Oster 1972; Oster and Salgo 1975). Accordingly, the rate of the dissolution of copper is proportional to the serum albumin concentration and for a given albumin concentration, the presence of saline increases the rate of formation of cupric ions. Further, oxygen participates in the formation of cupric ions in solution by generating copper oxide, on the surface of the metal, which is then removed by aminoacids. Experiments show that the disulphide bond is also critical in the copper dissolution process, since it too acts as an oxidizing agent in the transition from metallic copper to cupric ions. Consequently, if the copper in an IUD before insertion is dark due to an oxide or sulphide layer, it merely enables the dissolution process to start immediately.

II. DEPOSITS

The corrosion of metals usually begins where a different material is present on the surface. The potential of foreign material differs from that of the base metal, and an anodic-cathodic reaction is created between them. If a deposit or thick oxide partially covers the surface, a similar condition arises due to different aeration between these areas and the base metal (Leidheiser 1971). This different aeration initiates a local dissolution, which leads to the so-called 'pitting corrosion'. Figure 1 illustrates the process, showing a partially cracked cuprous oxide layer initiating an anodic-cathodic reaction. In IUDs, the organic deposit on the surface of the copper creates conditions for the process described (Figure 2).

The deposit on the metal is normally dark and contains mostly organic compounds. However, as shown in Figure 1, $CaCO_3$ is formed as a natural result of the corrosion process and therefore exists in the deposit. In some cases, the quantity of $CaCO_3$ is so great that the deposit becomes greyish or white in appearance. In one exceptional case, the deposit of $CaCO_3$ on a device used 35.5 months was nearly as thick as the copper wire (Figure 3). In such cases, the $CaCO_3$ is not a result of corrosion, but is a precipitation from uterine fluids; it will exist all over the device, even on the plastic far from the copper. Calcium carbonate is hard, but due to its porosity it does not prevent dissolution, although the progress

E.S.E. Hafez and W.A.A. van Os (eds.), Medicated Intrauterine Devices, 22–29.

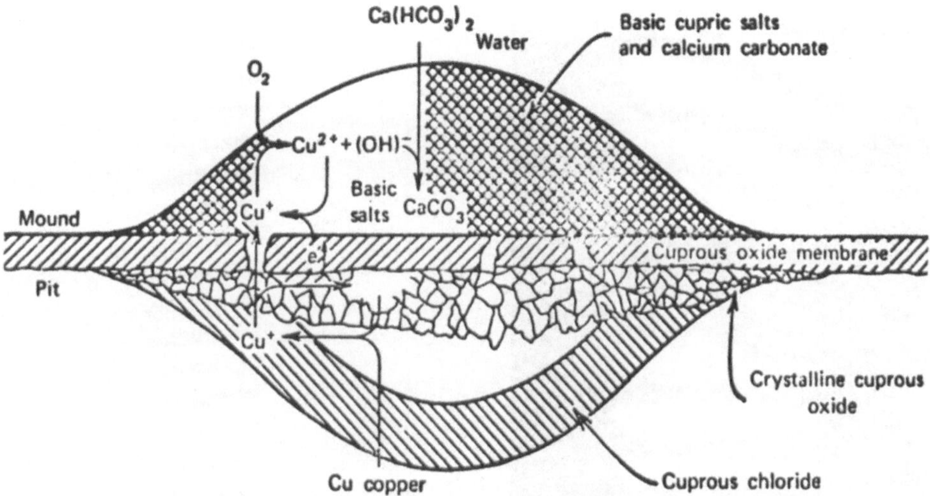

Figure 1. Diagrammatic representation of the arrangement of corrosion products and of the reactions involved in the pitting corrosion of copper. (1) Reaction occurring within the mound above a pit: $4CuCl + Ca(HCO_3)_2 + O_2 \rightarrow CuCO_3 \cdot Cu(OH)_2 + CaCO_3 + 2CuCl_2$. (2) Cathodic electrode reaction occurring on the outer surface of the oxide membrane: $Cu^{++} + e \rightarrow Cu^{+}$. (3) Anodic electrode reaction occurring on the inner surface of the oxide membrane: $Cu^{+} - e \rightarrow Cu^{++}$. (4) Reaction between the anodic product and the copper within the pit: $Cu + Cu^{++} \rightarrow 2Cu^{+}$.

of the corrosion observed is then slower than that which would normally be expected. The penetration of corrosion in this case was only 65 percent of the least that could normally be expected in copper wire after the same length of use. In another sample with thick calcareous deposits, corrosion after six years of use corresponded to that normally found in a device after 3.5 years of use. The slower dissolution could be related to an exceptional composition of uterine secretions, their being less corrosive than usual, rather than to the calcium carbonate reducing the rate of copper release.

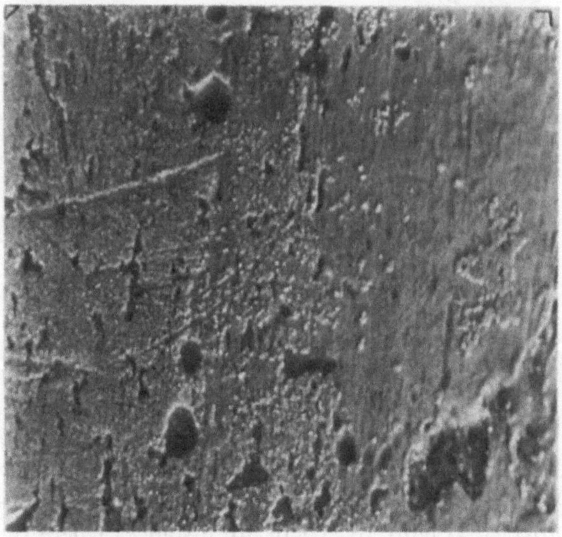

Figure 2. A scanning electron microscope picture showing deposit on the surface of the copper wire and small corrosion pits. The device had been 202 days in utero (× 1000).

III. THE PROGRESS OF CORROSION

The pits continue to grow in width and depth in the metal as time passes. The corroded areas are filled with 'corrosion products' when the copper atoms are replaced by foreign atoms present in uterine secretions. The corrosion products analyzed in an electron probe X-ray microanalyzer consisted of copper-rich areas which also included oxygen and chlorine. There were also areas where no copper could be detected, where sodium, chlorine and oxygen dominated (Kosonen 1978; Gosden et al. 1977). The further dissolution of copper continues by diffusion through this insoluble porous layer, the corrosion products remaining on the wire until a mechanical force such as bending causes them to crack and flake off (Kosonen 1978; Timonen 1976). Consequently, the wire appears to remain unaffected even rather a long period of use (Figure 4). This is why, in most cases, it is impossible to determine the progress of the corrosion by visual inspection, by examination of the surface with

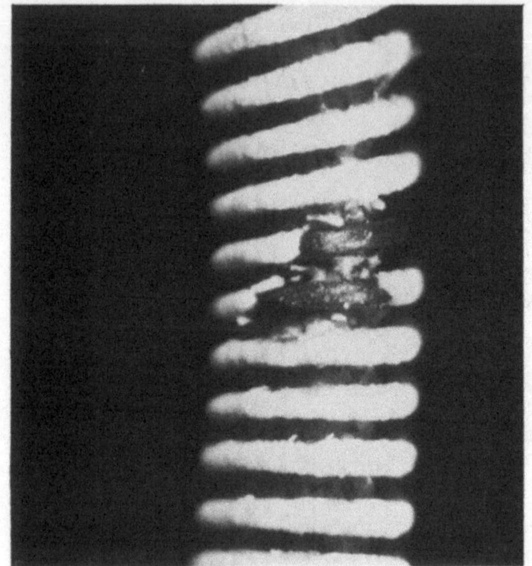

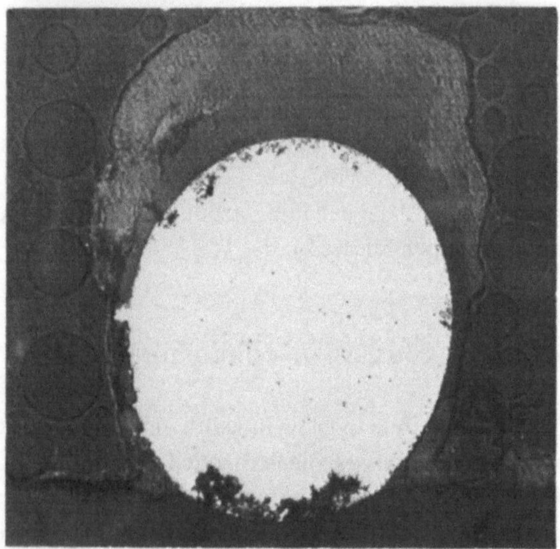

Figure 3. Heavy calcareous deposit on copper wire in Cu-7 device after 35.5 months in use. *Bottom:* cross section of the same wire. Clear corrosion under the deposit and more pronounced corrosion in the area which has been against the plastic body can be observed.

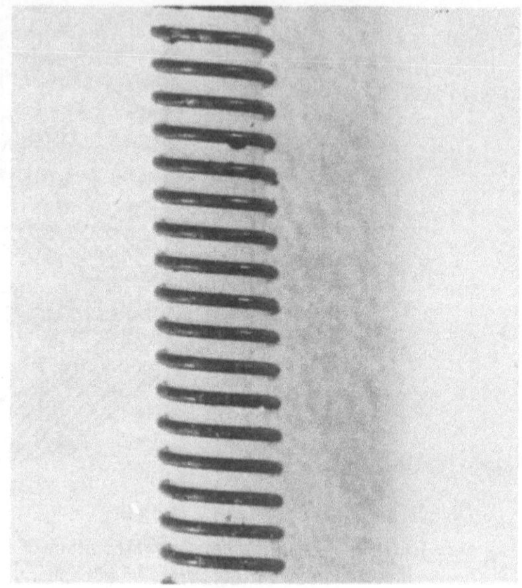

Figure 4. General appearance of the wire of the Cu-T200 after 22.7 months of use (stereomicroscopic picture, × 8). In a cross section of the wire, a corrosion depth of 18.2 percent of the diameter was detected.

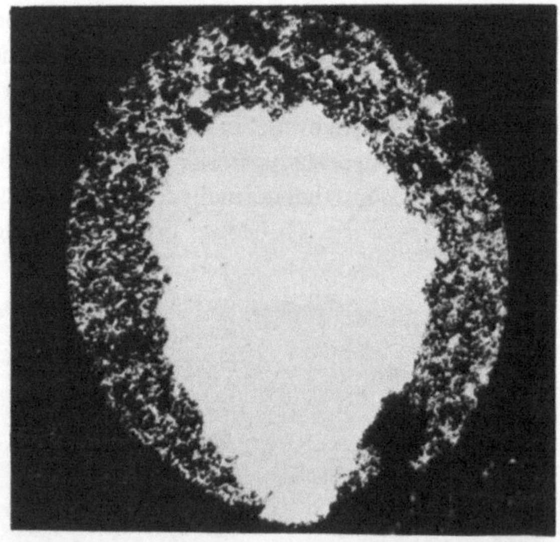

Figure 5. A cross section of copper wire showing an insoluble layer of corrosion products. The layer is porous and contains copper. The part against the plastic (bottom) is not corroded. The device had been 18.6 months in utero (× 300).

SEM, or by measuring the reduction of the diameter of the wire. The best method is to examine a cross section of the wire with a light microscope, after careful preparation of the sample to preserve the corrosion products on the metal, thereby making it possible to measure the depth of the pit (Figure 5).

The most remarkable characteristic of the corrosion process is the extreme variability of its location. The dissolution seems to concentrate only in narrow areas, where the corrosion progresses rapidly, leaving the neighbouring areas almost unaffected (Figure 6). There are instances where the wire has corroded completely through with pieces missing (Figure 7), while other areas show very little corrosion.

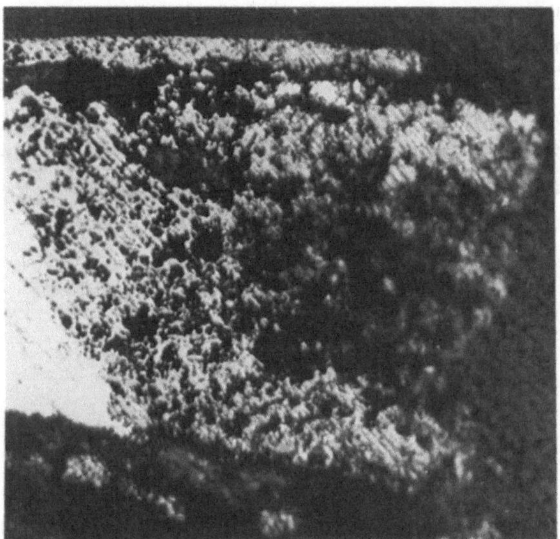

Figure 6. Longitudinal section of the broken wire of a device after 17.5 months of use (light microscopic picture, × 350).

The reason for the local character of the corrosion is unknown. Oxygen, among other oxidizing agents, plays an important role in the dissolution process (Oster 1972; Oster and Salgo 1975). The locality of the corrosion may, therefore, depend on differences in oxygen concentrations in the endometrium and on variations in the protection of the copper surface against corrosion. Oxygen enters the uterine cavity mainly through the cervix – devices which have been displaced to the lower part of the endometrium or to the cervix are severely corroded within a very short time (Figure 7), and it can be expected that the copper nearest to the cervix will always be the most severely corroded. Examination of about fifty devices showed that the area of deepest corrosion existed as often in the middle of the stem as in the lower part. Unexpectedly, some devices also showed the concentration of corrosion on the upper part of the stem; rarely did the corrosion occur uniformly along the stem. It may be possible that, during the menstrual period, hemoglobin carrying oxygen causes corrosion on the copper situated far from the cervix, or that oxygen is not the only dissolving medium. Heavy bleeding increases copper release (Timonen 1976).

Because the original contour of the wire in cross section can nearly always be clearly detected under the light microscope (Figure 5), the depth of the corrosion in the cross section of the wire can be

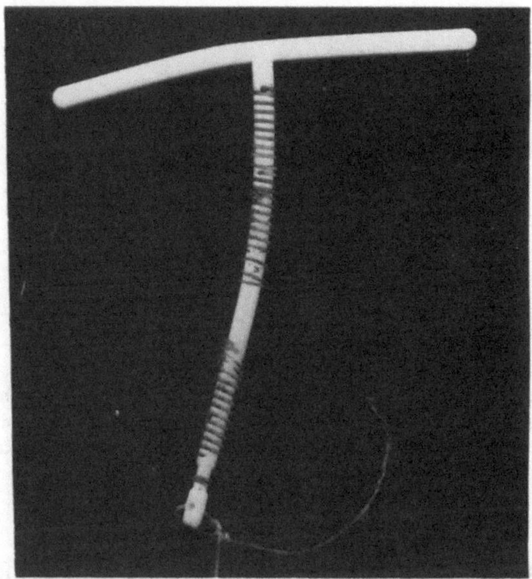

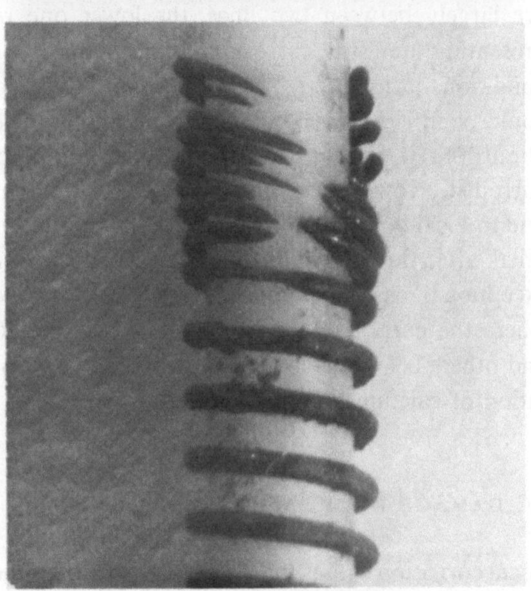

Figure 7. Top: a device used only eight months (× 2.5). The distorted appearance and the short plastic threads are evidence of a too-low position of the device in utero. *Bottom:* detail of the same device (× 18).

measured and compared with its original diameter. This enables us to express the progress of the corrosion numerically. In Figure 8, the relation between time of use and maximum observed corrosion in the device is shown. The deepest observed pit is measured and expressed as a percentage of the diameter of the wire. It was decided that corrosion reaching the centre of the wire from one side represented breakage of the wire: this is shown in

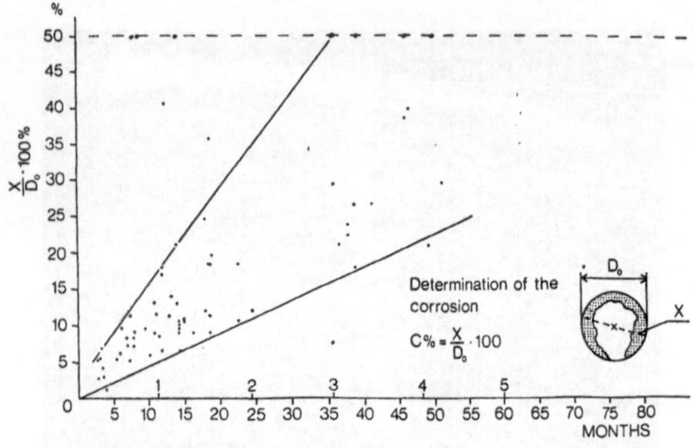

Figure 8. The corrosion depth as compared with the original diameter of the copper wire. The value 50% represents the point at which the corrosion reaches the middle of the wire and is taken to show wire breakage. The diameter of the wires was 0.2 mm.

the diagram by a value of fifty percent. The points are largely between two lines, the lower one representing uniform corrosion and/or favourable conditions in the uterus, indicating that the device could be in situ at least six years, whereupon only about thirty percent of the diameter would be corroded. However the upper line indicates that, due to local corrosion, the wire can be expected to break after three years of use. There are also some exceptional cases falling outside the upper line, where the corrosion has been grossly accelerated, and others below the lower line, where the precipitation of calcium has been observed.

IV. DAMAGE IN THE WIRE

Local corrosion causes the breakage of the wire and the loss of copper in the form of metallic fragments. Tests with monkeys show that the metal fragments are expelled from the uterus relatively soon (Tatum 1973). Although there is no evidence that these fragments are harmful, they at least accelerate the copper loss and quickly diminish the lifetime of the device. The earliest wire breakage reported by the Population Council was after 5.5 months of use (Population Council 1973). Figure 7 shows one device, originally inserted low in the uterus, after eight months of use.

The number of cases in which the wire is broken increases with time; when the time of use exceeds 3.5 years, breakage appears to increase more rapidly. The risk of breakage or fragmentation can be indicated by comparing the number of cases with broken wires to the number of devices observed. Combining our results (Kosonen 1978) with those of others (Timonen 1976; F.H. Schmidt 1977, personal communication), the relation of fragmentation to the time of use can be tabulated:

Time of use (years)	*Number of IUDs having fragmented wire (%)*
2	5
3	21
4	33

These figures are valid when the diameter of the wire is 0.2 mm. For the Cu-T200, which nowadays has a wire diameter of 0.25 mm, the figures will perhaps be somewhat lower. Wire fragmentation is the main reason for limitation of the period of use of a copper-bearing IUD; when the wire begins to break, the risk of pregnancy increases and the possibility exists that needle-sharp wire fragments may cause complications. For the Cu-T200, three years of use is recommended, which according to the above means a 20% risk of fragmentation.

V. COPPER RELEASE

The rate of dissolution of the copper is directly proportional to the surface area, so the risk of pregnancy decreases with increasing copper area in a device (Tatum 1973). The other determinant of the rate of dissolution is the quantity of dissolving agents present. When the surface area exceeds 300 mm^2, the dissolution rate seems to become constant (Timonen 1976).

It would be useful to know the average amount of copper being released daily after long-term use and to calculate the time needed for complete dissolution of the copper, but there are several factors, for example individual differences in patients, the limited number of devices available for study after many years of use, wire fragmentation, and uncertainties in the calculations due to the lack of knowledge of the exact original metal weight, which influence the calculation and cause variations in the results.

However the following rates have been reported as being the average copper release rate after three years of use: 43.8 μg/day (Timonen 1976), 20 μg/day (Zielske et al. 1974), 14.3 μg/day (F.H. Schmidt 1977, personal communication). On the basis of measurements from seventeen devices, we calculated a release rate of 23 μg/day after three years of use. Possible variations in the original copper weight could be estimated fairly accurately, as we manufactured the devices. None of the devices had a broken wire when removed.

The average of the figures referred to above gives a rate of release of around 25 μg/day of copper after three years of use. Accordingly, if uniform corrosion with no occurrence of fragmentation could be arranged, it would take thirteen years for all the copper to be dissolved in, for example, the Cu-T200, which initially contains 120 mg of copper. It has to be noticed that this calculation does not indicate the functional lifetime of the device. Due to the decreasing surface area of wire and the increasing diffusion path for copper atoms the copper release rate most likely decreases with time, but there is no information on the amount of copper release sufficient to prevent pregnancy.

VI. PREVENTION OF FRAGMENTATION

There is evidence that under some conditions alloys behave differently, and from some aspects have a better resistance to corrosion than pure metals. In order to verify that an analogous effect is also created using alloys in IUDs, a test of the following seventeen alloys was arranged in vitro.

Cu: oxygen-containing copper
Cu: oxygen-free copper
Cu: oxygen-free copper of high-grade purity
Cu: 9% Sn
Cu: 5.8% Al
Cu: 5.2% Al, 1.9% Fe
Cu: 0.5% Fe
Cu: 1% Ag
Cu: 5.1% Ag
Cu: 4.8% Ag, 5.2% Al
Cu: 5.0% Ag, 1% Fe
Cu: 1.9% Fe, 5.5% Ag, 5.5% Al
Ag: 17% Cu
Ag: pure silver
Cu: 25% Au
Cu: 50% Au
Cu: 75% Au

Elements for the alloys were chosen from metals which were known to be neither allergenic nor carcinogenic. Uterine conditions were simulated with an aminoacid solution, the composition of which is indicated in Table 1. Thin wires of 0.2-0.25 mm diameter from each respective alloy were incubated in a solution of 1:1 Levamin 70 and Levamin Essential Oxygen was added by bubbling 5 l/min air through the solution.

Table 1. Compositions of aminoacid infusion solutions.

	*Levamin® Essential**	*Levamin® 70**
Histidin acet. respond 1 – histidin	0.55 monochlorid	2.2
Isoleucin	0.7	2.8
Leucin	1.1	4.4
Lysin acet. respond 1 – lysin 0.8 monochlorid		3.2
Methionin	1.1	4.4
Phenylalanin	1.1	4.4
Threonin	0.5	2.0
Thyptophan	0.25	1.0
Valin	0.8	3.2
Alanin		16.0
Acid. aminoacet.		16.0
Sorbitol		50
Aq. steril. ad.	100 ml	1000 ml

* Manufactured by Leiras Pharmaceutical Company, Turku, Finland.

Within three days severe corrosion occurred in alloys containing Al, Fe or Sn, while Au-rich and Ag-rich compositions showed very slight corrosion. Copper containing 5 percent Ag, which indicated moderate corrosion (Figure 9), was chosen for clinical testing. Before the in-vivo study began, the antifertility effect of the alloy was tested in animals. For the in-vivo study, the wire was wound onto the prototype of the newly patented Nova T device. The results, as indicated in Table 2 (Skouby and Tabor 1978), were favourable. However, microscopic examination of removed devices showed no improvement in corrosion over that of pure copper. It might be possible to find copper alloys having better corrosion characteristics in IUDs than pure

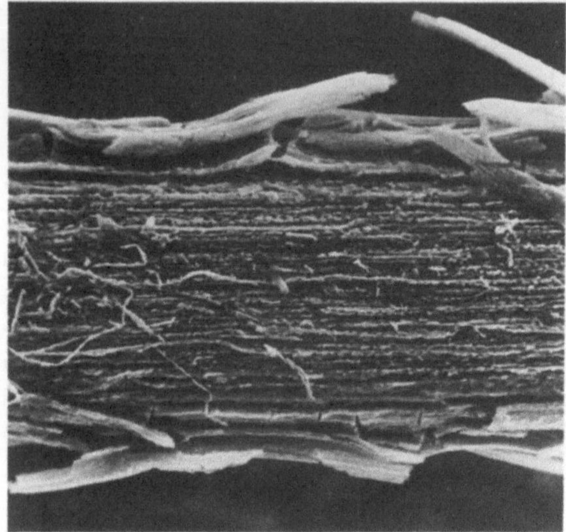

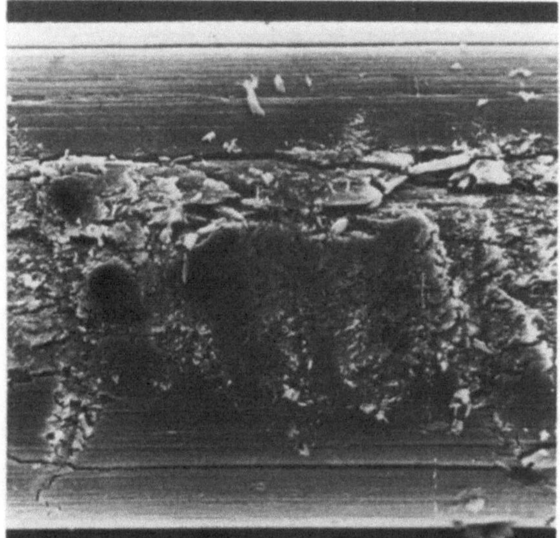

Figure 9. Oxygen-free copper of high grade purity (*top*) and Cu with 5.1 percent Ag (*bottom*) after 12 days incubation in Levamin solution (SEM picture, × 400).

copper, but there is always the risk of increased pregnancy rate when dissolution of the metal is suppressed.

Another possibility to eliminate the disadvantage of local corrosion is to arrange a thin core, inside the copper, which does not dissolve in the uterine secretions. This kind of wire remains unbreakable, although all the copper is dissolved around it. We developed a wire in which pure silver was processed inside a copper covering to serve as a noncorrodible core. We have subjected this wire to clinical

Table 2. Net cumulative rate of events and closures per 100 cases by type of termination after twelve months of use (Nova-T prototype).

Reason for termination	*Nulliparous*	*Parous*
Accidental pregnancy	0.0	0.0
Expulsion	8.1	1.6
Removals	35.1	15.3
Bleeding disturbances	5.4	1.7
Bleeding and pain	16.2	1.7
Adnex inflammation	5.4	1.7
Other medical	0.0	0.0
Planned pregnancy	5.4	5.9
Total terminations	43.2	16.9
Continuous rate	70.0	
Number of women	37	

testing since 1976. Silver-core copper wire is used in a new IUD, the Nova-T (Figure 10). This device has been tested in a multicentre study which was well randomized and of a double-blind nature (Luukkainen et al. 1979). The most important result was that the Nova-T had a statistically significant lower pregnancy rate than the Cu-T. The silver-core wire (Figure 11) in Nova-T has a diameter of 0.3 mm, of which the silver inside is 0.1 mm. Because the core keeps the wire coherent and prevents fragmentation, the functional lifetime of this device can be prolonged up to five years.

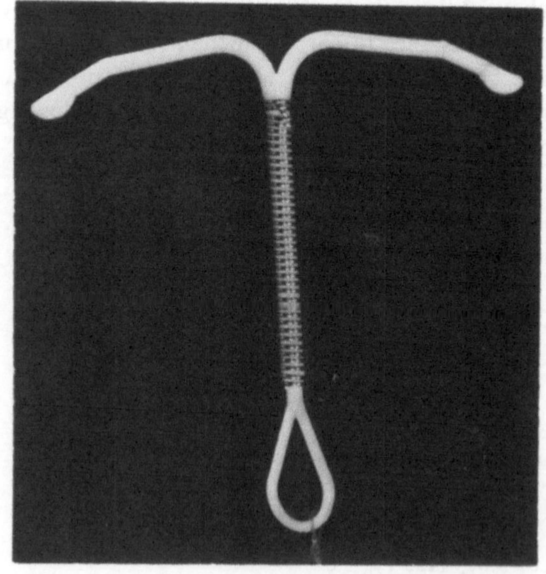

Figure 10. Nova-T. US Patent No. 3937217.

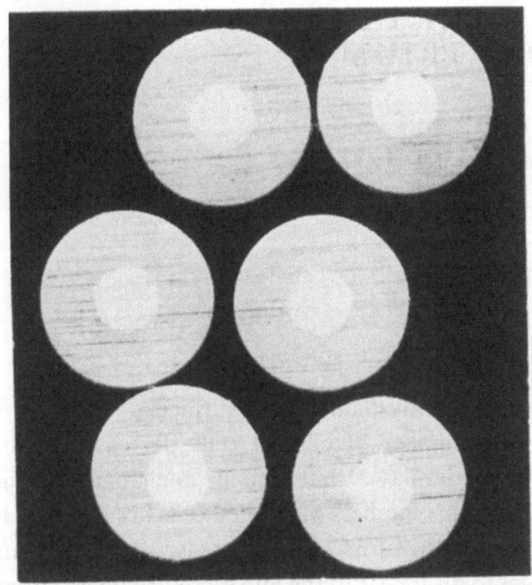

Figure 11. Copper wires, 0.30 mm diameter, with 0.10 mm silver core.

REFERENCES

Bank HL, Williamson HO, Manning K: Scanning electron microscopy of copper-containing intrauterine devices: long-term changes in utero. Fertil Steril 26: 503, 1975.

Gosden C, Ross A, Loudon NB: Intrauterine deposition of calcium on copper-bearing intrauterine contraceptive devices. Br Med J 1: 202, 1977.

Hagenfeldt K: Intrauterine contraception with the copper-T device I: effect on trace elements in the endometrium, cervical mucus and plasma. Contraception 6: 37, 1972.

Johnson AB, Maness RF, Wheeler RG: Calcareous deposits formed on IUDs in human exposures. Contraception 14: 507, 1976.

Kosonen A: Corrosion of copper in utero. Fertil Steril 30: 1, 1978.

Leidheiser H Jr: The corrosion of copper, tin and their alloys. New York, John Wiley and Sons, 1971, p 100ff.

Luukkainen T, Nielsen NC, Nygren KG, Pyörälä T, Kosonen A: Randomized comparison of clinical performance of two copper-releasing IUDs, Nova-T and Copper-T 200, in Denmark, Finland and Sweden. Contraception 19: 1, 1979.

Oster G: Chemical reactions of the copper intrauterine device. Fertil Steril 23: 18, 1972.

Oster G, Salgo M: The copper intrauterine device and its mode of action. N Engl J Med 293: 432, 1975.

Population Council: Report on Copper-T 200: 121: wire fragment. New Drug Application, March 1973.

Sikov MR, Devine JR, Hackett PL: Studies of Dublex (copper-coated) wires for use in intrauterine devices. Contraception 13: 55, 1976.

Skouby SO, Tabor A: Erfaringer med en kobber-sølvspiral, Cu-T2200W. Ugeskr. Laeger 140: 31, 1978.

Tatum HJ: Copper-bearing intrauterine devices. Clin Obstet Gynecol 17: 93, 1974.

Tatum HJ: Metallic copper as an intrauterine contraceptive agent. Am J Obstet Gynecol 117: 602, 1973.

Timonen H: Copper release from copper-T intrauterine devices. Contraception 14: 25, 1976.

Van Eyck J, Lagasse A, Thiery M: Scanning electron microscopy of inert and copper-bearing intra-uterine devices. Contraception 13: 65, 1977.

Zielske F, Koch UJ, Badura R, Ladeburg H: Studies on copper release from copper-T devices (T-Cu 200) and its influence on sperm migration in vitro. Contraception 10: 651, 1974.

4. THE EFFECT OF THE IUD ON THE ULTRASTRUCTURE OF THE ENDOMETRIUM

H.H. El-Badrawi and E.S.E. Hafez

I. THE SURFACE ULTRASTRUCTURE OF THE NORMAL ENDOMETRIUM

The surface epithelium of the endometrium is smooth with no mucosal folds. It is composed of columnar ciliated and nonciliated cells. Endometrial gland openings, apparent within the surface, have different shapes and distribution throughout the menstrual cycle. The surface epithelium of the normal endometrium undergoes cyclical alterations in cell shape, apical microvilli, ciliation and secretory activity (Daniel et al. 1973, 1975; Ferenczy and Richart 1973; Johannisson and Nilsson 1972; Morgenroth and Verhagen 1972; Nilsson and Nygren 1972).

I.A. Ciliated cells

Ciliated cells are less abundant in the endometrium than in the oviductal apithelium (Figure 1.) They are found singly or in clusters, and are present from the beginning of the epithelial regrowth, tending to remain concentrated near the gland orifices. By the early proliferative phase, 4-8 days postmenstrual, the endometrial surface becomes completely reepithelized and is covered by closely packed, dome-shaped cells mined with numerous ciliated cells in an approximate ratio of 30: 1 (Ferenczy et al. 1972a). The cilia at that time are well-developed, being morphologically similar to those seen in the oviduct (Ferenczy et al. 1972b). During the late proliferative and early secretory phases, the number of ciliated cells increases and the cell's individual cilia increase in length and density (Hafez et al. 1975). The ratio of nonciliated to ciliated cells becomes approximately 15: 1 (Ferenczy et al. 1972a). Ciliated cells are also noted in the gland opening and in the deeper glandular epithelium, but less frequently than on the surface.

The number of ciliated cells decreases slightly from about day 21 but remains unchanged through to day 28. Numbers of ciliated cells are reported by some investigators to be decreased markedly and even to disappear in the late secretory phase (Wynn and Harris 1967; Wynn and Wolley 1967; Fleming et al. 1968; Fruin and Tighe 1967; Schueller 1968). The discrepancy may have arisen because most previous studies were principally concerned with endometrial glands rather than surface epithelium.

Since cellular modifications in the uterine mucosa are hormone-dependent, it is possible that the surface epithelium has a different sensitivity to hormonal stimuli than does the glandular epithelium, a possibillity which is supported by the longer persistence of intracytoplasmic glycogen and RNA synthesis in secretory cells of the uterine lining as compared to the glandular epithelium.

I.A.1. Ciliogenesis

The morphogenesis of cilia in the endometrial epithelium has been studied by means of light and phase contrast microscopy (Schueller 1961, 1968), but there have been no systematic studies of human endometrial ciliogenesis (Figure 2). The structure of the cilium, including basal body and ciliary bud formation, is similar to that of cilia found in the mammalian oviduct (Anderson and Brenner 1971). The cilia of the endometrium are typical kinocilia (motile) with nine peripheral and two central filaments (Hafez et al. 1975). The turnover of endometrial cilia must be considerably greater than that of the oviductal epithelial cells, with a peak of ciliogenesis immediately following the menstrual period (Ferenczy et al. 1972a). Ciliogenesis in the uterine glands bears a close resemblance to that in the oviductal mucosa, in which ciliogenesis and

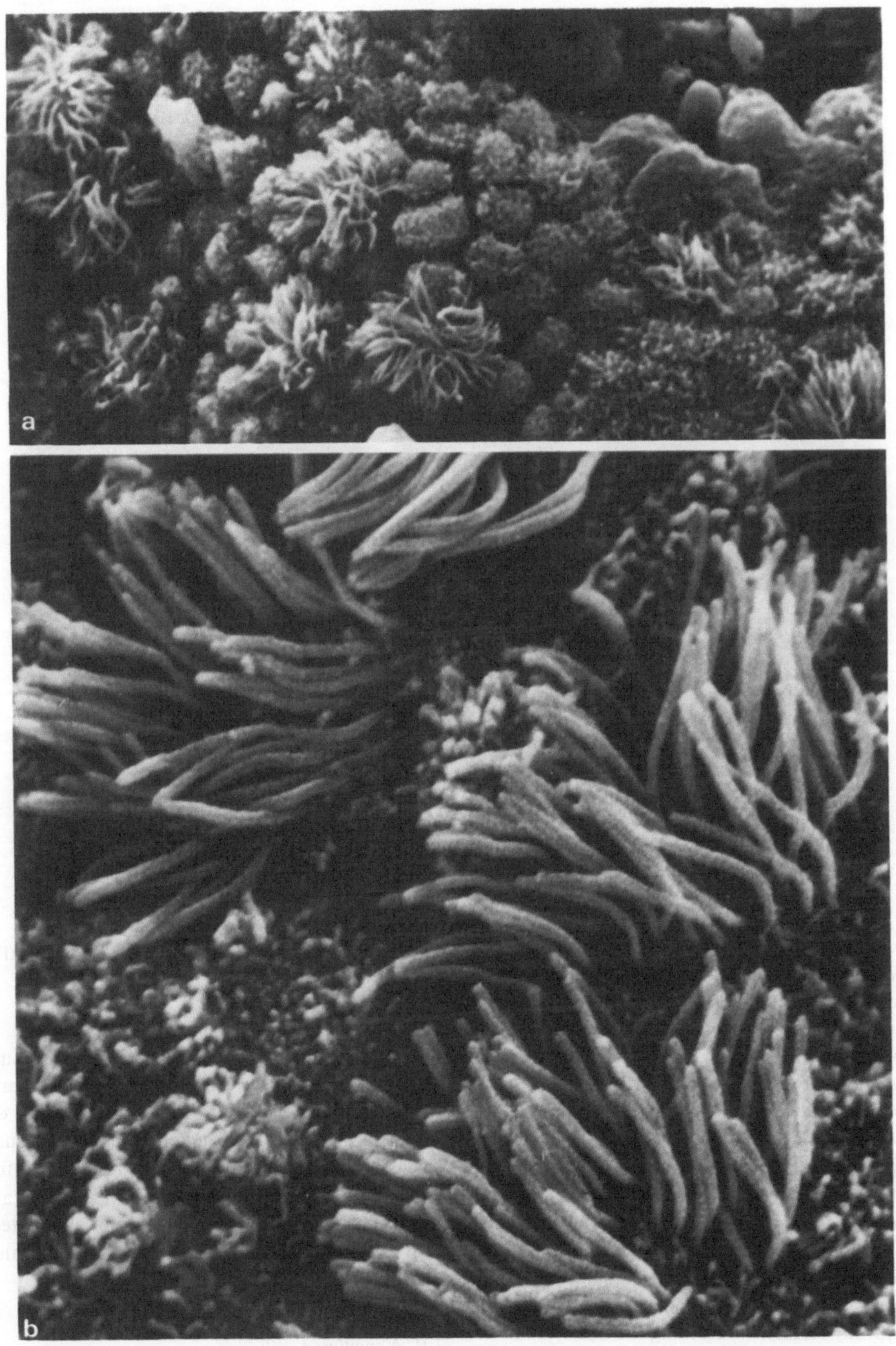

Figure 1. Scanning electron micrographs of normal endometrium. Note ciliated and nonciliated cells and normal distribution of endometrial gland openings (a- × 3,000; b- × 7,500).

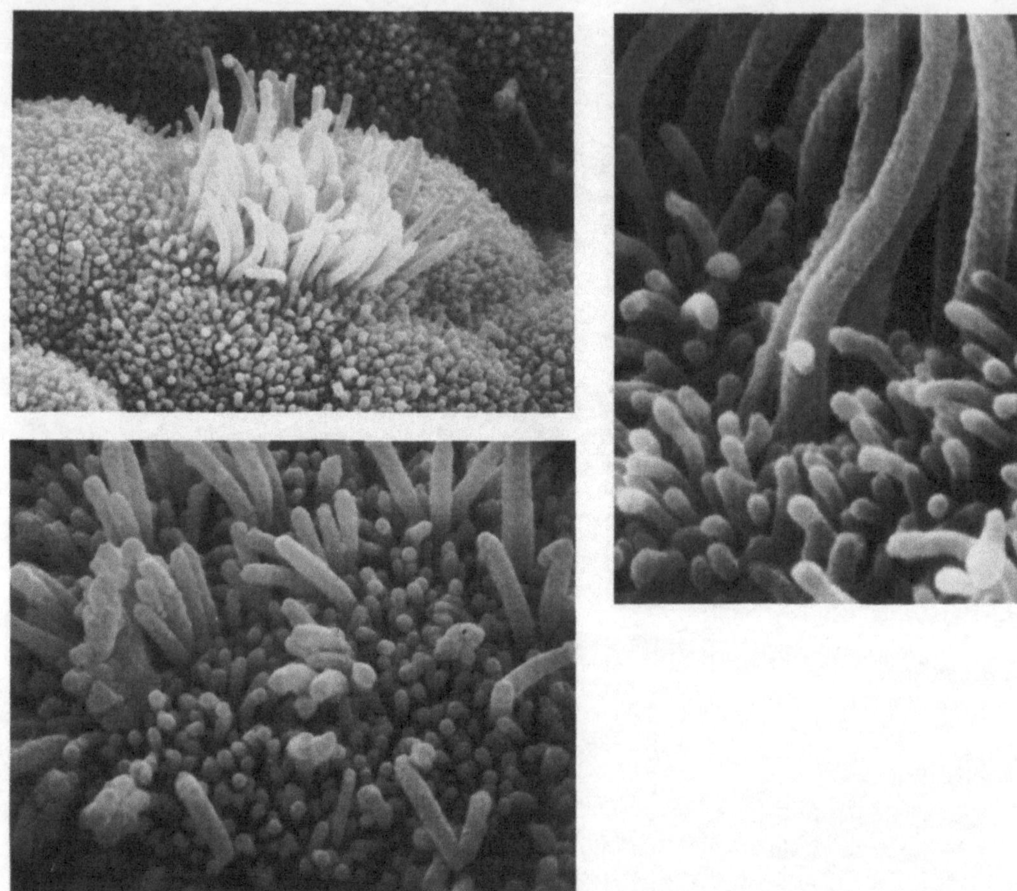

Figure 2. Scanning electron micrographs of normal human endometrium showing ciliated and nonciliated cells in mid and late proliferative phases of the menstrual cycle. *Upper left, lower left:* note the process of ciliogenesis; the cilia are healthy and erect towards the endometrial cavity. The nonciliated cells, dome-shaped, are more numerous, with a normal microvillous pattern covering their apical surfaces (upper left: ×6020; lower left: ×11410; right: ×50000).

secretory activity undergo minimal cyclic changes (Wynn and Wooley 1967). Development and maintenancy of ciliated cells in both types of epithelia, however, seem to be under estrogenic control, since an absence of estrogen results in deciliation and cessation of secretory activity (Ferenczy et al. 1972b; Schueller 1968).

Ludwig et al. (1976) have defined three different types of ciliated cells: (1) ciliated cells which remain intact from cycle to cycle within the glandular epithelial layer through some unknown preservation process; (2) ciliated cells within the surface epithelial layer which are desquamated with the menstrual breakdown of the tissue and are subsequently reestablished during the first week of the menstrual cycle; (3) solitary cilia sprouting from enlarged cuboidal cells within the lining surface epithelium. The possible significance of the last type is unknown.

I.A.2. The function of ciliated cells

The precise significance of cilia in the endometrium, especially on the surface, is not understood. Ciliary motion in the endometrium is in the form of uniform stroke and counterstroke movements (Schueller 1968), most probably promoting fluid circulation or sperm and egg transport (Hafez et al. 1975). In this regard, the concentration of ciliated cells around gland openings may facilitate the distribution of glandular secretions.

I.B. Nonciliated cells

The dome-shaped nonciliated cells contain a profuse array of short, occasionally branching, hairlike projections, the *microvilli* (Figure 2). In the early proliferative phase, with reepithelization of the surface epithelium, growth of the microvilli is very apparent. They cover the apical surface of the cells and are dispersed and to form ridgelike patterns. The density of cells increases during this phase. They become columnar, with slightly protruding apices. The length and density of microvilli on the cell surface also increase (Hafez et al. 1975).

Cytoplasmic blebs, connected to the cell apex by narrow stalks, begin to appear in the late proliferative, becoming widespread in the secretory phase. When observed with transmission electron microscopy, they are seen to possess glycogen granules and numerous vesicles (Nilsson 1962; Themann and Schunke 1963). These secretory domes, generally attributed to a macroapocrine secretory process, are implicated to pinocytotic activity as well.

The microvilli seem to give some rigidity to the cell membrane and may be concerned with some forms of movement under the influence of the contractile protein action (Hafez et al. 1975). Cell membranes are hormonally controlled, as inferred from the cyclic changes in the distribution, shape, and the number of apical microvilli in the secretory cells throughout the menstrual cycle.

I.C. Endometrial gland openings

In the early proliferative phase of the cycle, with complete reepithelization of the surface endometrium, the epithelial cells are arranged spirally around the gland openings. The glandular gaps being wide enables observation of the pattern of the epithelium. With regard to cell volume, cell boundaries, cilia and microvilli, there are differences between the surface ultrastructure of the endometrial epithelium and the epithelium lining the glands (Figure 3). Ciliogenesis in the glandular epithelium can be observed during the early proliferative through to the mid-proliferative phase, but by then it is completely terminated. The ciliated cells are more abundant in the surface than in the glands; they decrease in number or disappear in the postovulatory phase of the cycle.

From the early proliferative phase to midcycle, the endometrial surface changes drastically. In the late luteal phase the narrow, small gland openings lose their round shape and appear like a cleft, especially in the lower uterine segment. Along the margin of the glandular clefts there is a remarkably smooth transition from surface to glandular epithelium. With the increase in the endometrial surface convolutions at this stage, the endometrial gland openings become difficult to distinguish.

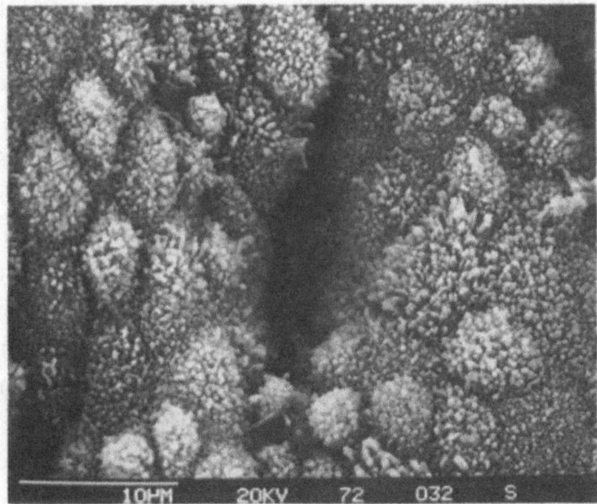

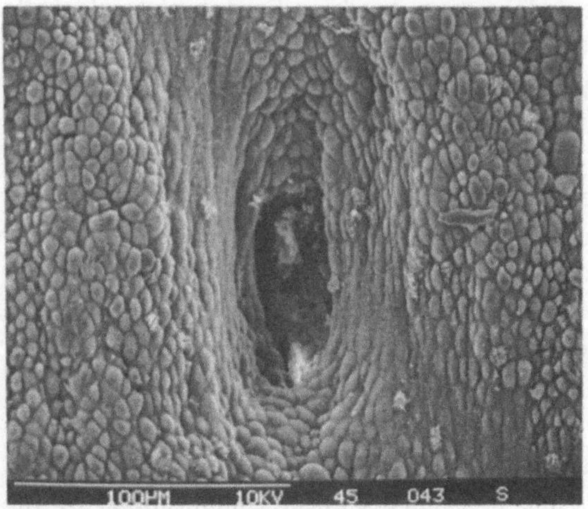

Figure 3. Scanning electron micrograph of endometrium showing endometrial gland openings. Right: note the spiral arrangement of cells around the gland with inflammatory material coming out from it (× 1330). Left: note abundance of ciliated cells around gland opening. Ciliated cells are also seen with the glandular epithelium (× 2170).

II. ULTRASTRUCTURE OF THE ENDOMETRIUM IN THE PRESENCE OF AN IUD

The interaction between an IUD and the endometrium is primarily a surface phenomenon and is therefore well suited to investigation by scanning electron microscopy (Daniel et al. 1973, 1975). In order to exert its contraceptive action, the IUD must be placed properly in the uterine cavity so that its local mechanical effects might operate on a larger area of the endometrium (Elstein and Sparks 1977). The device must come into close contact with the endometrial surface to provide a basis for interplay between the IUD and the epithelium (Hafez et al. 1975).

In the areas of contact, the mechanical pressure caused by the IUD leads to atrophy of the endometrium underlying the device. When IUD contact areas are compared with other areas of the endometrium the histological differences are striking (Moyer and Shaw 1973). The possible effect of the IUD and the associated histological changes on the endometrium are discussed in Chapter 5. The surface ultrastructural alterations and the morphological changes from inert and medicated IUDs are discussed in this chapter.

There is a great morphological difference between the epithelium at the site of IUD impression and away from it. The indentation of the IUD on the endometrial surface can be seen even by the naked eye (Figure 4), but this depends on whether the endometrium has been fixed in glutaraldehyde with the IUD in situ or after its removal. The depressions left by the IUD are shallow in the proliferative phase, but become considerably deeper with tissue growth around the device during the secretory (Daniel et al. 1973, 1975; Moyer and Mishell 1971). The combination of pressure and restricted growth leads to morphological alteration of the surface epithelium (Hafez et al. 1975). This alteration is also affected by the types of medication used with the IUD, namely copper and progesterone. At the same time, the surface ultrastructural changes of the endometrium are influenced by the possible associated clinical complications of the IUD and how long the IUD has been used.

II.A. Scanning electron microscopy of endometrium with inert IUD

II.A.1. The site of IUD impression

At the site of IUD impression, the surface epithelium shows multiple areas of superficial loss of cells and exposure of the basement membrane (Figure 4). Some of the erosive areas may touch each other. The basement membrane is occasionally destroyed in these eroded areas, exposing the endometrial stroma (Ludwig et al. 1976; Ludwig and Metzger 1976). The disrupted areas are unevenly distributed thoughout the entire IUD contact zone. Endometrial gland openings can be seen in a normal pattern and number (Figure 5).

There is great variation in the size of the nonciliated cells, with a decrease in the number of microvilli (Figure 6). With the progress of the menstrual cycle from the proliferative to the secretory phase, the epithelial cells become more flattened and compressed, tending to be elongated and cuboidal, with slightly protuberant surfaces (Daniel et al. 1975). The microvilli are shorter and more diffuse over the cell surface than in areas not in contact with the IUD.

There would seem to be two types of secretory mechanism in the epithelial cells: macroapocrine secretion (Morgenroth and Verhagen 1972; Themann and Schunke 1963) and microcrine secretion (Daniel et al. 1975). The normal secretory pattern with inert IUD is altered: there is no secretion within the gland lumina at the area of IUD contact; the apical cytoplasmic protrusions of the secretory cells are rare, despite the abundant glycogen within the cytoplasm of endometrial cells – this indicates a disturbed secretory function at these sites (Gonzalez-Angulo et al. 1973). The secretion pattern, if present, is in the form of an amorphous sheet, rather than of secretory droplets, covering the cells and partially obscuring the surface. This is explained by the fact that the contact pressure from the IUD, may prevent the secretions from retaining their shape (Daniel et al. 1975).

The ciliated cells are markedly reduced in number at the contact zone. If present they are flattened, compressed, shorter, and unhealthy (Figure 6), only

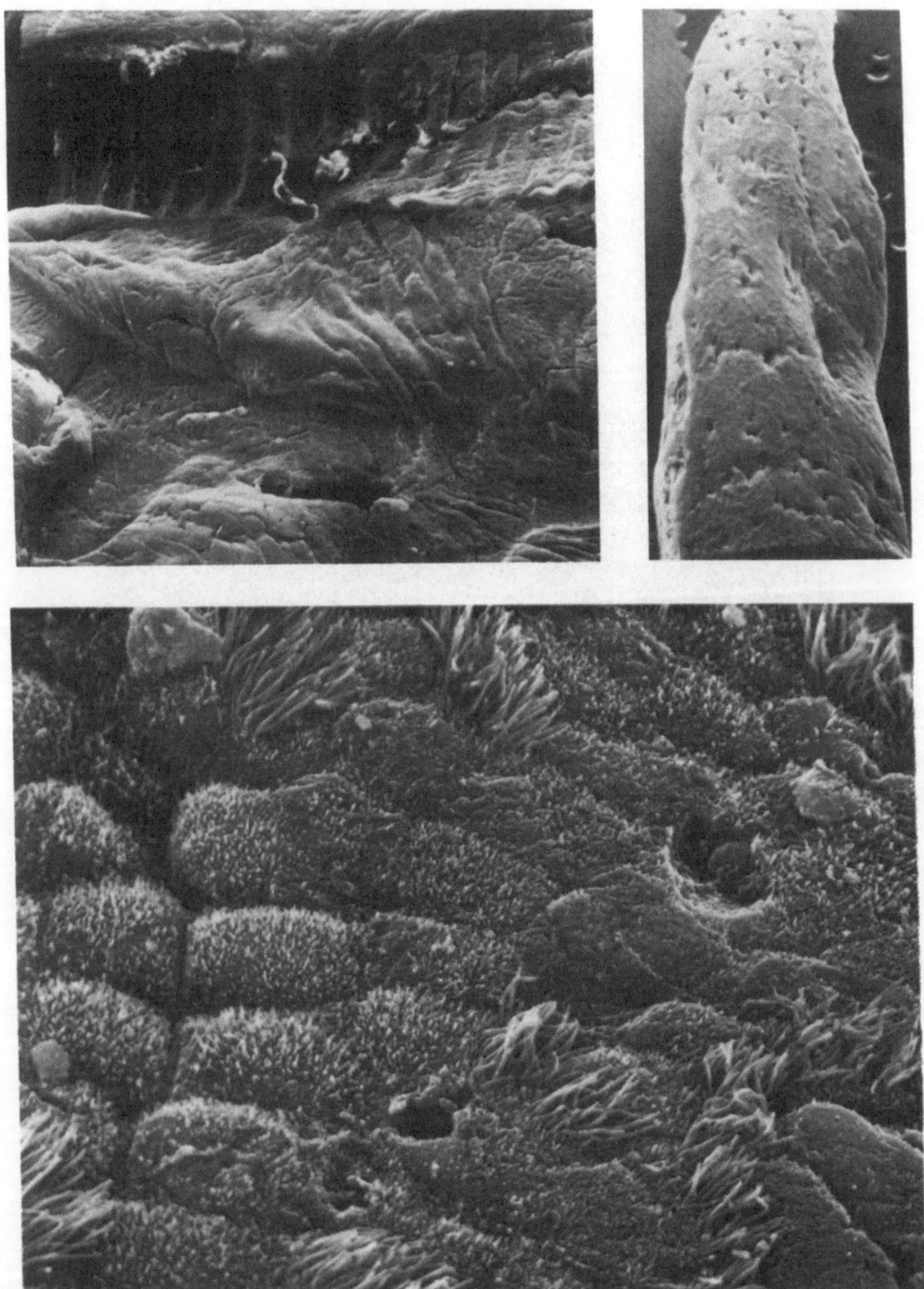

Figure 4. Scanning electron micrographs of endometrium. *Top left:* the indentation of the ML Cu-250 IUD on the surface endometrium. Note site of impression of copper and inert parts of IUD (×20). *Top right:* overview of curettage sample showing endometrial gland openings (×20). *Bottom:* note the loss of superficial cellular components near the site of impression of a Lippes inert IUD during the early secretory phase (×2160).

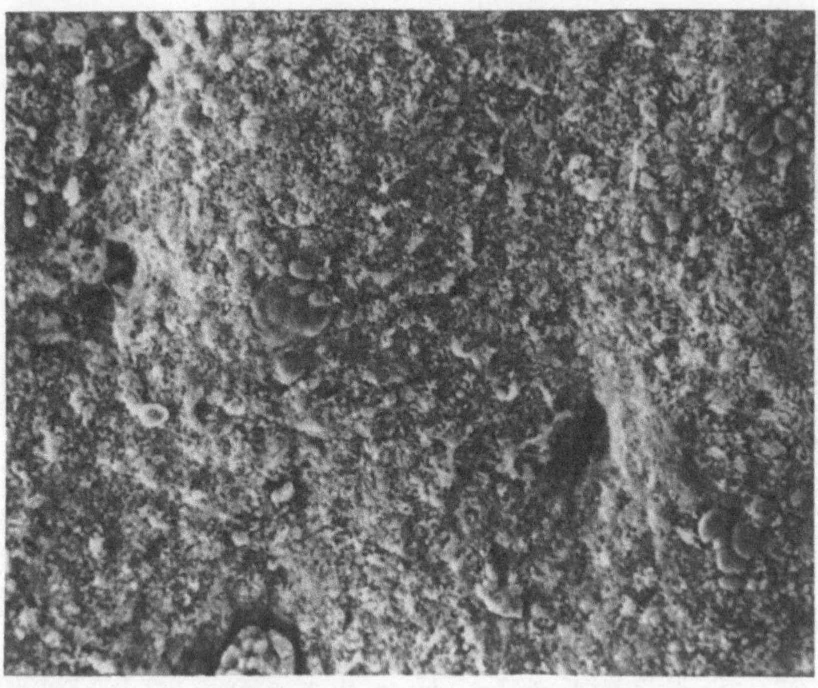

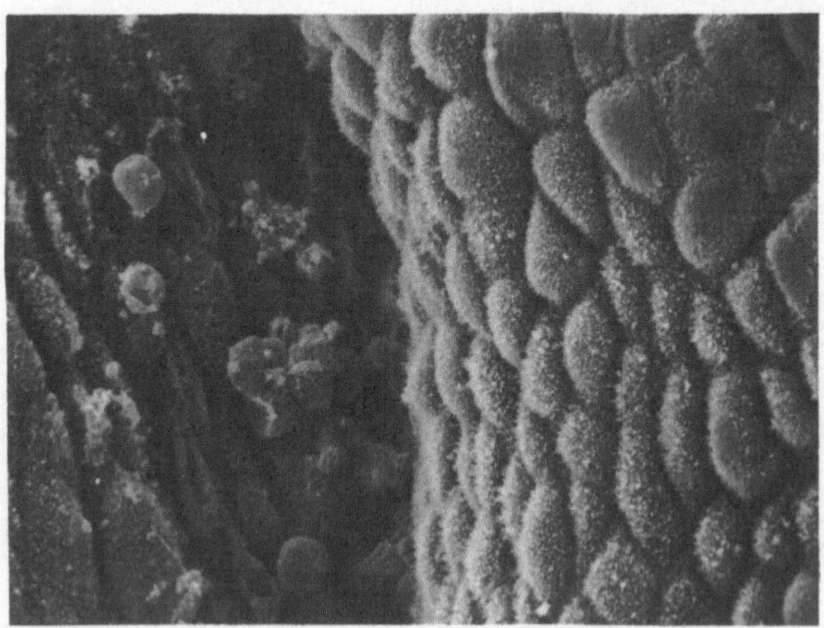

Figure 5. Scanning electron micrograph of endometrium. Note endometrial gland openings at the site of inert IUD impression. The glands are normally distributed with inflammatory material extruding from them (top: × 1000; Bottom: × 1900).

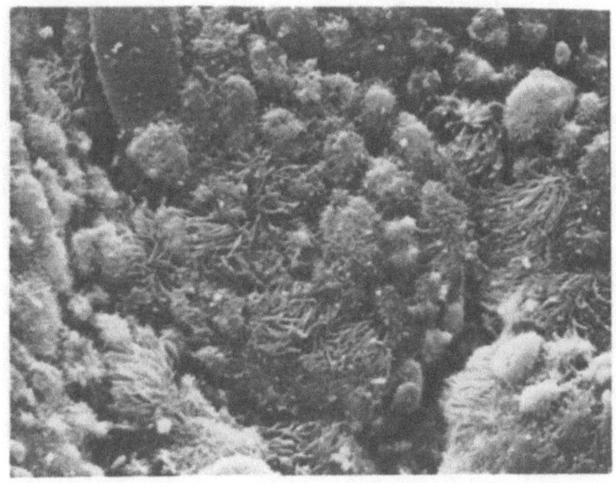

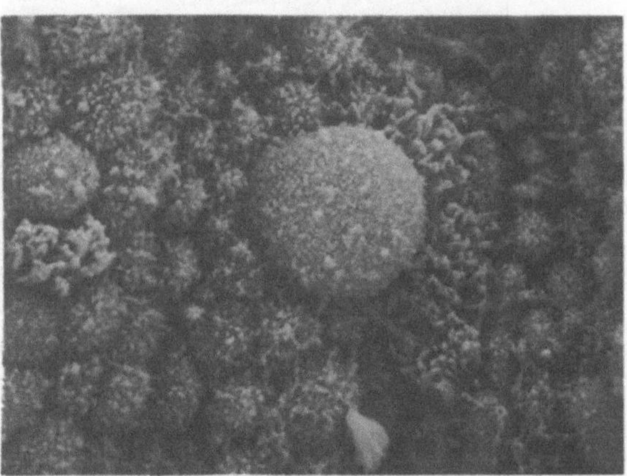

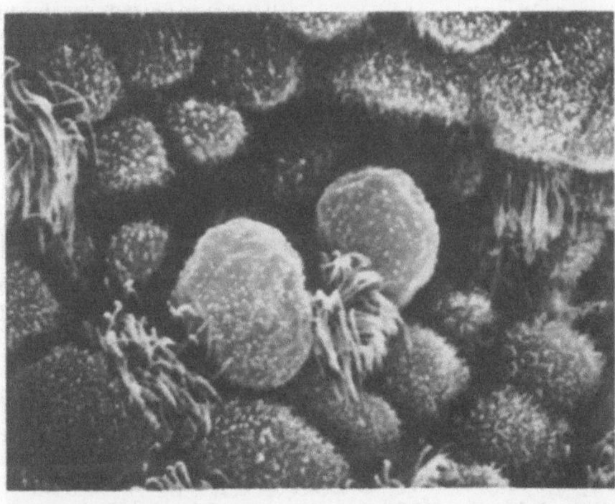

Figure 6. Scanning electron micrographs of endometrium at the site of impression of an inert IUD. *Top:* the ciliated cells are compressed, not erect, with indistinct intercellular boundaries (×1400). *Middle, bottom:* note variability in size of nonciliated cells, the well-developed intercellular connections and the short and diffused microvilli (middle: ×3500; bottom: ×6020).

occasionally being found as healthy as in the normal endometrium. However, the variability of the changes in ciliated and nonciliated cells at the contact zone may be attributed to the fact that, microscopically, the device does not touch the endometrium in all the areas of the macroscopic contact zone. This may also explain the more extensive effect on the cilia, their tips being in contact with the device throughout the contact zone. Some investigators reported the complete absence of cilia at the site of inert IUD contact (Ludwig et al. 1976).

II.A.2. Away from the site of IUD impression

The surface ultrastructure of the endometrium away from the site of an inert IUD impression has almost the character of the normal endometrium at the equivalent phase of the menstrual cycle (Figure 7). There may be some focal defects in the surface epithelium close to gland openings. The only marked morphological difference between the epithelial cells away from the site of IUD impression and in the normal endometrium is seen during the luteal phase of the cycle, when there is extreme balloon distension of the upper portions of the nonciliated cells within the glands as well as around them (Ludwig and Metzger 1976). The membranes of the ballooned tops are porous, with no signs of deflation. These distended structures appear within the microvilli, with their bases connected to the surface of the cell, thus giving an impression of being distended microvilli. They may be secretory granules which fail to separate from the secretory cell, so indicating a defect in the secretory activity mechanism (Gonzales-Angulo et al. 1973; Wynn 1968), but in our opinion this needs more investigation.

The gland openings show the usual architecture and distribution. The ciliated cells around these openings correspond with those of the normal luteal endometrium.

II.B. Ultrastructural changes of the endometrium with copper IUD

For proper evaluation of the effect of copper IUDs on the surface ultrastructure of the endometrium, we have to consider some important factors: (1) the distribution and amount of copper on the device;

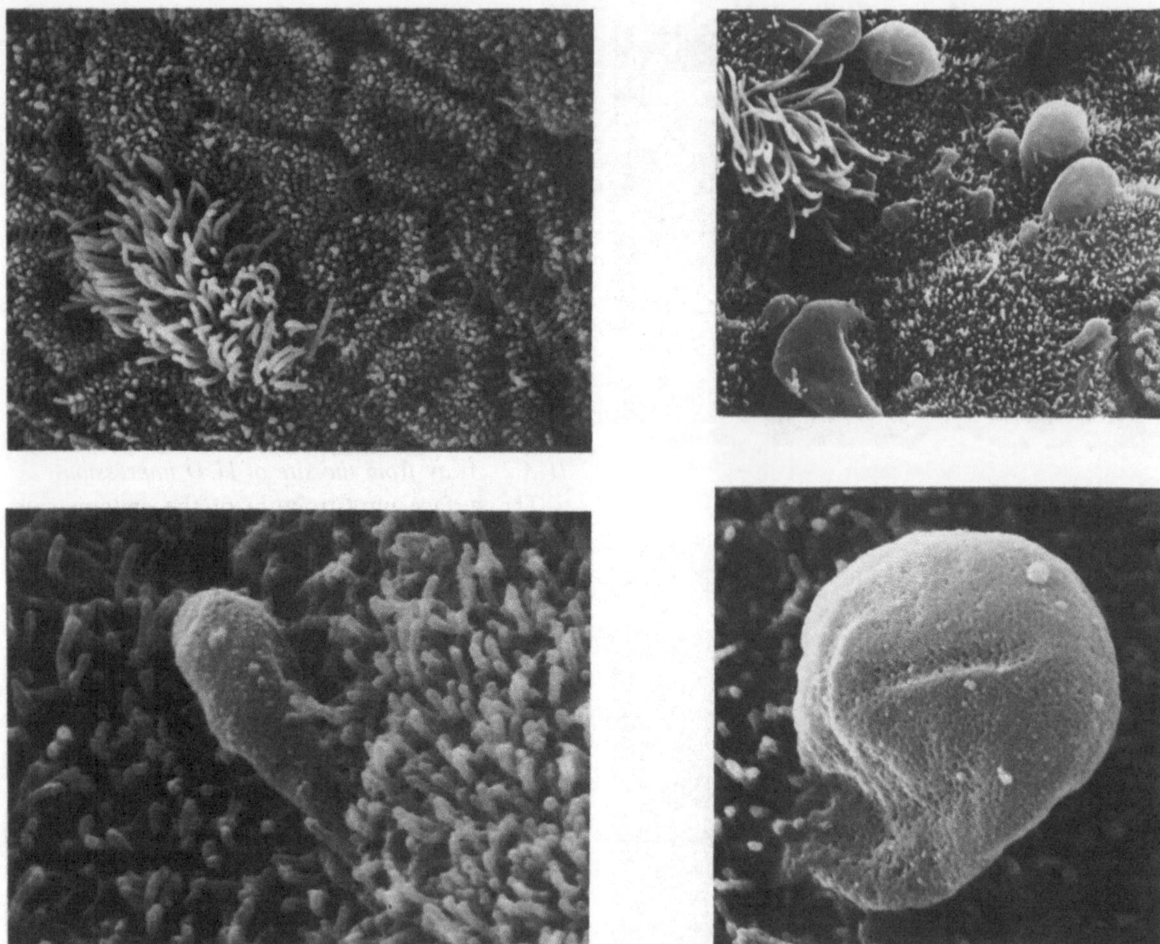

Figure 7. Scanning electron micrographs of endometrium with inert IUD in situ for 16 months, secretory phase, day 22, in areas not adjacent to the site of the IUD. *Above left:* normal appearance of the ciliated cell: well-developed microvillous pattern, well-developed intercellular connections. Secretory cells show depression of their domes (×3500). The other micrographs show the characteristic extruded structures commonly observed with an inert IUD. Note their connection with the surface of the cell and their spongy irregular surface indicating metabolic disturbance of secretory cells with defective secretory activity (above right: ×14000; below left: ×5500; below right: ×17500).

(2) the many areas of interaction with the endometrium: (a) endometrium in contact with the copper, (b) endometrium in contact with the plastic, (c) endometrium between these two zones, and (d) endometrium away from both zones; (3) the associated clinical complications with the device; (4) the duration of the device in situ; and (5) the stage of the menstrual cycle at the time of tissue examination.

II.B.1. Changes at the site of impression of a copper IUD

There is much more destruction of the cellular architecture at the site of copper-endometrium contact than that noticed with inert IUDs. There is also an increase in the extent of cellular morphological alteration with increase in the amount of copper incorporated in the device. Epithelial cells become abnormal in shape and distribution (Figure 8). Microvilli are either absent or very few per cell; they are shorter and are dispersed over the cell surface. Some of the cells may show rupture of their apical membranes. Flat erosions under the copper wire of the Cu-T200 are described by Ludwig et al. (1976); these are mostly covered by fibrin and cellular debris, including white blood cells. At the bottom of erosions not covered by debris, macrophages, lymphocytes, and red blood cells may be found.

The epithelial cells are forced to the side and

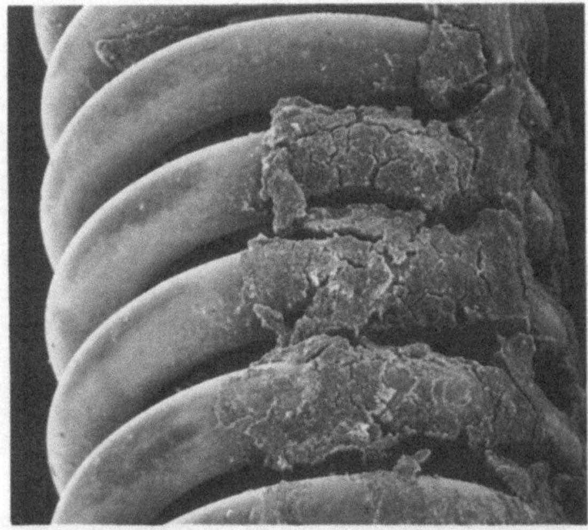

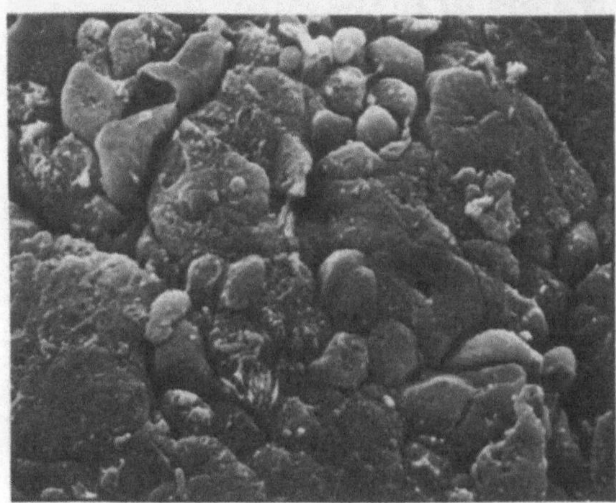

Figure 8. Scanning electron micrographs of endometrium. *Top:* The copper wire of ML Cu-250 – note attachment of endometrial tissue (×28). *Bottom:* endometrial surface at the site of impression of the copper IUD (ML Cu-250). Note the variability in the size of cells, the absence of ciliated cells and endometrial gland openings and the defective microvillous pattern (×1400).

sometimes overlap. Even in the proliferative phase, the apices of the cells are so flattened by the contact with the copper part of the device that the surface may appear nearly structureless. The cells may retain their columnar shapes, with stubby and depressed microvilli, in contact with Cu-200, but they show great individual variation, possibly with complete absence of microvilli, with ML Cu-250 and 375.

The ciliated cells are very infrequently seen in areas of contact with copper. The cilia, if seen, are crushed and lie flush with the surface rather than projecting up into the uterine cavity (Daniel et al. 1975). Subsequently, in the secretory phase, the pressure and restricted growth in IUD contact areas force cilia and microvilli to arise from between cells instead of from the exposed surface (Hafez et al. 1975).

There is complete absence of gland openings at the site of impression of ML Cu-250 and 375 in all phases of the menstrual cycle (Figure 8). Even with less copper incorporation, Cu-7 or Cu-T200 devices, no gland openings appear at the IUD site in the late proliferative phase or in the secretory phases. A few glands open within the impression site in the early proliferative are found on the ridges adjacent to the plastic support, but not in the depressions adjacent to copper coils.

The surface epithelium discloses no secretion to the lumen of the uterus. There is accumulation of glycogen, as well as of other secretory substances, such as glycoproteins, lipids, and mucopolysaccharides, within the cytoplasm (Gonzales-Angulo and Aznar-Ramos 1975; Nilsson and Hagenfeldt 1973).

II.B.2. Changes away from the device

Many investigators believed that the ultrastructural morphological changes resulting from the copper devices, as well as from the inert ones, were localized to the site of IUD impression (Hafez et al. 1975; Daniel et al. 1975), but our investigations, as well as those of Ludwig et al. (1976), have shown that the changes in the endometrium spread over areas not in contact with the IUD. These changes are marked near the copper wire, fading away from it. They are also directly related to the amount of copper incorporated in the device (Figure 9).

The lining epithelium seems to be without function near the copper. This is morphologically detected by the loss of microvilli, the wide intercellular clefts, and the absence of secretory cytoplasmic protrusions. If the surface ultrastructure is studied in the secretory phase of the cycle, the expected degree of endometrial maturation is not found. The distribution of the gland openings and their shapes, the ciliated cells, and the microvillous growth pattern are similar to those seen in the early proliferative phase, which indicates delayed maturation of the epithelium. This phenomenon is not seen at all in the epithelium away from the inert devices. The activity of the copper ions is not restricted to the area of contact and affects the rest

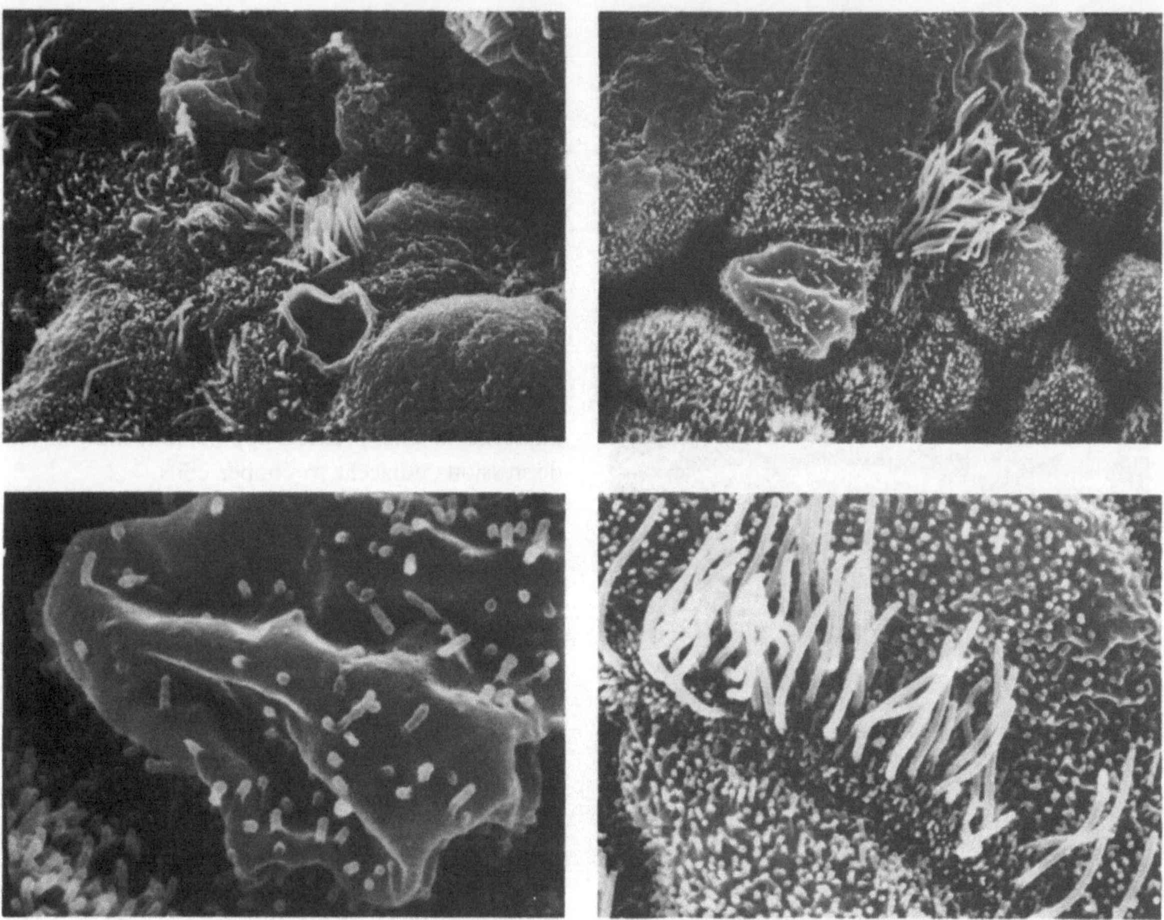

Figure 9. Scanning electron micrographs of human endometrium not adjacent to site of impression of ML Cu-250 (day 22 of menstrual cycle). Note abnormalities in cell topography, deflated cells, delayed microvillous growth and decreased number of cilia per cell (upper left: ×3080; upper right: ×3500; lower left: ×13300; lower right: ×7000).

of the endometrium (Oster and Salgo 1975). The ultrastructural changes in the endometrium as shown by transmission electron microscopy are summarized in Table 1.

II.B.3. Changes in the endometrium underlying the plastic part of the copper device

The surface alterations of the inert parts of the device are subject to the influence of the copper ions released. There is a mechanical impression on the endometrium comparable to that originating from inert IUDs. The ultrastructural changes at the inert part of the device include flattening of the surface epithelial cells, variability in cell shape and loss of normal microvillous pattern (Figure 10). Ciliated cells are scarce and have fewer cilia. The gland openings decrease in number. The modification of the lining epithelium at these areas almost reaches the gland openings; although the epithelium inside the gland is not compressed by the device, it is influenced by the copper ions in the endometrial secretion. This shows that the copper ions themselves may cause the delay in maturation of the endometrium, as will be discussed later (Ludwig et al. 1976).

III. GLYCOGEN AND CARBOHYDRATE METABOLISM WITH INTRAUTERINE DEVICES

Both synthesis and degradation of glycogen occur during the late luteal phase (Nilsson et al. 1974). It is difficult to analyze the ultrastructure of glycogen metabolism due to the fact that its metabolic

Table 1. Summary of some intracellular changes of endometrial cells during the proliferative and secretory phases of the menstrual cycle of women with copper IUDs, as shown by transmission electron microscopy (Ferenczy and Richart 1973; Gonzalez-Angulo and Aznar-Ramos 1975; Hsu et al. 1976; Wynn and Wooley 1967).

Cellular organelles	*Proliferative phase*	*Secretory phase*
Mitochondria	less numerous than those described for this phase of the cycle rounded or elongated vacuolation of the matrix with myelin figure formation in approximately 80% of mitochondria per cell in ciliated and nonciliated cells; mitochondria showing no alterations are rather small, which may indicate a degenerative damage leading to deficiency in the energy supplied to the cell	no giant mitochondria, which is characteristic of ovulation and implicated in steroid metabolism leading to interference with normal steroid effect on the cells
Golgi complex	unremarkable	prominent
Lysosomes	predominant toward to apical portion of the cell, which may reflect early disposal of degrading organelles and membrane material	more numerous
Glycogen metabolism	not prominent mainly of the mono-particulate type	accumulation of glycogen in the cell with impaired degradation and faulty secretion mono-particulate and clump fashions

products are to a certain extent dissolved during the preparatory steps and are therefore difficult to visualize by electron microscopy. It is also difficult to use microanalytical techniques for the detection of the enzymes involved in glycogen metabolism in the cytoplasm or those attached to the glycogen molecule. However, from the ultrastructural point of view, the glycogen granules generally are related to (1) glycogen vacuoles, (2) profiles of smooth membrane, (3) light areas (large vacuolelike structures having a maximum size of about 6 μm and observed in all parts of the cells) and (4) lysosomelike bodies (Nilsson et al. 1974). The glycogen granules of the uterine epithelium are mostly β-granules but are sometimes α-granules (Drochmans 1962). The α-granules are regarded as polymerized complexes of β-granules. The apocrine cytoplasmic projections, noted by SEM and TEM, are regarded as secretory structures; their presence indicates an active macroapocrine secretory mechanism in the endometrial cells (Gonzales-Angulo et al. 1973; Nilsson and Hagenfeldt 1973; Daniel et al. 1975).

A defective carbohydrate metabolism of the endometrial epithelial cells with inert IUD can be inferred from the absence of apocrine cytoplasmic projections in the secretory cells despite the abundant glycogen within their cytoplasm (Gonzales-Angulo et al. 1973). In our studies on the Lippes Loop, the cytoplasmic secretory projections are absent only at the site of contact of the IUD with the endometrium (El-Badrawi et al. 1980).

With copper IUDs there is a lack of large light areas in the cytoplasm of endometrial glandular and surface epithelial cells which might indicate an interference with the degradation of glycogen by an inhibition of some enzymes (Nilsson et al. 1974). This occurs all over the endometrial surface, even away from the IUD. The existence of a defective carbohydrate metabolism with copper IUDs (Nilsson and Hagenfeldt 1973) is supported by the finding that the insertion of a copper device results in a decrease of the amylase activity of the endometrium (Tobles et al. 1972). Furthermore, an increase in the endometrial content of glycogen in the secretory phase of the cycle follows the insertion of the copper devices (Lopez de la Osa et al. 1972). The disturbed glycogen metabolism detected by both scanning and transmission microscopy in both surface and glandular epithelium gives further support to the view that the mode of action of the IUD, especially the copper device, might be through interference with the blastocyst-endometrium interaction and blastocyst survival (Sawaragi and Wynn 1969).

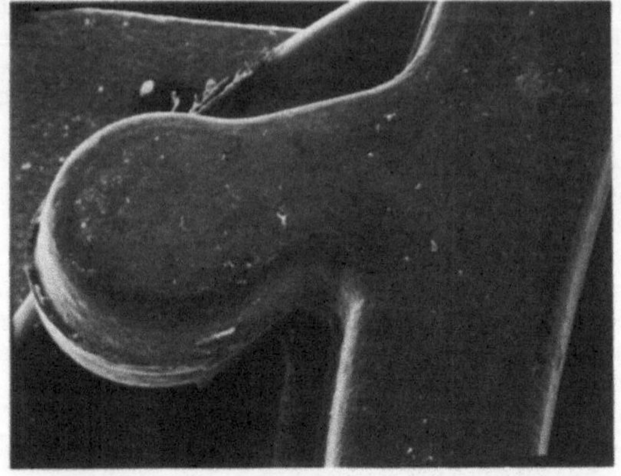

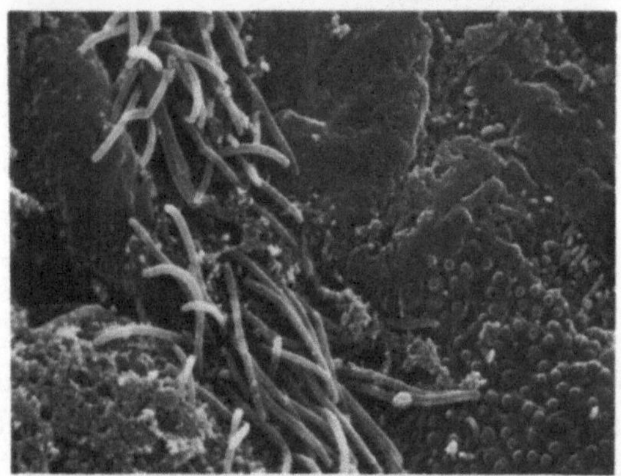

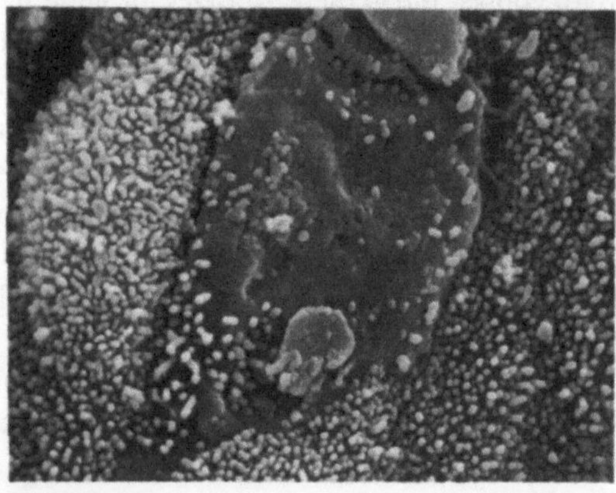

Figure 10. Scanning electron micrographs of endometrium. *Top*: the inert part of ML Cu-250 without attached tissues (×21). *Middle, bottom: endometrium of the site of* impression of the inert portion of a Cu IUD. Note the abnormality in ciliary and microvillous growth (middle: ×6000; bottom: ×4500).

IV. CONCLUDING REMARKS

In contrast to the extremely limited areas which can be examined by the conventional transmission electron microscope, scanning electron microscopy (SEM) offers a new approach to study the three-dimensional topographic surface of large fields of cells. It is not easy to standardize the patterns of surface ultrastructure of the normal endometrium because of the difficulties in obtaining the samples. Some investigators believe hysterectomy is the only method of obtaining uterine endometrium for SEM for proper evaluation (Ludwig et al. 1976). Others, including ourselves, believe that endometrial curettage can yield satisfactory samples and widen the scope of SEM studies (Ferenczy et al. 1972; Johannison and Nilsson 1972; Morgenroth and Verhagen 1972; Nilsson and Hagenfeldt 1973). This is particularly true since hysterectomy specimens may be associated with various gynecological pathologies whereas curettage samples can be obtained from normal carefully monitored device wearers. This difficulty is increased, however, with the study of the endometrium with an IUD in situ. The type of IUD, the incorporated medication and its amount, its position, shape and any associated local endometrial factors may change the ultrastructure characteristics of the endometrium.

The normal endometrial surface has a regular, smooth configuration penetrated by unevenly distributed endometrial gland openings. Endometrial surface regeneration appears to be completed by the early proliferative phase of the cycle. The surface is composed of an intermixture of cobblestone-shaped, nonciliated and ciliated cells in a ratio of 30: 1. During the early proliferative phase the ciliated cells characteristically are concentrated around the gland openings. The nonciliated cells are covered by numerous microvilli and show cytoplasmic projections of secretory products especially in the postovulatory phase. There is no striking surface modification of the surface ultrastructure pattern in the luteal phase. A number of ciliated cells with short microvilli display and apocrine secretory activity which is conspicuous between days 20 and 24 of the cycle. The secretory cells contain giant mitochondria and aggregates of supranuclear glycogen particles. The gland openings become cleftlike and difficult to detect because of the growth of the rest of the epithelium.

The inert IUD affects the local area of contact with the endometrium. Minimal changes are detected away from it. The copper ions incorporated with copper IUDs can affect areas of the endometrium not in direct contact with the IUD. These effects are increased and intensified with the increase *in amount of copper* incorporated. Intrauterine devices seem to be associated with a defective carbohydrate metabolism of the endometrial cells detected by the absence of cytoplasmic secretory projections, the accumulation of glycogen in the cellular cytoplasm and the decrease in the number of light areas within the cells. This may contribute in part to the antifertility effect of the IUD. The effect of copper IUDs, as detected by TEM, on the intracellular components are summarized in Table 1.

REFERENCES

Anderson RGW, Brenner RM: The formation of basal bodies (centrioles) in the rhesus monkey oviduct. J Cell Biol 50: 10, 1971.

Daniel JL, Riches WG, Gibor Y: SEM observations of the effects of an IUD on the endometrium of the human uterus. In: SEM/IITR/1973, Johaii O, Corvin I (eds), Chicago, IIT Research Inst, 1973, p 62ff.

Daniel JL, Gibor Y, Riches WG: The human endometrium and effects of intrauterine devices. In: SEM atlas of mammalian reproduction, Hafez ESE (ed), Igaku Shoin, Tokyo, 1975.

Drochmans P: Morphologie du glycogène: étude au microscope de colorations négative du glycogène particulaire. J Ultrastruct Res 6: 141, 1962.

Elstein M, Sparks RA: Intrauterine contraception, volume one, Annual reseach reviews 1, St. Albans, Vermont, Eden Medical Research, 1977.

Ferenczy A, Richart RM: Scanning and transmission electron microscopy of the human endometrial surface epithelium. J Clin Endocrinol Metab 36: 999, 1973.

Ferenczy A, Richart RM, Agate F Jr, Purkerson ML Dempsey EW: Scanning electron microscopy of the human endometrial surface epithelium Fertil Steril 23: 515, 1972a.

Ferenczy A, Richart RM, Agate F Jr, Purkerson ML, Dempsey EW: Scanning electron microscopy of the human fallopian tube. Science 175: 783, 1972b.

Fleming S, Tweeddale DN, Roddick J: Ciliated endometrial cells. Am J Obstet Gynecol 102: 186, 1968.

Fruin AH, Tighe JR: Tubal metaplasia of the endometrium. J Obst Gyn Br Comm 74: 93, 1967.

Gonzalez-Angulo A, Aznar-Ramos R: Ultrastructural studies on the endometrium of women wearing T Cu-200 intrauterine device by means of transmission and scanning electron microscopy and X-ray dispersive analysis. Am J Obstet Gynecol 121: 170, 1975.

Gonzalez-Angulo A, Aznar-Ramos R, Feria-Velasco F.: Ultrastructural changes found in endometrium of women using Lippes intrauterine device. J Reprod Med 10: 44, 1973.

Hafez ESE, Barnhart MI, Ledwig H, Lusher J, Joelsson I, Daniel JL, Sherman AI, Jordan JA, Wolf H, Stewart WC, Chrétien FC: Scanning electron microscopy of human reproductive physiology. Acta Obstet Gynecol Scand 40: 12, 1975.

Hsu C, Ferenczy A, Richart RM, Darabi K: Endometrial morphology with copper-bearing intrauterine devices. Contraception 14: 243, 1976.

Johannisson E, Nilsson L: Scanning electron microscopic study of the human endometrium. Fertil Steril 23: 613, 1972.

Lopez de la Osa E, Hagenfeldt K, Diczfalusy E: Effect of the Cu-T device on the glycogen content of the human endometrium. Contraception 6: 449, 1972.

Ludwig H, Metzger H: The human female reproductive tract: a scanning electron microscopic atlas, Berlin Springer, 1976.

Ludwig H, Metzger H, Gallies R, Walz KA, Kuppe G: The tissue surface of the human endometrium after the insertion of intrauterine contraceptive device (IUD). In: Scanning electron microscopy 1976: proceedings of workshop on SEM in reproductive biology, part six, Chicago, IIT Research Inst, 1976.

Morgenroth K, Verhagen A: Submicroscopic surface structure of the endometrium. Arch Gynaekol 212: 30, 1972.

Moyer DL, Mishell DR: Reactions of human endometrium to the intrauterine foreign body II: long-term effects on the endometrial histology and cytology. Am J Obstet Gynecol 111: 66, 1971.

Moyer DL, Shaw ST: Intrauterine devices: biological action. In: Human reproduction, conception and contraception, Hafez ESE, Evans TN (eds), New York, Harper and Row, 1973, p 309-334.

Nilsson O: Electron microscopy of the glandular epithelium in the human uterus. J Ultrastruct res 6: 413, 1962.

Nilsson O, Hagenfeldt K: Scanning electron microscopy of human uterine epithelium influenced by the T Cu intrauterine contraceptive device. Am J Obstet Gynecol 117: 469, 1973.

Nilsson O, Nygren KG: Scanning electron microscopy of human endometrium. Ups J Med Sci 77: 3, 1972.

Nilsson O, Hagenfeldt L, Johannisson E: Ultrastructural signs of an interference in the carbohydrate metabolism of the human endometrium produced by the intrauterine copper-T device. Acta Obstet Gynecol Scand 53: 139, 1974.

Oster G, Salgo MP: The copper intrauterine device and its mode of action. N Engl J Med 293: 432, 1975.

Robles F, Lopez de la Osa E, Lerner V, Johannisson E, Brenner PI, Hagenfeldt K, Diczfalusy E: Amylase, glycogen synthetase and phosphorylase in the human endometrium: influence of the cycle and of the Cu-T device. Contraception 6: 373, 1972.

Sawaragi I, Wynn RM: Ultrastructural localization of metabolic enzymes during the human endometrial cycle. Obstet Gynecol 34: 50, 1969.

Schueller EF: Epithelien und Stromazellen des menschlichen Endometriums. Arch Gynaekol 196: 49, 1961.

Schueller EF: Ciliated epithelia of the human uterine mucosa. Obstet Gynecol 31: 215, 1968.

Themann H, Schunke W: The fine structure of the glandular epithelium of human endometrium: electron microscopic morphology. In: The normal human endometrium, Schmidt-Matthiesen H (ed), New York, McGraw-Hill, 1963, p 99ff.

Wynn RM: Fine structural effects of intrauterine contraceptives on the human endometrium. Fertil Steril 19: 887, 1968.

Wynn RM, Harris JA: Ultrastructural cyclic changes in the human endometrium I: the normal preovulatory phase. Fertil Steril 18: 632, 1967.

Wynn RM, Wooley RS: Ultrastructural cyclic changes in the human endometrium II: Normal postovulatory phase. Fertil Steril 18: 721, 1967.

5. THE EFFECT OF A PROGESTERONE-RELEASING IUD ON THE MORPHOLOGY OF THE ENDOMETRIUM AND THE OVIDUCT

U.M. Spornitz, K.S. Ludwig, M. Mall-Haefeli, J. Werner-Zodrow and A. Uettwiller

In a combined clinical and morphological investigation the effects of the Progestasert IUD were studied in the endometrium and oviducts of over 100 women.

I. SAMPLING OF THE MATERIAL

As has been pointed out earlier by ourselves and by other investigators the effect of the IUD on the endometrium is of a rather heterogeneous nature and depends largely on the localization of the biopsy material with respect to the position of the IUD (Ludwig and Spornitz 1977; Pharriss 1977). The closer the biopsy was taken from tissue areas immediately adjoining the IUD, the more consistent were the results we had. Therefore it was tried whenever possible to obtain the material for our investigations through hysterectomy with the IUD still in situ. Thus we were able to compare tissue in direct contact with the IUD with other tissue areas. With the background of the hysterectomy results, interpretation of findings from biopsy material was greatly facilitated.

II. INITIAL RESPONSE CLOSE TO THE IUD

Because the initial response of the endometrium to the IUD was found to differ from the long-term response, changes which take place in the endometrium during the initial phase will be considered first.

The tissue in direct contact with the IUD exhibited the most drastic initial reaction, which, at least during the first weeks of exposure, is probably due more to hormonal stimulation than mechanical irritation.

II.A. Stromal cells

In the latter half of the proliferative phase of the first postinsertion cycle there is already a considerable decidual transformation of the stromal cells in the upper part of the functionalis. The decidual transformation of the stromal cells appears even in the secretory phase of the cycle to be primarily effected through the progesterone released from the IUD. It was found that the periarterial coats of predecidual cells which regularly occur under physiological conditions in the secretory phase (Dallenbach-Hellweg 1975) were missing. The wave of decidualization started from the cells lying directly underneath the superficial epithelium.

By the end of the first month the majority of the stromal cells in the tissue areas in direct contact with the IUD had been transformed into true decidual cells (Wynn 1974). The characteristic morphological features of these decidual cells are the low ratio of nuclear size to cytoplasmic size, the well-developed endoplasmic reticulum and Golgi apparatus, the high glycogen content and a strong basal-lamina-like extracellular coat (Figure 1). Another very characteristic feature of these decidual cells is the presence of cytoplasmic protrusions containing an osmiophilic granular material which appears to be secreted into the intercellular space. Preliminary results obtained while studying these vesicles indicate that their content is neither carbohydrate nor protein but rather of a lipid nature. Taking all the features of the decidual cells at the end of the first postinsertion month together they very closely resemble the decidual cells from about the tenth week of gestation (Liebig and Stegner 1977).

By the end of the first postinsertion month about

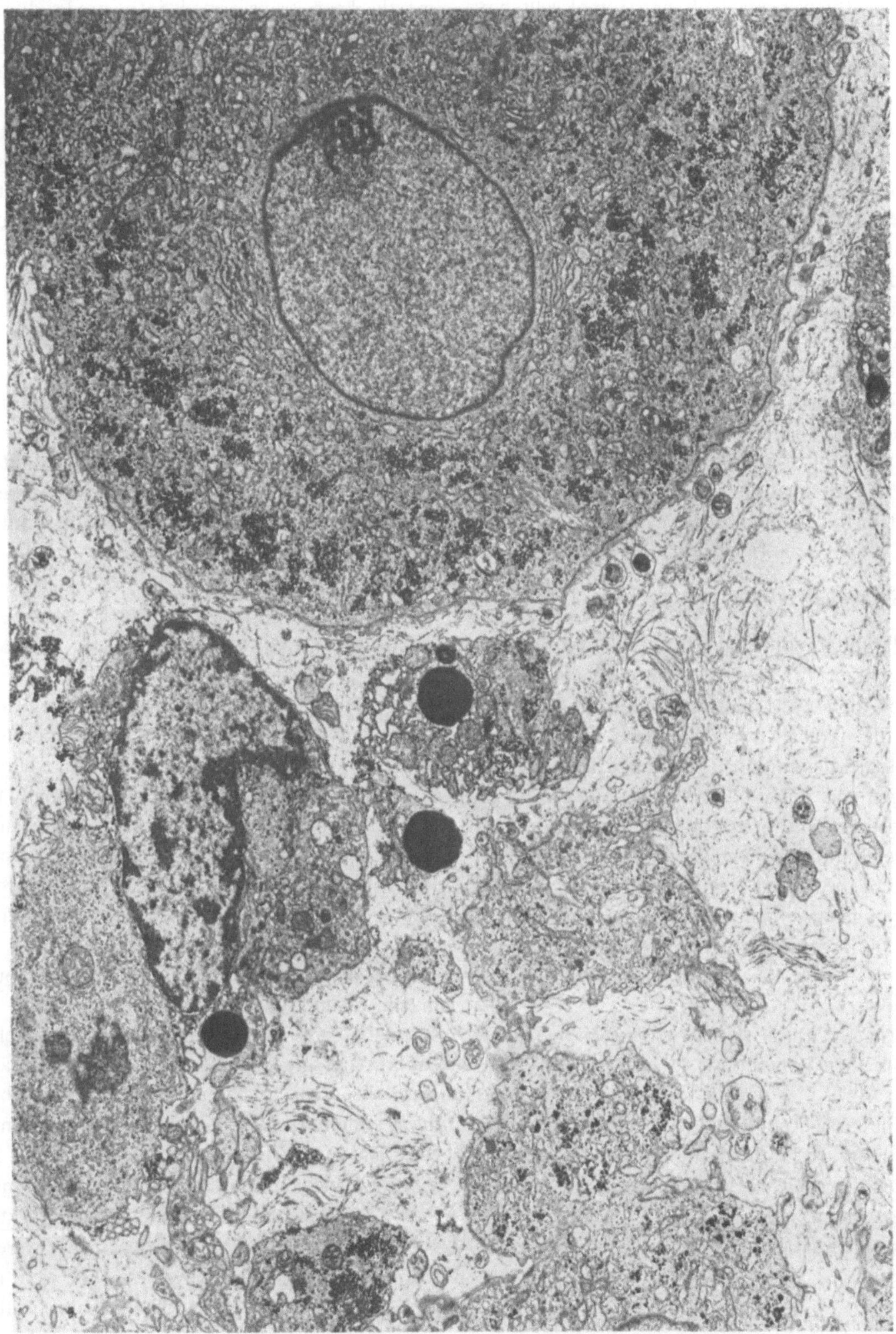

Figure 1. In the upper half of this micrograph of the third postinsertion month there is a decidual cell which, unlike other stromal cells, is surrounded by a basal lamina. Close to it are several 'decidual granules'. In the lower half there is an endometrial granulocyte (K-cell) apparently in the process of disintegration. Three large Relaxin granules are present: two seem to have been expelled from the endometrial granulocyte (×6756).

twenty to thirty percent of the stromal cells have been transformed into endometrial granulocytes or K-cells. In contrast to the K-cells which occur under physiological conditions during the secretory phase of the cycle, they seem to contain, however, only a relatively small number of relaxin granules (cf. Cardell et al. 1969). Moreover the K-cells very often exhibited morphological features which were suggestive of secretion or even disintegration. They seemed to be pinching off large areas of their cytoplasm which contained great amounts of glycogen, and occasionally mitochondria and relaxin granules (Figure 2). These cytoplasmic extrusions were found to disintegrate and to discharge their contents into the intercellular space. During the initial phase of response of the endometrium there is only a very small number of inflammatory cells present in the stroma.

II.B. Glandular cells

The glandular epithelial cells from the tissue in direct contact with the IUD seemed to have stopped most of their cycle-related activities and did not show the typical transformations found under physiological conditions (Wynn and Harris 1967). Glycogen was found still to be formed during the first postinsertion month, but very little seemed to be secreted into the glandular lumen (Figure 3). By the end of the second postinsertion month much of this glycogen in subnuclear regions had been replaced by large accumulations of lipid.

III. INITIAL RESPONSE IN DISTANT PARTS OF THE ENDOMETRIUM

In tissue areas not in direct contact with the Progestasert IUD the initial phase of response exhibited somewhat different morphological changes which were by no means as dramatic as those just described.

III.A. Stromal cells

The stroma generally exhibited a morphology which resembled different stages of the endometrial cycle, ranging from mid-proliferative to the early secretory phase. In these areas the fibrocytes had mostly been transformed into predecidual cells rather than true decidual cells. They were neither found to be coated with typical basal-lamina-like material nor did they seem to be secreting the osmiophilic lipid granules which are characteristic for decidual cells. The K-cells or endometrial granulocytes also showed a normal appearance and did not exhibit any signs of disintegration as did the ones in the decidualized areas.

III.B. Glandular cells

The glandular epithelial cells in the more distant areas of the endometrium not only seemed to elaborate considerable amounts of glycogen but also apparently secreted this glycogen into the glandular lumen. In the same areas stromal edema developed during the first postinsertion month and was found to be quite pronounced.

IV. LONG-TERM RESPONSE IN THE STROMA

After prolonged exposure of the endometrium to the delivery system, that is, for up to 15 months in our study, the decidual response spread over almost all of the endometrium and was occasionally found in the region of the tubal openings. But even after longer periods of exposure the endometrial stroma was found to be far from uniform. The areas in direct contact with the delivery system always showed the highest degree of decidualization, while stromal edema was found to be more pronounced in the distant parts of the endometrium. Most surprising was the finding that the K-cells or endometrial granulocytes were practically absent from the areas immediately surrounding the delivery system. Instead another group, inflammatory cells, had moved into these areas (Figure 4). Polymorphonuclear granulocytes were most numerous in the upper stromal parts directly underneath the superficial epithelium. In many cases we were able to observe these granulocytes as they were apparently crossing the layer of the superficial epithelium. Frequently the superficial epithelium was found to have become extremely thin and there were instances where it was even found to be missing.

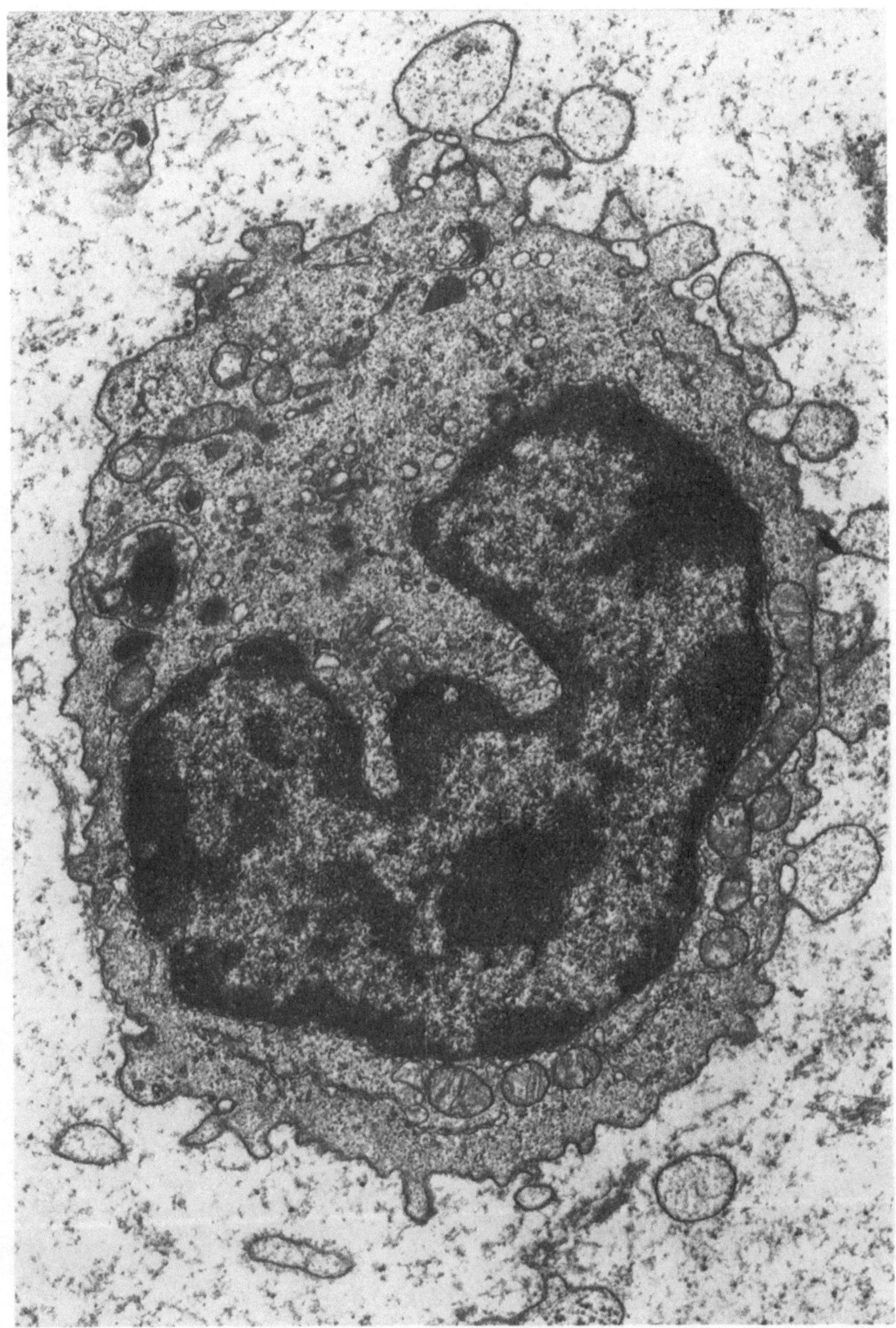

Figure 2. Micrograph taken from the tissue area directly underneath the IUD, showing an endometrial granulocyte (K-cell) which pinches off cytoplasmic protrusions. Note the disintegrating relaxin granule on the left side of the cell ($\times$ 18900).

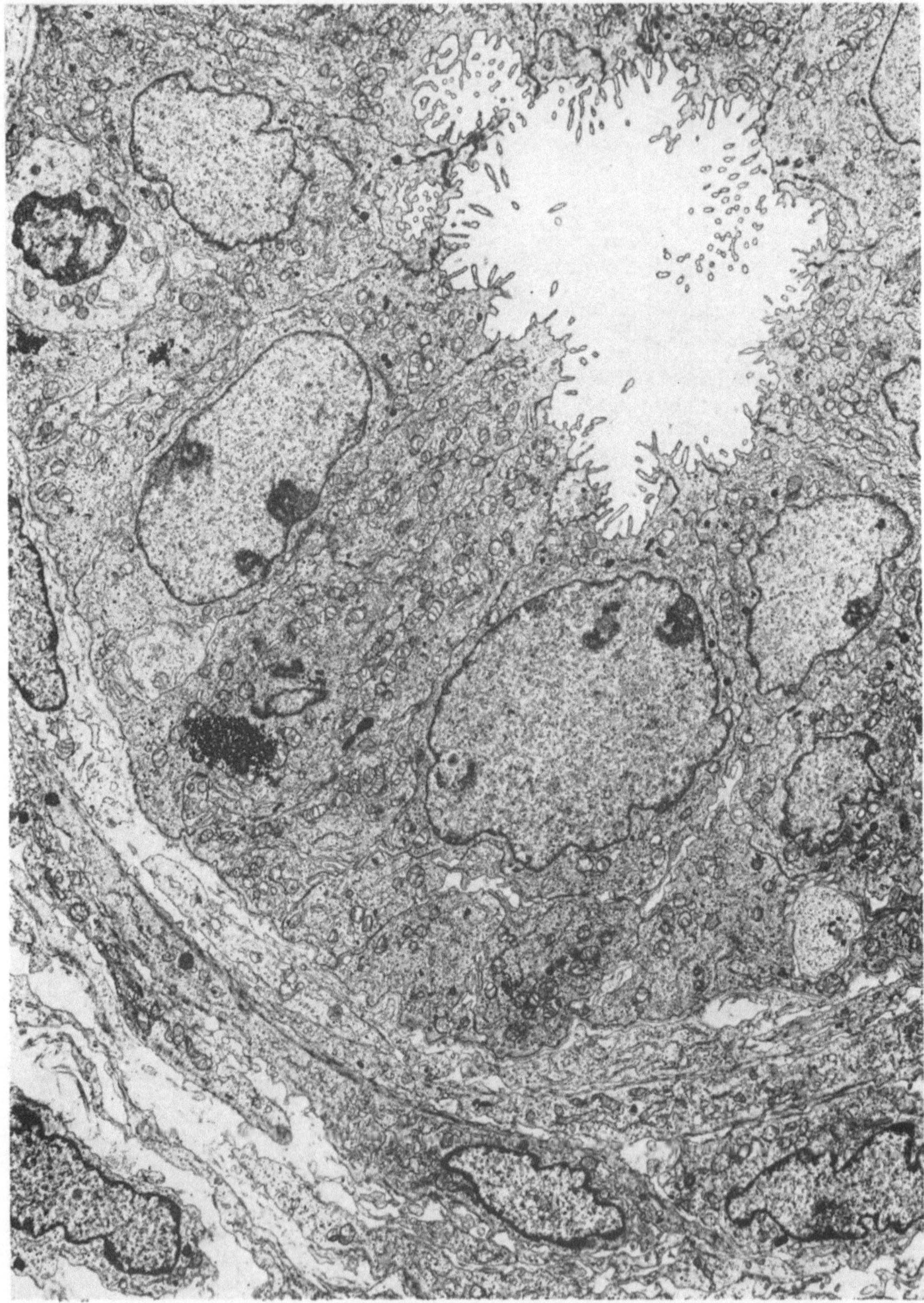

Figure 3. Glandular epithelial cells from the tissue area in direct contact with the IUD, middle of secretory phase of the first postinsertion month. The cells are relatively short, there is little glycogen, no basal giant mitochondria and the cells generally seem to be rather inactive (×5130).

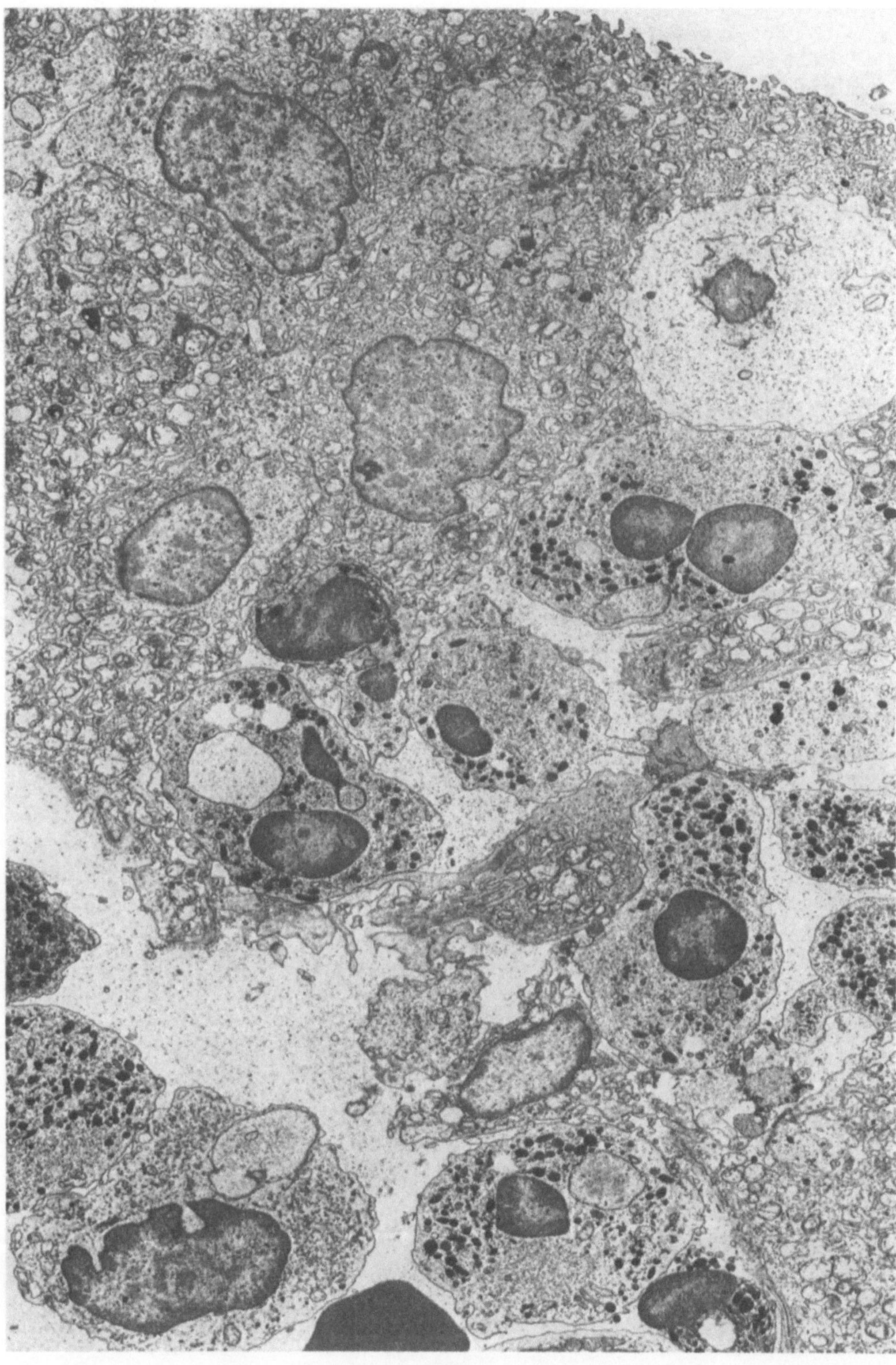

Figure 4. Micrograph showing numerous inflammatory cells, mostly polymorphonuclear granulocytes, located directly underneath the superficial epithelium. This section has been taken from the area in direct contact with the IUD during the late proliferative phase of the fifteenth postinsertion month ($\times$ 5130).

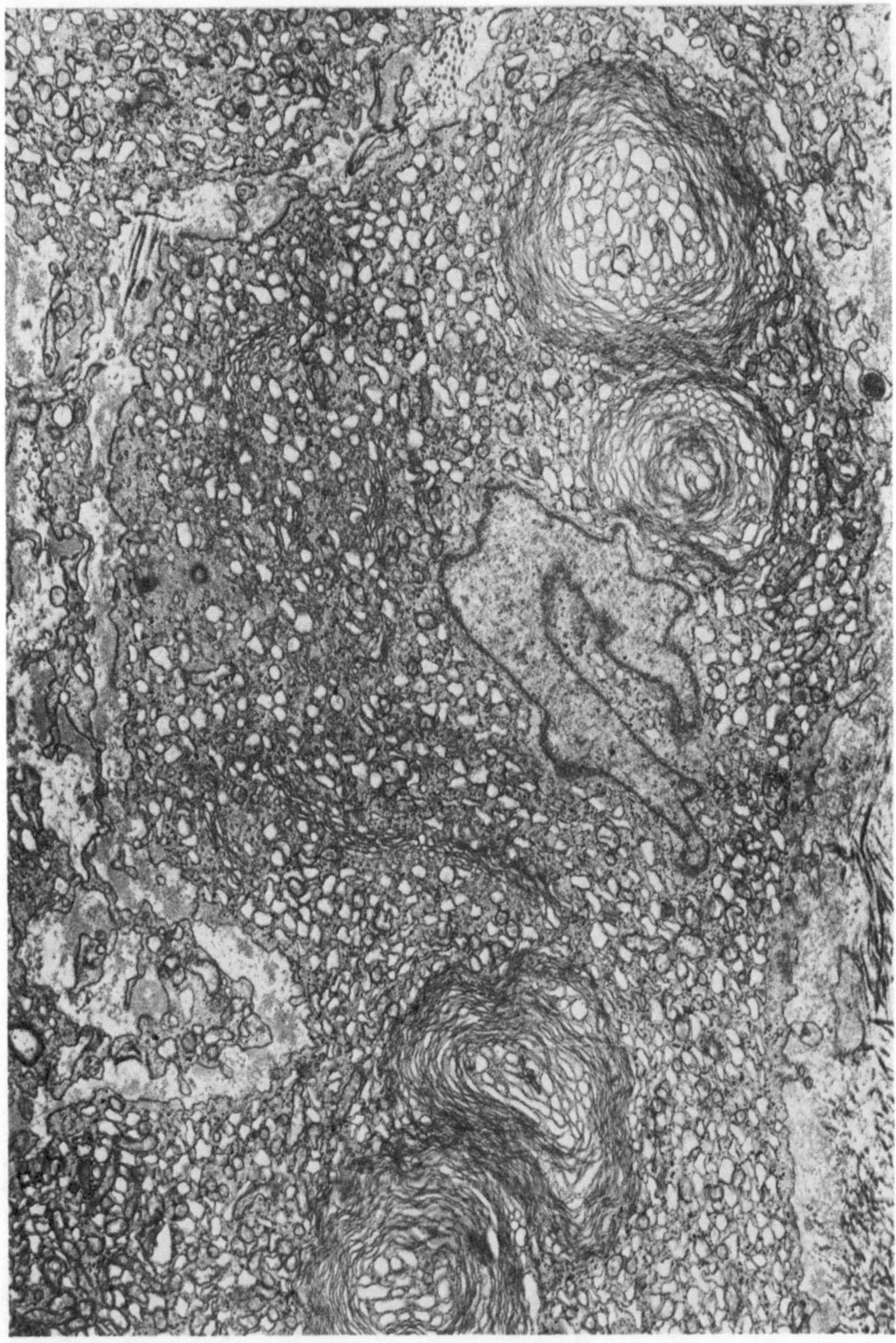

Figure 5. The cell on this micrograph shows the typical Arias-Stella transformation of decidual cells which can be found in the areas in direct contact with the progesterone-releasing IUD. In these cells the endoplasmic reticulum is very prominent and mostly forms lamellar whorls (×12150)

V. LONG-TERM RESPONSE OF THE GLANDULAR EPITHELIUM

The glandular epithelium in most areas of the endometrium seemed to be intensely suppressed after prolonged exposure to the IUD. The synthetic activity of the cells was found to have almost completely stopped. They showed all the features typical of glandular atrophy. We were not able to detect any signs of a response to cyclic variations of hormone concentrations in the blood. Particularly important seem to be three observations made during this study namely that: (1) the formation of the nucleolar channel system (Gordon 1975) is completely suppressed after the insertion of the IUD; (2) giant basal mitochondria formation (Gordon 1975) also never occurs with this type of IUD; (3) glycogen formation in the glandular cells was found to be drastically diminished.

Both the nucleolar channel system (NCS) and the presence of giant mitochondria are believed to be dependent on ovulation having occurred. Endocrinological data as collected in our laboratory show that from the fourth postinsertion month on, about half of the cycles are anovulatory. Since the NCS and the giant mitochondria are, however, absent in all tissue samples, that is also during the ovulatory cycles, the anovulatory cycles can certainly be ruled out as a possible explanation for this fact. In several cases a strong Arias-Stella reaction was found, which we believe to be due to a combination of a rather high endogenous level of progesterone and the sometimes very high rates of release from the delivery system. Ultrastructurally the Arias-Stella reaction is most obvious in the stromal cells, where it produces typical lamellar whorls, as demonstrated in Figure 5.

VI. MORPHOLOGICAL CHANGES IN THE OVIDUCTS: LOCAL OR SYSTEMIC EFFECT?

We still hesitate to put forward the hypothesis that there is a systemic action of the progesterone released from the IUD but as is evident on the hormonal profiles of Figure 6, there are several alterations to the hormonal cycle, the most obvious or drastic being the anovulatory cycles in about half of our patients (Figure 6, bottom). Because of these changes in the hormonal values the oviducts of these patients were also investigated. In our laboratory the lower part of the tubal ampulla is normally studied because this is the region were changes occurring during the course of the cycle are most evident (Spornitz et al. 1977). In this region it was found that the ratio of ciliated to nonciliated cells remained at about one throughout the cycle, which strongly contrasts with the cyclic deciliation and reciliation found under physiological condition (Mall-Haefeli et al., 1979). Moreover there were always some cells which contained an excessive amount of secretory granules, comparable to the amounts found in the mid-luteal or late luteal phases of the normal cycle (Figure 7). In addition there were always many cells, both ciliated and non ciliated, which contained large numbers of lysosomes, resembling those found regularly during the first trimester of pregnancy (Ferenczy and Richart 1974). Because of the changes we observed in the morphology as well as in the hormonal values, we are convinced that there are of course several factors on the side of the endometrium but also on the side of the oviduct which participate in the contraceptive action of the progesterone-releasing IUD.

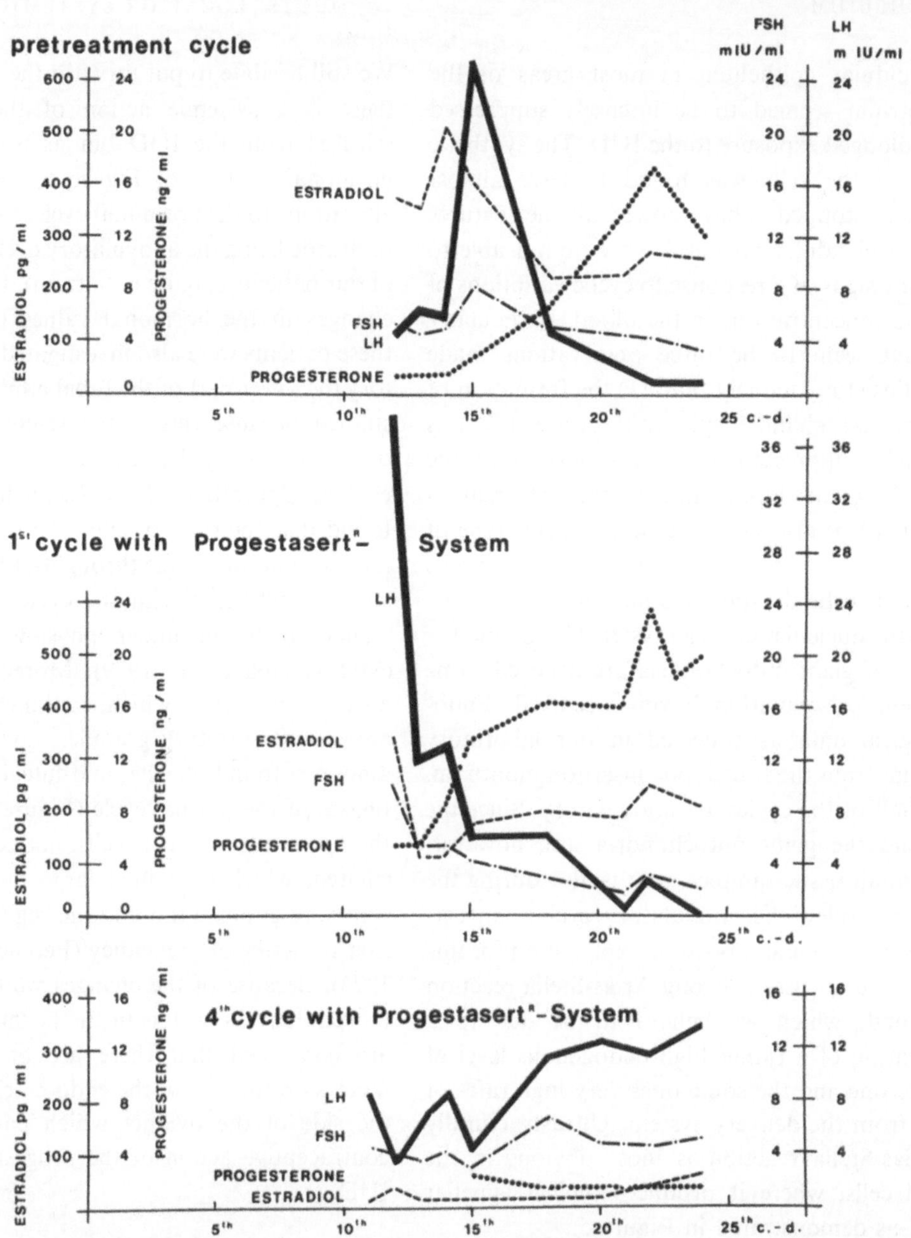

Figure 6. Three hormonal profiles found to be typical for the progesterone-releasing IUD. Note the bottom profile with the lowered steroid values in the second half of the cycle (from Mall-Haefeli 1978).

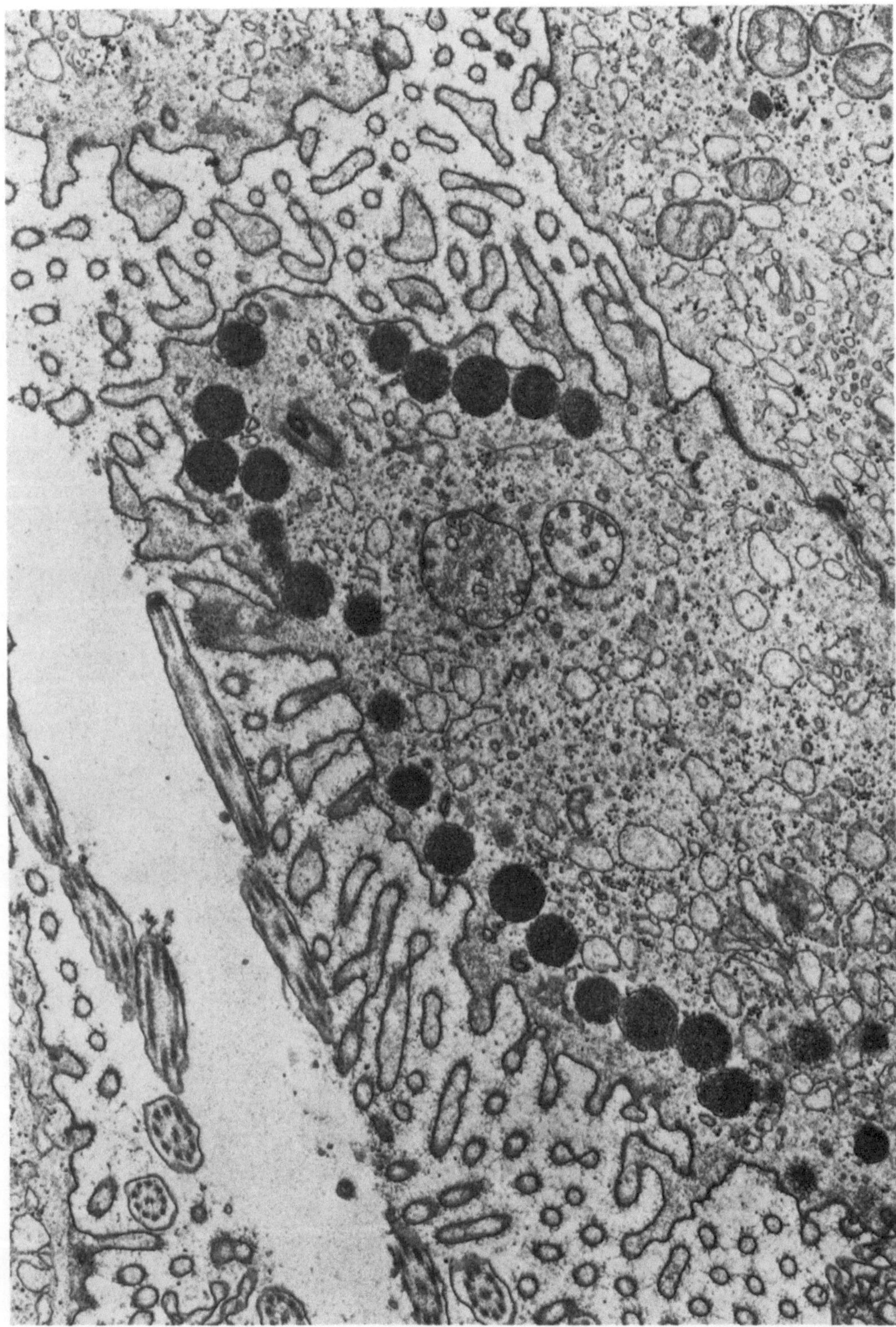

Figure 7. Detail of a secretory cell taken from an oviduct in the early proliferative phase of the cycle. The cell contains an excessive number of secretory granules similar to those present in the untreated oviduct in the mid-secretory phase of the cycle (× 27000).

ACKNOWLEDGEMENT

The authors gratefully acknowledge the excellent technical assistance of Ms. C. Kunz and Ms. E. Weber

REFERENCES

Cardell RR, Hisaw FL, Dawson AB: The fine structure of granular cells in the uterine endometrium of the rhesus monkey (*Macaca mulatta*) with a discussion of the possible function of these cells in relaxin secretion. Am J Anat 124: 307, 1969.

Dallenbach-Hellweg G: Histopathology of the endometrium, Berlin, Springer, 1975.

Ferenczy A, Richart RM: Female reproductive system: dynamics of scan and transmission electron microscopy, New York, John Wiley and Sons, 1974.

Gordon M: Cyclic changes in the fine structure of the epithelial cells of human endometrium. Int Rev Cytol. 42: 127, 1975.

Hamperl H, Hellweg G: Granular endometrial stroma cells. Obstet Gynecol 11: 379, 1958.

Liebig W, Stegner HE: Decidualisation of the endometrial stromal cell. Arch Gynaekol 223: 19, 1977.

Ludwig KS, Spornitz UM: Veränderungen des Endometriums beim Progestasertsystem. Acta Anat 99: 237, 1977.

Mall-Haefeli M: Das Progestasertsystem. Gynaekol Rundsch 18: 253, 1978.

Mall-Haefeli M, Ludwig KS, Spornitz UM, Uettwiller A, Werner-Zodrow I: Tubal secretion: ultrastructure related to endocrinology. In: The biology of the fluids of the female genital tract, Beller FK, Schumacher GFB, (eds), Amsterdam, Elsevier/North-Holland, 1979.

Pharriss BB: Local treatment of the endometrium with progesterone. Ann NY Acad Sci 286: 226, 1977.

Spornitz UM, Ludwig KS, Mall-Haefeli M: Morphologic alterations in the epithelium of the human oviduct induced by a low dosis gestagen. Arch Gynaekol 223: 269, 1977.

Wynn RM: Ultrastructural development of the human decidua. Am J Obstet Gynecol 118: 652, 1974.

Wynn RM, Harris JA: Ultrastructural cyclic changes in the human endometrium. Fertil Steril 18: 632, 1967.

6. THE EFFECT OF THE IUD ON THE GLYCOGEN METABOLISM OF THE ENDOMETRIUM

M.S. Buckingham, E. Chantler and M. Elstein

The principal function of the endometrium is to provide an environment suitable for blastocyst embedding. The cyclical nature of female fertility results in a recurrent process of proliferation and differentiation in the endometrium with subsequent shedding if pregnancy does not occur.

The cellular metabolism of the endometrium may be observed during the menstrual cycle by a number of techniques. Histochemical examination will reveal the presence of a variety of enzymes and metabolites. However the information thus obtained tends to be qualitative rather than quantitative and the processes involved in the preparation of samples may alter the levels of substances present in the tissues being examined (Cohen et al. 1964).

Quantitative assay of various metabolites may be undertaken to provide information not available from histochemical studies but the dynamic synthesis and breakdown of these substances may not be revealed by these methods. An indication of the metabolic activity of the endometrium may be obtained by the assay of various enzymes. This provides a dynamic rather than a static view of the metabolic processes under investigation.

Research into the biochemistry of the endometrium has made use of all these techniques, in particular in relation to glycogen metabolism. Although the precise role of the glycogen in the endometrium is difficult to establish, it seems reasonable to suppose that it is involved in providing an environment suitable for implantation. Having established the normal glycogen metabolism of the endometrium, changes induced by the presence of IUDs may subsequently be observed. In this way it is possible that the biochemical method of action of IUDs may ultimately be described.

I. NORMAL ENDOMETRIAL CARBOHYDRATE METABOLISM

I.A. Glucose metabolism

The accumulation of carbohydrate within the endometrium is dependent upon there being adequate blood supply and upon the levels of circulating glucose. The transfer of glucose across the cell membrane is an active process. Free plasma glucose will diffuse slowly across cell membranes but the transfer rate is increased by the enzyme hexokinase which catalyses the reaction:

$$\text{glucose} + \text{ATP} \xrightleftharpoons{\text{hexokinase}} \text{glucose-6-P} + \text{ADP}.$$

The glucose-6-phosphate so formed will not diffuse out of the cell although it may be converted back to glucose by the activity of the enzyme glucose-6-phosphatase, this enzyme having been demonstrated in the endometrium (Sawaragi and Wynn 1969; Ockerman 1969). Alternatively the glucose-6-phosphate may be metabolized via the pentose phosphate shunt, may undergo glycolysis or may be converted to glycogen.

Aerobic glycolysis via the tricarboxylic acid cycle is important as a source of adenosine triphosphate (ATP). Investigation of selected enzymes gives an indication of the metabolic flux of the endometrium. A progressive increase in succinate dehydrogenase activity from early to late in the menstrual cycle has been demonstrated both histochemically (Stuermer and Stein 1952) and by direct assay (Hackl 1973) although additional small peaks in activity in the proliferative and secretory phases, corresponding to the peak levels of estrogen and progesterone, have also been found (McKay et al. 1965). This variation in enzyme activity has also

Table 1. Mean endometrial glycogen levels, at various stages of the menstrual cycle, as estimated by different workers (g glycogen per 100g wet weight of tissue).

Authors	*Proliferative phase*	*Days 16-18*	*Secretory phase*
Zondek and Stein (1940)	0.1. (n=4)	0.61 (n=2)	0.36 (n=11)
Payne and Latour (1955)	0.23 (n=11)	0.94 1n=16)	0.66 (n=39)
Arronet and Latour (1957	0.31 (n=25)	1.13 (n=32)	0.64 (n=39)
Hughes (1964)	Days 17-19: 1.02 (n not stated)		
Rubulis et al. (1965)		days 7-12: 7-12 (n=15)	days 16-21: 0.87 (n=15)
Lopez de la Osa et al. (1976)		days 8-13: 0.14 (n=10)	days 18-27: 0.24 (n=10)

been found to occur with the enzyme isocitrate dehydrogenase (Spellman et al. 1974).

I.B. Glycogen metabolism

The glucose which enters the endometrial cells may alternatively be converted to glycogen. A number of investigations into the glycogen content of the endometrium have been undertaken. Although there is not complete agreement in the quantities of glycogen present there does appear to be a rise in glycogen content around midcycle. A summary of the findings appears in Table 1.

The enzymes which control the synthesis and breakdown of glycogen are glycogen synthetase (uridine diphosphoglucose [UDP-glucose]: glycogen-4-glycosyltransferase E.C.2.4.1.11) and glycogen phosphorylase ($\alpha - 1 \rightarrow 4$ glucan: orthophosphate glucosyltransferase E.C.2.4.1.1). These en zymes have been identified in human liver, muscle and brain and their biochemical characteristics established.

The incorporation of glucose into glycogen proceeds as follows:

1. Glucose crosses the endometrial cell membrane by conversion to glucose-6-phosphate under the action of hexokinase.
2. The glucose-6-phosphate is converted to glucose-1-phosphate by the action of phosphoglucomutase.
3. The glucose-1-phosphate is bonded to the nucleotide coenzyme uridine triphosphate (UTP) by the action of UDP-glucose pyrophosphorylase.
4. Finally the UDP-glucose is incorporated into the glycogen molecule by the action of glycogen synthetase.

The overall reaction may be summarized:

1. $\text{glucose} + \text{ATP} \xrightarrow{\text{hexokinase}} \text{glucose-6-phosphate} + \text{ADP}.$

2. $\text{glucose-6-phosphate} \xrightarrow{\text{phosphoglucomutase}} \text{glucose-1-phosphate}.$

3. $\text{UTP} + \text{glucose-1-phosphate} \xrightarrow{\text{UDP-glucose pyrophosphorylase}} \text{UDP-glucose} + \text{PPi}.$

4. $(\text{glucose})_n + \text{UDP-glucose} \xrightarrow{\text{glycogen synthetase}} (\text{glucose})_{n+1} + \text{uridine diphosphate (UDP)}$

Glycogen synthetase itself exists in two forms, first described in studies on rat diaphragms (Larner et al. 1964). The two forms differ in their degree of phosphorylation but are interconvertible. The dephosphoenzyme, which is enzymically active, can be phosphorylated by the specific enzyme glycogen synthetase kinase to form the phosphoenzyme. The latter is less active but is markedly stimulated by glucose-6-phosphate. Because of the influence of glucose-6-phosphate the phospho- and dephospho-forms of the enzyme are termed D (dependent) and I (independent) respectively.

Glycogen breakdown is governed by the enzyme glycogen phosphorylase which splits glucose molecules from glycogen by the cleavage of $\alpha - 1 \rightarrow 4$ bonds. The enzyme was first described in muscle extract (Gori et al. 1939) and subsequently identified in human endometrium (Zondek and Hestrin 1947). The action of glycogen phosphorylase may be represented thus:

$$(\text{glucose})_n + \text{Pi} \xrightarrow{\text{glycogen phosphorylase}} (\text{glucose})_{n-1} + \text{glucose-1-phosphate}.$$

In vivo the action of glycogen phosphorylase is unidirectional in favour of glycogen breakdown although in vitro, under certain conditions, the enzyme will stimulate glycogen synthesis (Cori et al. 1955).

The control of glycogen phosphorylase activity is highly complex. The enzyme, like glycogen synthetase, exists in two forms, each with a different activity. The dimeric form, (phosphorylase) *b*, with a molecular weight of 250,000, is active only in the presence of AMP – adenosine monophosphate (Sutherland and Rall 1958) and is inhibited by ATP and glucose-6-phosphate. The tetramic form, phosphorylase *a*, with a molecular weight of 500,000, is active in the absence of AMP. An increase in activity of the enzyme may thus occur by the conversion of phosphorylase *b* to phosphorylase *a* or by a change in the concentrations of AMP, ATP and glucose-6-phosphate leading to an activation of phosphorylase *b* without its conversion to phosphorylase *a* (Hales 1967).

The interconversion of glycogen phosphorylase is in turn controlled by enzyme activity (Krebs et al. 1966):

$$2\ \text{phosphorylase}\ b + 4\text{ATP} \xrightarrow{\text{phosphorylase}\ b\ \text{kinase}} \text{phosphorylase}\ b + 4\text{ADP}.$$

$$\text{phosphorylase}\ a + 4H_2O \xrightarrow{\text{phosphorylase phosphatase}} 2\ \text{phosphorylase}\ b + 4\text{Pi}.$$

The phosphorylase *b* kinase in turn exists in inactive and active forms, conversion to the active form being accelerated by cyclic AMP (Vilar-Palasi et al. 1971). A chain reaction thus exists which, in muscle, may be stimulated initially by adrenaline, as shown in Figure 1.

As with the other forms of cascade reaction, biological amplification occurs, so that very small quantities of adrenaline ultimately promote a wide spread breakdown of glycogen.

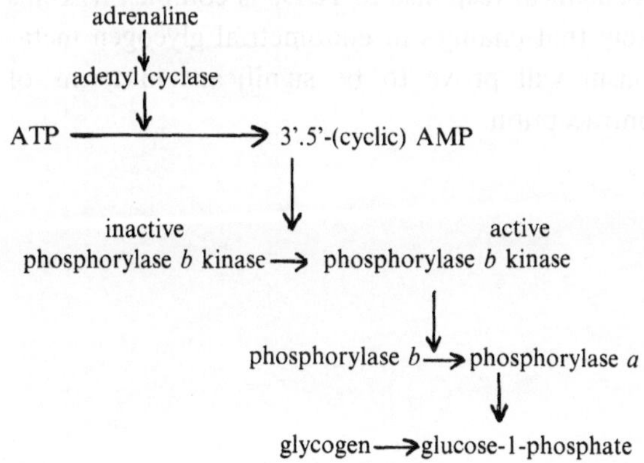

Figure 1. Cascade reaction illustrating the effect of adrenalin on glycogen breakdown.

The precise function of the glycogen found in the endometrium is uncertain. It is found in the greatest quantities in the gland cells, with smaller quantities present in the stroma. It has been suggested that the glycogen present is not important in term of implantation (Arronet and Latour 1957) as the peak of glycogen concentration does not coincide with the timing of implantation and because a pregnancy may become established in sites other than the uterine cavity. While there is no doubt that ectopic pregnancies do occur, the rate of failure to implant in sites other than the uterine cavity is not known and data relating to the changes in endometrial glycogen metabolism in the early days of pregnancy are lacking.

In other organs the function of glycogen is to provide a source of energy over and above that required for the normal metabolism of the organ storing the glycogen. Although a reduction of the glycogen content of the endometrium has been related to infertility (Zondek and Stein 1940; Hughes et al. 1969), the treatment of such patients with estrogens (Hughes 1964) has so many other effects which may increase fertility that evaluation of results becomes extremely difficult.

II. CHANGES INDUCED BY INTRAUTERINE DEVICES

II.A. Inert devices

Once IUDs had become accepted as a form of contraception twenty years ago, considerable efforts were made to determine the local effects produced on the endometrium. However, these efforts were directed mainly toward the histological and microbiological changes which occurred and few studies were made of the biochemistry of the endometrium in relation to IUDs. A study of the uterine fluid (Kar et al. 1968) showed that the presence of a Lippes Loop had little effect on the quantities of acid or alkaline phosphatase, glucose or glycogen, although the total protein content was found to be increased. To date, information regarding the changes in endometrial glycogen metabolism in relation to inert IUDs is curiously lacking.

II.B. Copper-bearing devices

The finding that copper attached to an IUD greatly enhanced its contraceptive efficiency (Zipper et al. 1971, 1976) has stimulated interest in the local endometrial effects of such devices. The very low release rate of copper from such devices, of the order of 45 μg/day (Hagenfeldt 1972a), gives rise to local rather than systemic effects. Ovulation is unimpaired (Nygren and Johansson 1973) and plasma copper levels remain unchanged.

The presence of copper has been found to have an inhibitory effect on a number of endometrial enzymes including alkaline phosphatase (Hagenfeldt 1972b). This is an important enzyme in terms of cellular metabolism and it has been suggested that alterations in its activity might affect the endometrium sufficiently to prevent implantation.

The effect of copper-bearing IUDs on endometrial glycogen levels has been shown to change with time after insertion (Lopez de la Osa et al. 1972), levels of glycogen rising between the fourth and fifteenth months. However a conflicting report of a decrease in the conversion of glucose to glycogen has also been made (Rosado et al. 1976). If alterations in endometrial glycogen content are the result of release of copper ions then it might be expected that the greatest change would be seen in the first weeks after insertion when copper release is at its highest level.

The enzymes glycogen synthetase and glycogen phosphorylase have been assayed in normal women and following insertion of a Cu-T device. Glycogen synthetase activity appears to increase during the menstrual cycle (Robles et al. 1972), although a premenstrual decrease in activity has also been found (Hughes et al. 1969). Glycogen phosphorylase activity has been described as being constant throughout the cycle (Robles et al. 1972), and as following a similar variation in activity during the cycle to that of glycogen synthetase (Hughes et al. 1969).

Changes in the activity of these enzymes following the insertion of Cu-T devices include the abolition of the rise in glycogen synthetase activity which occurs in normal women but no change in glycogen phosphorylase activity (Robles et al. 1972). These studies were made in the first three cycles after insertion. Studies to investigate the long-term effects of copper-bearing IUDs in relation to endometrial glycogen metabolism are clearly required.

III. CONCLUSIONS

A great deal is known of the normal biochemistry of the endometrium and of the changes which take place following insertion of an IUD. However the significance of these changes in relation to contraception is difficult to evaluate.

Investigation of changes in endometrial glycogen metabolism in relation to IUDs appears to be a promising field for research. Comparisons need to be made of the effects of inert and copper-bearing devices to determine the specific effects of copper. The effects of the decrease in copper release with time need also to be determined. Further studies of the activities of glycogen synthetase and glycogen phosphorylase may clarify the changes that take place during the cycle in the presence of IUDs.

The mechanism of action of IUDs, and whether inert and copper-bearing devices have the same effects, remains to be established. Although the biochemical response to IUDs is complex it seems likely that changes in endometrial glycogen metabolism will prove to be significant in terms of contraception.

REFERENCES

Arronet GH, Latour JPA: Studies on endometrial glycogen. J Clin Endocrinol Metab 17: 261, 1957.

Cohen S, Bitensky L, Chayen J, Cunningham GJ, Russell, JK: Histochemical studies on the human endometrium. Lancet 2: 56, 1964.

Cori CF, Schmidt G, Cori GT: The synthesis of a polysaccharide from glucos-1-phosphate in muscle extract. *Science* 89: 464, 1939.

Cori CT, Illingworth B, Keller PJ: Muscle phosphorylase Methods Enzymol 1: 200, 1955.

Hackl H: Metabolism of glucose in the human endometrium with special reference to fertility and contraception. Acta Obstet Gynecol Scand 52: 135, 1973.

Hagenfeldt K: Intrauterine contraception with the copper-T device I: effect of trace elements in the endometrium, cervical mucus and plasma. Contraception 6: 37, 1972a.

Hagenfeldt K: Intrauterine contraception with the copper-T device II: influence on endometrial acid and alkaline phosphatase, beta-glucuronidase and lactic dehydrogenase activities. Contraception 6: 191, 1972b.

Hales CN: Some actions of hormones in the regulation of glucose metabolism. Essays biochem 3: 73–104, 1967.

Hughes EC: Effect of treatment for sterility and abortion upon the carbohydrate pathways of the endometrium. Am J Obstet Gynecol 89: 59, 1964.

Hughes EC, Demers LM, Csermely T, Jones DB: Organ culture of human endometrium: effect of ovarian steroids. Am J Obstet Gynecol 105: 707, 1969.

Kar, AB, Engineer AD, Goel R, Kamboj VP, Dasgupta PR, Chowdhury SR: Effect of an intrauterine contraceptive device on biochemical composition of uterine fluid. Am J Obstet Gynecol 101: 966, 1968.

Krebs, EG, DeLange RJ, Kemp RG, Riley WD: Activation of skeletal muscle phosphorylase. Pharmacol Rev 18: 163, 1966.

Larner J, Rosell-Perez M, Friedman DL, Craig JW: Insulin and the control of UDP α-glucan Transglucosylase activity In: Control of glycogen metabolism Whelan WJ, Cameron MP (eds), Boston, Little, Brown, 1964.

Lopez de la Osa E, Hagenfeldt K, Diczfalusy E: Effect of the Cu-T device on the glycogen content of the human endometrium. Contraception 6: 449, 1972.

McKay DG, Hertic AT, Bardawil WA, Velardo JT: Histochemical observations on the endometrium. Obstet Gynecol 8: 22, 1956.

Nygren K, Johansson EDB: Premature onset of menstrual bleeding during ovulatory cycles in women with an intrauterine contraceptive device. Am J Obstet Gynecol 117: 971, 1973.

Ockerman PA: Glucose-6-phosphatase in human endometrium. Acta Obstet Gynecol Scand 48: 229, 1969.

Payne HW, Latour JPA: Quantitative estimations of endometrial glycogen, using the anthrone method. J Clin Endocrinol Metab 15: 1106, 1955.

Robles F, Lopez de la Osa E, Lerner U, Johannisson E, Brenner P. Hagenfeldt K, Diczfalusy E: α-Amylase, glycogen synthetase and phosphorylase in the human endometrium: influence of the cycle and of the Cu-T device. Contraception 6: 373, 1972.

Rosado A, Hernandez O, Aznar R, Hicks JJ: Comparative glycolytic metabolism in the normal and in the copper-treated endometrium. Contraception 13: 17, 1976.

Rubulis A, Jacobs RD, Hughes EC: Glycogen synthetase in mammalian uterus. Biochim Biophys Acta 99: 584, 1965.

Sawaragi I, Wynn WM: Utrastructural localization of metabolic enzymes during the human endometrial cycle. Obstet Gynecol 34: 50, 1969.

Spellman, CM, Fotrell DF, O'Dwyer EM, Clinch JD: Abnormal endometrial enzyme levels in primary infertility. Fertil Steril 25: 774, 1974.

Stuermer VM, Stein RJ: Cytodynamic properties of human endometrium. Am J Obstet Gynecol 63: 359, 1952.

Sutherland EW, Rall TW: Fractionation and characterization of a cyclic adenine ribonucleotide formed by tissue particles. J Biol Chem 232: 1077, 1958.

Villar-Palasi C, Larner J, Shen LC: Glycogen metabolism and the mechanisms of action of cyclic AMP Ann NY Acad Sci 185: 74, 1971.

Zipper JA, Tatum HJ, Medel M, Pastene L, Rivera M: Contraception through the use of intrauterine metals I: copper as an adjunct to the 'T' device. Am J Obstet Gynecol 109: 771, 1971.

Zipper J, Medel M, Pastene L, Rivera M, Torres L, Osoria A, Toscanini C: Four years experience with the Cu-7 200 device: endouterine copper in fertility control. Contraception 13: 7, 1976.

Zondek B, Hestrin S: Phosphorylase activity in human endometrium. Am J Obstet Gynecol 54: 173, 1947.

Zondek B, Stein L: Glycogen content of the human uterine mucosa glycopenia uteri. Endocrinology 27: 395, 1940.

7. PHYSIOLOGICAL MECHANISMS OF IUDs

H.H. El-Badrawi and E.S.E. Hafez

I. INTRODUCTION

The increasing worldwide utilization of the intrauterine contraceptive device (IUD) has been associated with intensive investigation into the physiological mechanisms of its actions. One of the main problems has been the variety of antifertility effects the device causes in different species (Eckstein 1970). Inert IUDs today are primarily made of polyethylene and polypropylene. The constituents of inert IUDs play a major role in its function. Most of the studies have indicated that medicated IUDs have different and often better efficiency than inert ones (Chang et al. 1970).

The Ypsilon-Y and the intrauterine contraceptive membrane (IUM) are the most recent models of the inert IUD, designed to increase efficacy and minimize side effects (Batar et al. 1979), but the new models did not represent an improvement in efficacy over the Lippes Loop. The performance of inert IUDs may not be improved and further progress can be expected only in development of bioactive and medicated devices (Batar et al. 1979).

In order to exert their contraceptive action, inert IUDs must be placed at the uterine fundus so that their local mechanical effects might operate on the total area of the endometrium, leading to delay in its maturation, or by producing an inflammatory response detrimental to implantation (Elstein and Sparks 1977).

The complications associated with the utilization of the nonmedicated IUDs may be attributed to the size or shape of the device. Considerable effort has been directed toward achieving a suitable balance between contraceptive effectiveness and side effects – as is evidenced by the variety of devices currently available for clinical use. The new types of devices, known as *bioactive (IUDs)*; or medicated *intrauterine delivery systems*, were developed in an attempt to alleviate the side effects while still maintaining a high antifertility effect.

Chemical compounds or metals are either incorporated directly into the body of the device (progesterone) or placed on its surface (copper). The most active inflammation-inducing metals include iron, nickel, copper and zinc (Hersh and Bodey 1970). There is no need therefore to rely on the large surface area of a device to provide chemotactic attraction for polymorphonuclear leukocytes in order to produce the desired antifertility effect. In clinical practice it is therefore possible to reduce the size and vary the configuration of IUDs in order to reduce the side effects significantly.

Two major factors are of importance in the selection of the medication-carrier combination utilized for IUDs. The first is that the drug be highly effective as an antifertility agent when administered in low concentration without producing localized side effects. The second is the capability of the delivery system to produce a long-term continuous release of the lowest dosage of medication needed to produce 100-percent contraception. If the medication is incorporated into a synthetic carrier material, it is possible to produce devices with varying diffusion rates, thus affording the opportunity to control the release of medication within the uterine cavity to the minimal therapeutic dose level (Moyer et al. 1977).

Different components have been successfully utilized in this type of IUD, including progesterone (Seshadri et al. 1971; Vickery et al. 1970), copper (Polidoro et al. 1974), and nonsteroidal compounds because of their action on the fertilized ovum or their spermicidal effects in comparison with compounds currently in use (Moyer et al. 1977).

Emetine hydrochloride is an example of a compound which is an effective antifertility agent in humans and in rats (Khanna et al. 1962; Moyer et al. 1977). It has a pharmacologic effect in interfering with cellular protein synthesis (Chakrabarti et al. 1972), reducing the size of the Golgi complex (Flickinger 1971), and interfering with the oxidative phosphorylation normally occurring in the mitochondria (Lietman 1970).

The two commonly used medicated IUDs are the copper-releasing and the progesterone-releasing devices. The copper IUD is less often spontaneously expelled from the uterus, produces fewer cases of irregular bleeding, and causes less pain than the inert devices (Zipper et al. 1971). The effectiveness of IUDs is usually proportional to their size, but the copper device is effective in a relatively small size, a factor which is presumably one of the reasons for the reduction of the undesirable side effects (Oster 1972).

The copper IUD produces both biochemical and morphological changes (Figure 1) in the female reproductive tract (Oster 1971, 1972; Middleton and Kennedy 1975). The relative importance of each of these changes in producing an antifertility effect is still unresolved, but it is likely that the numerous biochemical changes may be cumulative in producing the antifertility effect. More research in this area will elucidate why copper is preferable to other metals such as zinc, iron, gold and silver in producing an antifertility effect (Moyer and Shaw 1980). In general, the copper IUD is a highly effective contraceptive method in both experimental animals and in man (Zipper et al. 1969a, 1969b, 1971).

The chemical state and the release rate of copper from the IUD are influenced by pH, O_2 tension, amount of blood loss, and protein components of

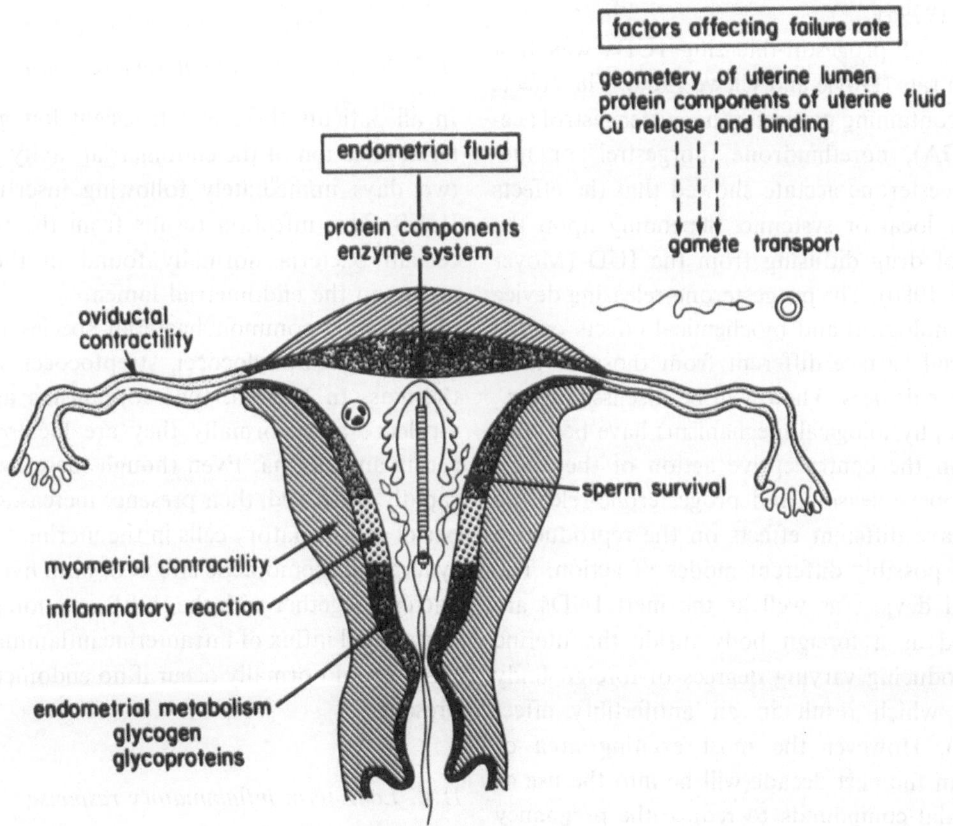

Figure 1. Physiological mechanism of action of Cu IUD. Note effect of copper on endometrial secretion and protein content, enzymatic activity, sperm transport and activity, oviductal motility, endometrial foreign body reaction, and uterotubal motility.

the endometrial secretions. Copper serum levels of IUD users are normal, and the endometrium of Cu IUD users is shown by X-ray dispersive analysis not to contain copper. Increased endometrial levels of copper, magnesium and calcium have been recorded with a depression of endometrial zinc, suggesting that copper and zinc may compete for binding sites. Nevertheless, serum copper and ceruloplasmin levels remain within the normal range (Hagenfeldt 1976).

Although a systemic action of copper from copper IUDs is generally discounted, Barkoff (1976) reported a case of copper allergy presenting with urticaria, joint pains and angioneurotic edema one month after insertion of a copper IUD. The diagnosis of sensitivity to copper was confirmed by positive scratch tests. The antifertility effect of copper IUDs depends partially on the copper surface area exposed in the uterine lumen, but it is stated that amounts of copper larger than 250 mm^2 are not expected to increase the contraceptive effect (Wagner 1979a).

The use of progestin-releasing IUDs was first studied in rats (Doyle and Clewe 1968). The effects of IUDs containing progesterone, melengestrol acetate (MGA), norethindrone, norgestrel, or medroxyprogesterone acetate showed that the effects are either local or systemic, depending upon the amount of drug diffusing from the IUD (Moyer and Shaw 1980). The progesterone-releasing device has morphological and biochemical effects on the endometrial surface different from those of inert and copper devices. These will be discussed later.

Several physiological mechanisms have been implicated in the contraceptive action of the IUD. Inert, copper-releasing and progesterone-releasing devices have different effects on the reproductive tract and possibly different modes of action. The medicated devices as well as the inert IUDs are considered as a foreign body inside the uterine cavity producing varying degrees of foreign body reactions which result in an antifertility effect (Table 1). However the most exciting area of research in the next decade will be into the use of nonsteroidal compounds to reduce the pregnancy rate (Moyer et al. 1977).

This chapter deals with the endometrial reactions, endocrine mechanisms, biochemical mechanisms, and immunological mechanisms which may be involved in the mode of action of inert and medicated intrauterine devices.

II. FOREIGN BODY REACTION

Extensive investigations in experimental animals have resolved some of the important questions regarding the physiological significance of the foreign body reaction and inert IUDs. It is a biological principle that whenever foreign material is inserted into the body biochemical and cellular reactions occur to dispose of the foreign body. These reactions vary in severity and appear to be partly related to the type of material of which the foreign body is composed (El Sahwi and Moyer 1970).

The cellular and biochemical responses to the intrauterine foreign body (IUFB) placed in the sterile environment of the endometrial lumen involve two reactions: one short-term and the other long term (Mishell et al. 1966).

II.A. Short-term inflammatory response

In all patients there is a transient low-grade bacterial infection of the endometrial cavity for one to two days immediately following insertion of an IUFB. This infection results from the transfer of certain bacteria normally found in the cervical mucus to the endometrial lumen.

The most common bacterial species in cervical mucus are staphylococci, streptococci, and diphtheroids. In general, these organisms are of low virulence and normally they are localized in the cervix and vagina. Even though these bacteria are rapidly destroyed, their presence increases the number of inflammatory cells in the uterine cavity. The synergistic chemotactic effects of both live and dead bacteria together with the IUFB reaction produce a more rapid influx of intrauterine inflammatory cells than would normally occur if no endometritis were present.

II.B. Long-term inflammatory response

The long-term reaction is due to the presence of the IUD, persisting as long as the IUD remains in utero. These responses involve morphological, ultrastructural, physiological and biochemical

Table 1. Summary of the possible modes of action of inert and medicated IUDs, based on studies on laboratory animals and man.

Reaction	*Antifertility mechanism*
I. Foreign body reaction (FBR)	1. Production of toxic cellular component from macrophages and neutrophils which affect preimplanted implanting blastocyst 2. Asynchronous development of endometrium → defective implantation 3. Phagocytosis of spermatozoa and/or blastocyst
II. Biochemical alteration in uterine secretions	4. Modification of structure of protein content of uterine secretion (effect of copper): A. precipitation of albumin → change in endometrium → defective implantation B. loss of stickiness of uterine secretion → defective implantation C. lysis of mucoid material → defective sperm transport D. inactivation of specific enzymes needed for implantation process (carbonic anhydrase, alkaline phosphatase) 5. Alteration of mucopolysaccharides on surface of blastocyst → defective implantation
III. Enzymatic changes in luminal fluids	6. In cervical mucus ↓ amylase activity → ↓ sperm survival ↓ alkaline phosphatase → ↓ sperm motility 7. In uterine secretions ↓ carbonic anhydrase ↓ alkaline phosphatase → ↓ implantation ↑ protease → survival and implantation of blastocyst
IV. Sperm transport and survival	8. Defective transport via the uterine lumen because of lysis of mucoid material A. direct effect of copper B. toxic cellular inflammatory products 9. Phagocytosis of spermatozoa by macrophages
V. Egg transport and survival	10. Delayed or accelerated pattern of transport due to altered oviductal or uterine motility
VI. Blastocyst survival and implantation	11. Direct lethal effect on the embryo by A. copper B. toxic cellular component 12. Defective implantation due to: A. endometrium not prepared for implantation a. direct effect of copper or progesterone b. asynchronous development B. defective enzymatic action C. disturbed biochemical interaction with endometrium
VII. Hormonal response	13. ↑ Prostaglandin release from neutrophil and macrophages → antifertility effect (inert and copper) 14. ↑ Prolactin → no significance 15. No changes in steroid hormone
VIII. Immunological reaction	16. Loss of immunologic tolerance → inability of blastocyt to implant or to resist phagocytosis 17. ↑ Inflammatory response to IUD A. production of antibodies of endogenous cellular component, e.g. ALG → ↑ inflammatory cell turnover B. IgG acts as a chemotactic factor → ↑ migration of polymorphonuclear leukocytes to the site of the inflammatory lesion

changes in the epithelial and subepithelial layers. The inflammatory responses of the tissue depend on several factors such as size and flexibility of device, interaction of the device with geometry of the uterine lumen, and the type of medication of the IUD – copper or steroid. Because of the cyclic decidualization of the endometrial surface, the foreign body reaction is continually renewed. This cyclic chronic inflammation may well explain the nonprogressing endometritis produced by the IUD (Halub et al. 1971). On the other hand, it is also stated that the sloughing of tissue and the biochemical events associated with menstruation do not in themselves eliminate these chronic inflammatory cells. The basalis of the endometrium as well as focal areas of superficial endometrium may remain during menstruation (McLennan and Rydell 1965; Flowers and Wilborn 1977; Nogales-

Ortiz and Nogales 1978) so it is likely that foci of chronic inflammatory cells may remain in the endometrial tissue which does not slough at menstruation.

In an effort to expel the IUD, the myometrium exerts a contractile force, and the foreign body is displaced within the uterine cavity (Bengtsson and Moawad 1967; Behrman and Burchfield 1968). This myometrial action varies in different patients, with a significant number of patients expelling the IUD during the first few months (Tietze 1970). The mechanical movement of the foreign body over the surface of the endometrium is partially responsible for some of the associated histological alterations. The formation of a small bleb on the surface of the endometrium with fluid formation elevating the superficial epithelium appears similar to formation of a cutaneous blister (Moyer and Mishell 1971). As the bleb ruptures and expels the fluid, the superficial epithelium is denuded with formation of an ulcerated area, exposing the superficial stroma. The superficial erosions are detected by scanning electron microscopy (Chapter 5).

II.B.1. Tissue and cellular changes

A series of morphological and physiological changes occur in the endometrial tissues and cells in response to the insertion of an IUD. Although the tissue damage to the superficial endometrium appears to be minor in histological sections, superficial and stromal endometrial cells appear in the flushings of the uterine cavity. The superficial epithelium may undergo reepithelization whereas the ulceration may persist for some time. In a study by Sagiroglu and Sagiroglu (1970a) relatively large numbers of endometrial stromal cells were present in cytologic smears taken directly from the IUD after its removal from the patients.

Under normal conditions, there are no inflammatory cells in the endometrium, except for a few scattered mononuclear cells in the stroma at the late luteal and menstrual phase of the cycle. Apart from these cells any inflammatory infiltration should be considered an abnormal occurrence. The inflammatory cells found in the late postpartum endometrium are the result of a noninfective physiological restorative process (Sharman 1966). The presence of plasma cells in the endometrium at any time of the cycle is abnormal, although the significance of these cells remains in doubt. Myometrial cellular infiltrates at any stage of the menstrual cycle should be considered abnormal(Moyer et al. 1970b).

The tissue trauma that results from the contact of an IUFB with the endometrium may be considered a minor tissue injury which causes a series of vascular and cellular events. This type of injury is similar to the multiple nonspecific episodes of mechanical trauma which occur to other portions of the body almost daily.

An early manifestation of tissue injury is an increase in vascular permeability. Changes were noted in the relative percentages of various types of inflammatory cells present in the endometrium at different times following the insertion of an IUD. During the early phase of injury, neutrophils (polymorphonuclear leukocytes) immigrate to the tissues of the injured area (Jessen et al. 1963). Both an immediate (thirty minutes) and delayed (several hours) immigration of leukocytes have been described (Hurley 1964; Sedlis and Reyniak 1970; Sagiroglu and Sagiroglu 1970a). The emigration of neutrophils from the vessels into an inflamed or injured area usually takes place within the first hour; the emigration of mononuclear cells takes place within three hours.

II.B.1.a. Polymorphonuclear leukocytes. The increased number of neutrophils in the uterine flushings and tissues following IUD insertion indicates an accelerated movement of neutrophils into the endometrial stroma with subsequent migration into the uterine cavity (Moyer and Mishell 1971). This migration takes place through the superficial ulcerations as well as the intact superficial epithelium and glands (Potts and Pearson 1967). Although the concentration of Neutrophils and macrophages is greatest at the ulcerated areas, these cells are present in smaller numbers in surrounding tissue and uterine fluids (Moyer and Shaw 1980). It would appear that neutrophils are distributed diffusely throughout the uterine cavity whereas macrophages adhere in significantly larger numbers to the plastic IUD than do neutrophils. Smaller numbers of macrophages are also present throughout the uterine cavity (Moyer and Mishell 1971).

II.B.1.b. Mononuclear cells: macrophages and lym-

phocytes. Sagiroglu and Sagiroglu (1970a) have noted large numbers of macrophages adhering to the surface of Lippes Loop that have been in the uterine cavity for 24 hours to 36 months. No significant reduction was observed in the number of mononuclear cells (macrophages and lymphocytes) during the time following the initial two years after insertion (Moyer and Mishell 1971). Sedlis and Reyniak (1970) reported the presence of neutrophils 72 months after insertion. The differences between different studies are most likely related to the differences in the technique of preparing the specimens.

Experimental studies have shown that the presence of neutrophils at the site of inflammation stimulates lymphocytic emigration and that substances are released which induce circulating lymphocytes to transform into macrophages which in turn participate in the inflammatory reaction. The long lifespan of lymphocytes and their ability to undergo mitosis in tissue contribute to their prolonged residence in the endometrium when appropriate stimuli are present (Little et al. 1962).

The secretory activity of macrophages having plasma membrane receptors includes the elaboration of extracellular lysosomes in response to the appropriate stimulation. They have a variety of cellular recognition responses to the appropriate stimulation (Gordon et al. 1975). They also have a much longer lifespan than do neutrophils, whereas the rate of their migration and mitosis differs in response to different foreign bodies (Spector and Ryan 1969). These macrophages are capable of releasing proteases and prostaglandins in vitro (Moyer and Shaw 1980). The inflammatory cells are noted also around blood vessels and lymphatics in the superficial myometrium as well as in areas of adenomyosis.

II.B.1.c. Plasma cells. Relatively high concentrations of plasma cells are present in the endometrium from the second to the fifteenth week following insertion and are greatly reduced in numbers thereafter. It is likely that these plasma cells represent a cellular response to the transient endometritis occurring immediately following insertion of the device. The plasma cells disappear completely in 80-90 percent of the patients six months following insertion and do not contribute significantly to the cellular decomposition by-products in the uterus (Moyer and Mishell 1971).

II.B.2. Endometrial inflammatory response and possible antifertility mechanism

Several mechanisms of foreign body response have been postulated as modes of action of IUDs.

II.B.2.a. Premature maturation and asynchronous development of endometrial epithelium and stroma. Both the stage of endometrial maturation and the age and development of the blastocyst should be synchronous in a special harmony for a successful implantation. The foreign body reaction in response to the presence of an IUD, inert or copper-medicated, is suggested to affect the rate of growth and maturation of the endometrium with asynchronous development of it and the implanting blastocyst. Wynn (1967), using transmission electron microscopy, has shown that the nucleolar channel system of glands and stroma is well-developed in a high percentage of preovulatory endometrium associated with an IUFB, whereas previously it was seen only after ovulation. Using routine histology of the endometrium, it has been suggested that there is an alteration of the cyclic pattern of endometrium in the presence of an IUFB. This observation was not confirmed by Moyer and Mishell (1971) and Hall et al. (1965), who were unable to detect significant differences in the maturation of endometrium or the timing of the luteal phase when the histologic findings were correlated with the date of onset of the last menstrual period. Further studies are necessary to determine the exact changes in the nucleolar channel system and the significance of their early appearance in the preovulatory period of their absence in the early luteal phase as detected by others.

II.B.2.b. Hostile uterine milieu. It is possible that the continuous release of inflammatory cells creates a uterine milieu hostile to the embryo (Parr 1969), or the spermatozoa (Hawk 1969). These secretory products are primarily derived from the neutrophils and macrophages and to a lesser degree from endometrial cells and lymphocytes. The cellular products enter the uterine cavity either by secretions of intracellular substances or by the cytolysis of the inflammatory cells. Previous studies in organ systems other than the female reproductive tract have shown that cells participating in an inflammatory response release cytotoxic substances which result in damage to target cells. Cytotoxicity may result from leukocytes (Behrman et al. 1969) and lymphocytes (Shorter et al. 1970). However, the relative toxicity of each cell type to the blastocyst deserves further study.

The antifertility action of the IUFB may be directly related to the presence of increased numbers of intrauterine neutrophils and macrophages (Parr 1969; Sagiroglu and Sagiroglu 1970b; El Sahwi and Moyer 1971). Greenwals (1965) proposed that the increased numbers of neutrophils in the rat uterus associated with the IUFB were responsible for its antifertility effect.

The decline in pregnancy rate in rabbits with a silicone IUFB follows a dose-response curve which is directly related to the number of neutrophils present in the uterine lumen (El Sahwi an Moyer 1971). As these cells enter the uterine cavity, their cellular constituents are continuously released into the uterine milieu and thereby come into contact with both the ascending sperm and the ovum.

The increased cellular decomposition products cause a more acidic environment, as suggested by the slight lowering of the intrauterine pH (Sedlis et al. 1967). This alteration may have a role in changing the biochemical reactions at the time of implantation of the blastocyst. The toxicity of the intra-uterine cell decomposition to the preimplanted and implanted blastocyst as well as its effect on the ascending spermatozoa is one of the probable mechanisms of action of the IUD.

II.B.2.c. Phagocytosis of blastocyst or spermatozoa. Besides their toxic secretory products, the macrophages, may interfere with implantation by spreading over the superficial surface of the endometrium, isolating the blastocyst from it. Having phagocytosis capability, these macrophages may play an important role in the antifertility effect of the IUD by phagocytosis of the spermatozoa, reducing their number in the uterine cavity. The same action against the blastocyst during the preimplantation period may also be involved in the mechanism of action.

II.B.3. Medicated IUDs and the foreign body reaction

II.B.3.a. Copper Devices. Even though the copper IUD is smaller than the Lippes Loop, the copper IUD stimulates a sterile inflammatory response (Moyer and Shaw 1980). Leukocyte migration to the stroma is more evident in association with the copper IUD than with other devices (Bonnar and Sheppard 1979).The magnitude of the increased inflammatory response of the endometrium to copper IUDs over that of inert devices has been variable in different studies (Hagenfeldt et al. 1972). It is likely that the copper IUD exerts its antifertility effect primarily as the direct effect of copper on the blastocyst, and secondarily through a foreign body reaction. This is in contrast to inert IUDs in which the sterile inflammatory reaction is the basis of the mode of action.

II.B.3.b. Progesterone-releasing devices. The foreign body response is minimal in the presence of a progesterone IUD constructed of ethylene with vinyl acetate copolymer. (Moyer and Shaw 1980). The predominant effect of intrauterine progesterone is its ability to atrophy the glands and stimulate a pseudodecidual stromal reaction. Secondarily, progesterone in the uterine fluid may alter blastocyst metabolism. The morphological alterations of the endometrium vary according to the dose of progesterone released daily from the device. With a device releasing 65 μg progesterone per day the characteristic endometrial changes are present in approximately ninety percent of the women three months following insertion. Progesterone IUDs releasing only 10-25 μg progesterone per day show a typical suppressed endometrial reaction (pseudodecidual stromal reaction with inactive glands) in less than fifty percent of patients (Moyer and Shaw 1980). In contrast, an IUD releasing 120μg progesterone daily shows a suppressed type of endometrium in all patients within a short period after insertion (Martinez-Manautou et al. 1975). However the endometrial response to progestasert devices when fully developed creates an environment that is not conducive to implantation of the embryo (Lifchez and Scommegna 1970).

III. ENDOMETRIUM-BLASTOCYST INTERACTION

Little is known about the action of the IUD on the human blastocyst, but extensive animal experimentation has been conducted to detect the possible action. In some animal species the contraceptive effect of an IUD may occur both before and after implantation. If only minimal depression of DNA synthesis occurs during the preimplantation period, the embryo may implant, but the continuing low level of DNA synthesis during the postimplantation period will cause resorption of the implanting blastocyst (Mizumoto et al. 1976). Exposure of rodent embryos to the copper IUD suppresses their growth or renders them nonviable, depending on the period of exposure aroud the time of implantation (Chang et al. 1970) In the rabbit, the increased concentration of neutrophils and macrophages in the uterine lumen is associated with a decrease in the number of blastocysts that implanted. Both homogenates and intact cells, when introduced into the uteri of rabbits during the preimplantation phase, markedly reduce the number of pregnancies (El Sahwi and Moyer 1977)

Human chorionic gonadotropin (HCG) is produced by the human blastocyst at 8–10 days after fertilization. Using sensitive and specific techniques. such as the radioreceptor assays (RRA) and radioimmunoassays (RIA) for HCG, it has been claimed that it may be produced by the blastocyst prior to implantation. It is usually detectable in the blood 8-10 days after ovulation and in the urine approximately 12 days after ovulation.In one clinical trail to estimate HCG using both RRA and RIA some 15 percent of IUD patients showed an increased amount of HCG in the serum during the luteal phase (Landesman et al. 1976). This finding was interpreted as an IUD-stimulated degeneration of the blastocyst both before and after the time of implantation. In another study urinary-HCG was estimated in 131 patients wearing IUDs (Beling et al.1976). Some fourteen patients showed higher levels of HCG after day 21 of the cycle. However the RIA studies of Sharpe et al. (1977) using 201 women wearing IUDs did not show a midcycle peak of luteinizing hormone (LH). Several technical difficulties are encountered in interpreting RRA/RIA assays in serum at the time of midcycle. It may be concluded that there is no substantial evidence to indicate that implantation occurs in women wearing IUDs. However it is possible that if fertilization and cleavage of the embryo take place in some women wearing IUDs, the preimplantation blastocyst undergoes cytolysis or expulsion.

III.A. Endometrium-blastocyst interaction as mechanism of IUD function

Several studies support the proposition that the main action of the IUD is to prevent implantation of the fertilized ovum (Elstein and Sparks 1977; Landesman et al. 1976). However, the IUD may possibly affect the implantation process through the following suggested mechanisms (see Table 1).

III.A.1. Direct lethal effect on the embryo

The direct effect of copper on the blastocyst represents the primary antifertility effect of these types of devices. This is proved by normal development and growth of rat embryos transferred on day 4 from the uterine horn with copper to the horn without copper. When they are transferred at day 5 the embryos degenerate (Chang et al. 1970).

Toxic cellular degeneration products from neutrophils and macrophages are injurious to the unimplanted as well as the implanted blastocysts, and if present in adequate amounts they are lethal to it (Parr 1969; Kar et al. 1968). This toxic substance may directly affect the DNA synthesis of the preimplantation blastocyst, leading to its lysis and death.

III.A.2. Effect of medication on the endometrium

The copper concentrations, as judged by energy-dispersive X-ray microanalysis, decrease to the periphery of the endometrium. Copper ions induce surface reaction in the endometrium sufficient to prevent implantation (Wagner 1979b). The progesterone-releasing IUD also produces drastic changes in the endometrium that render it hostile to implantation.

III.A.3. Asynchronous development of the endometrium

Implantation fails to occur when conditions of maturation of the preimplantation blastocyst and of the endometrium are asynchronous. Failure of implantation because of asynchronous development of endometrium and blastocyst was supported by Noyes et al. (1963) Margulies (1964) and Nygren and Johansson (1973). On the other hand, Hall et al. (1965) and Moyer and Mishell (1971) have recorded that the endometrium of women wearing IUDs appears to develop at the same rate as in women who are not wearing them. More details on this aspect will be discussed.

III.A.4. Defective egg transport

The data indicate that oviductal contractility is increased in patients with Cu-IUDs, an effect which can also be demonstrated in an in-vitro model utilizing $CuCl_2$ or metallic copper (Figure 2). Data from a variety of species suggest that pharmacological agents which are potent stimulators of oviductal motility may also accelerate ovum transport (Lindblom et al. 1979). The suggestion has been made that if the ferilized ovum is rapidly transported through the oviducts, arriving prematurely in the uterus, the endometrium will not have sufficient time to undergo the full progestational transformation necessary for the implantation of the blastocyst (Margulies 1964). However this possibility was not proven by the studies done on rhesus monkeys (Marston et al. 1969; Mastroianni et al. 1967).

III.A.5. Defective enzymatic action

Proteolytic enzymes necessary for the implantation are inhibited by the action of copper. Carbonic anhydrase, a zinc-containing enzyme, undergoes significant modification as a result of its association with copper ions. Carbonic anhydrase is thought to be essential for the adhesion of the blastocyst to the superficial endometrium.

The possibility also exists that alterations of the mucopolysaccharides on the surface of the balstocyst modify the protective role of the endometrial mucus to the trophoblast.

IV. SPERM TRANSPORT AND SURVIVAL

There is a controversy about the effect of the inert and medicated IUDs on the sperm transport in animals and man. In sheep, sperm transport into uterine horns and oviducts in the presence of an IUD is inhibited (Hawk 1970; Warren and Hawk 1971). However, sperm transport in the female genital tract of the rhesus monkey is not affected by the presence of an inert IUD (Marston et al. 1969).

In-vitro studies on copper IUDs showed that the copper-incubated cervical mucus causes complete inactivation of the sperm within two hours of incubation at 37.5°C. Spermatozoa show increased motility just prior to their loss of activity. Washed sperm brought into contact with cervical mucus which had not been treated with copper showed no comparable inactivation (Oster 1971, 1972).

The presence of spermatozoa in the uterine and oviductal lumen of patients wearing an IUD has been documented (Malkani and Sujan 1964; Morgenstern et al. 1966). The majority of sperm in the uterine washings have normal morphology, although the abnormalities included swollen midpieces, broken necks or tails, cytoplasmic droplets on the neck, and abnormal heads.

It appears that the number and activity of penetrating spermatozoa (Figure 3) decrease with increasing levels of copper on the device (Aref et al. 1979). Two factors may affect sperm transport and activity with a copper IUD: (1) lysis of the mucoid material, which may no longer provide a supporting medium for sperm transport (Oster and Salgo 1974);

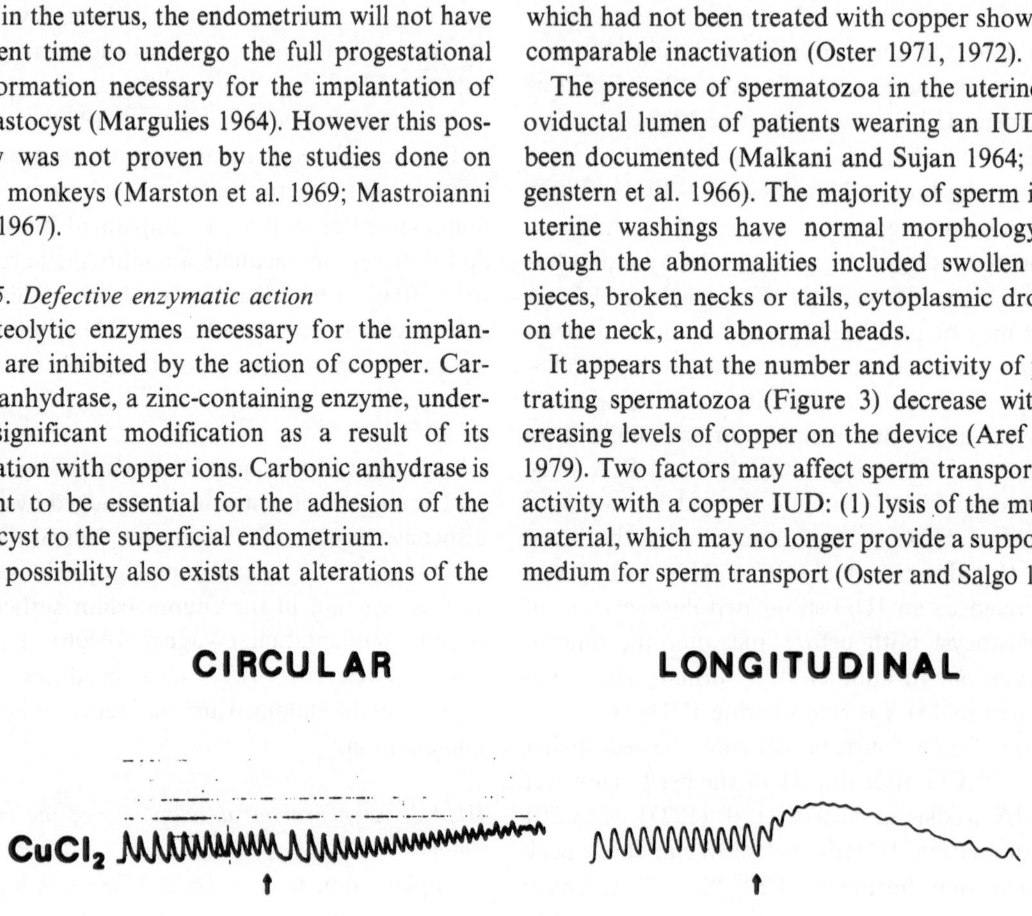

Figure 2. Influence of copper in vitro on the contractile pattern in the human oviductal isthmus.

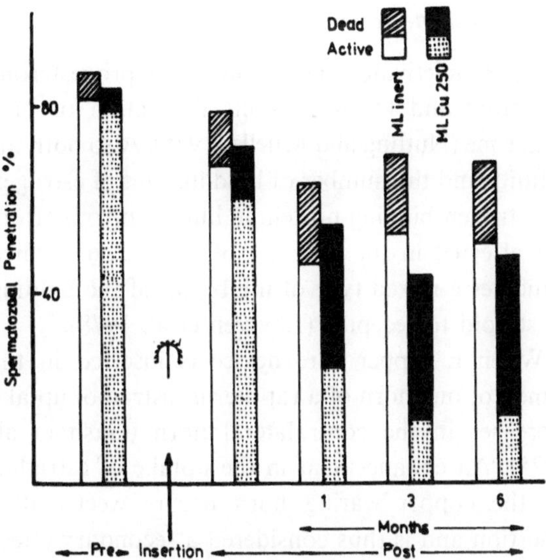

Figure 3. Sperm penetration in cervical mucus in users of ML Cu-250 and ML inert IUDs (Aref et al. 1979).

and (2) decreased activity of amylase and alkaline phosphatase enzymes which may play a role in sperm metabolism and energy production (Kandil et al. 1979).

On the other hand, phagocytosis of spermatozoa by neutrophils and mononuclear cells was reported in both vaginal and cervical fluids. In the uterine lumen, phagocytosis of the ascending spermatozoa would decrease their number and minimize the incidence of pregnancy. It would appear that disturbance in sperm transport and survival is partly involved in the antifertility effect of the IUD (Koch and Vogel 1979).

V. HORMONAL MECHANISM

V.A. Steroid hormones

There is evidence of altered endocrine profile in farm animals as a result of the presence of intrauterine devices (Bhalla and Casida 1970a 1970b). For example, IUDs cause an increase in pituitary LH of goats (Janakiraman et al. 1969) and interfered with gonadotropin secretion in cattle (Bhalla et al 1969). The luteolytic effect of an ipsilateral IUD in the live sheep was prevented by injection of human chorionic gonadotropin. This finding gives evidence that there is a deficiency of circulating LH in association with an IUD in some animal species (Stromshak et al. 1967).

Divergent results have been presented from studies on the effect of the IUD on ovarian function in women. It has been argued that ovulation is suppressed, that the lifespan of the corpus luteum is shortened (Sammour et al. 1967), and that the production of ovarian steroids is affected (Faucher et al. 1969). On the other hand, evidence has been presented of essentially normal levels of gonadotrophins (Vorys et al. 1965), of an essentially unchanged histologic maturation of postovulatory endometrium (Moyer and Mishell 1971), and of no effect on ovulation or fertilization in man (Noyes et al. 1965; Polidoro and Black 1970; Nygren and Johansson 1973; Abdalla et al. 1979).

Nygren and Johansson (1973) stated that while the ovarian function is unaffected by the IUD, its presence causes a premature onset of the menstrual bleeding in most women. In relation to the patterns of the ovarian steroids, menstruation starts on an average some two days earlier in the Cu-T cycles than in the control cycles and earlier than would be expected from the plasma levels of the ovarian steroids. This is of importance in studies where dating the cycles is necessary. This phenomenon is not restricted to the first few cycles after insertion, since it occurred also in cycles where the IUD had been in situ for up to eighteen months (Nygren and Johansson 1973). Nygren and Johansson also stated that the menstrual bleeding starts at about the same hormonal levels with both copper and inert devices and the lack of difference in this respect between the two IUDs seems to indicate that the distension of the uterine cavity is not a major factor. This phenomenon has been proposed as an effect of the IUD on the hormonal profile, but more likely leukocyte infiltration and other local changes which have been shown to occur within the endometrium in the presence of an IUD are the main causes of the premature onset of menstrual bleeding (Nygren and Johansson 1973).

However, using light microscopy techniques, other investigators have shown that maturation of the endometrium of women using IUDs appears to occur at the same rate as in women with no IUDs (Hall et al. 1965).

It is interesting also to know that copper IUDs cause an increase in prolactin levels in their users

(Mehta et al. 1977). No relationship was found between prolactin levels and duration of IUD use or between those who had previously used oral contraceptives and those wo had not. The mechanism behind the increased levels needs evaluation.

V.B. Prostaglandins

Measurable concentrations of prostaglandin-E (PGE) and prostaglandin-$F_{2\alpha}$ $(PGF)_{2\alpha}$ have been observed in normal endometrium without IUD. There is small rise of prostaglandin-concentrations in the late proliferative phase of the menstrual cycle. At the time of menstruation, the content of PGE and $PGF_{2\alpha}$ in menstrual blood is high. Inert and copper IUDs result in prostaglandin release, either by tissue trauma of from the induction of an inflammatory response to the device. Neutrophils and macrophages produce prostaglandins and can be recovered, either by flushing the uterine cavity or by examining the removed devices for adherent leukocytes (Elstein and Sparks 1977).

The role of prostaglandin intermediates (endoperoxides, PGG_2 and PGH_2), thromboxanes and prostacycline (PGI_2) has not yet been evaluated in relation to the mechanism of action and extent of side-effects of IUDs. It seems possible that the absolute production rates and the delicate balance between prostaglandins may be crucial elements in the development of side-effects and the establishment of the contraceptive effect of IUDs. Data support the role of prostaglandins since the biosynthesis of their inhibitors could interfere with the antifertility effect of IUDs and have been used with success to alleviate uterine pain and bleeding problems due to IUDs, which implies prostaglandin overproduction in the pathogenesis (Chapter 8).

On the other hand, Elstein and Sparks (1977) did not confirm the role of prostaglandins in the mechanism of side effects of IUDs. They did not detect any evident difference in prostaglandin production between inert and copper devices and between devices removed for medical or nonmedical reasons. This suggests that prostaglandins released by leukocytes are not responsible for side effects such as bleeding and pain. However the role of prostaglandins released by the endometrium still needs further evaluation (Elstein and Sparks 1977).

V.C. Hormone receptors

Copper inactivates the cytoplasmic progesterone receptors and locally inhibits the action of progesterone (Nutting and Mueller 1975). Also both the affinity and the number of binding sites of estrogen to estrogen-binding protein in human myometrium are affected in the presence of CU^{++} ions, which indicates a mixed type of inhibition of the binding of steroid to receptor (Lövgren et al. 1978).

When a copper wire device is inserted in the lumen of one horn of a rat uterus, estradiol uptake increases in the contralateral horn (Gash et al. 1975). An enhancement in the uptake of estradiol by the copper-bearing horn occurs weeks after insertion and is thus considered a secondary effect (Adedevoh and Dada 1973). The in-vitro inhibition of incorporation of ^{3}H-uridine into uterine RNA in copper-bearing horns compared with control horns (Dada and Adedevoh 1976) supports the hypothesis that the estrogen receptor complex is influenced.

Concentrations of Cu^{++} ions above 10 μM are required before remarkable alterations in the binding characteristics are established. As the copper level in the uterine fluid of women using a Cu IUD is in the range of 20 μM, the interaction of Cu^{++} ions with the binding of estrogens to their specific receptors is responsible for the uterine changes in the presence of the device (Lövgren et al. 1978).

Since several biochemical changes occur in the uterus in the presence of a Cu IUD (Middleton and Kennedy 1975; Oster and Salgo 1975), the influence of Cu^{++} ions on estrogen binding cannot be considered as the sole mechanism responsible for the contraceptive effect of the device, but it is one important possibility (Lövgren et al. 1978).

VI. BIOCHEMICAL REACTION

VI.A. Endometrial secretions

In the presence of an IUFB there is an increase in the total protein density of the uterine fluid which is related directly to the white blood cell count in uterine secretion (Kar et al. 1968; Moyer and Mishell 1971). This suggests several possibilities:

1. High levels of intrauterine protein may result from the cellular degradation of neutrophils and macrophages;

2. The blood proteins may transverse the vascular walls more rapidly than in patients without an IUFB in situ; and
3. Exudation of serum may occur through the superficial ulcerations of the endometrium.

At the same time, there is a modification in the structure and the protein content of uterine secretion in the presence of copper (Oster 1971). The copper-incubated albumin has less SH content than unincubated albumin. Apparently Cu^{++} ions formed during the incubation catalyze air oxidation of the SH groups originally present or formed by reduction with copper metal. This oxidized albumin, however, is different from normal albumin (Oster 1971).

The reduction of S-S groups in proteins by metallic copper must be a general phenomenon resulting in change of the conformation of the molecule and may have a role in the antifertility action of the copper devices. It was suggested by Oster (1971) that such a modification may cause several reactions in the uterus:

1. Precipitation of albumins which may change the uterine wall in such a way as to prevent implantation;
2. Loss of 'stickiness' of the uterine secretions, which may interfere with implantation;
3. Lysis of the mucoid materials which may no longer provide a supporting medium for sperm transport (Oster and Salgo 1974); and
4. Inactivation of specific enzymes crucial in reproductive processes, notably carbonic anhydrase and alkaline phosphatase.

The copper ions also inhibit the incorporation of hexoses into the glucosaminoglycans of the endometrium and blastocyst. Changes in glucosaminoglycan (GAG) have been reported in response to the presence of IUDs; such changes have been called 'estrogenlike'. The GAGs studied have included carboxymucins, sulphomucins other than heparin, and heparin per se (Moore and Rosenquist 1979b). The alteration of mucopolysaccharides on the surface of the blastocyst may modify the protective role of endometrial secretions on the trophoblast and disturb its survival and implantation.

Glycogen, normally present on the apical protrusions of endometrial cells, is lost, indicating metabolic disturbance of cells, which can affect the implantation process (Moyer and Shaw 1980). On the other hand, Moore and Rosenquist (1979a) reported that the myometrial glycogen content of the uterine horns of cycling, castrated, and castrated hormone-treated hamsters was basically unaffected by the presence of an IUD. The disturbed glycogen metabolism is discussed in Chapter 6.

VI.B. Enzymes of luminal fluids

Inert and copper IUDs bring about various effects on the enzymatic activity of cervical and uterine secretions. There is loss of activity of some enzymes such as alkaline phosphatase and carbonic anhydrase following in-vitro incubation with metallic copper (Moyer and Shaw, 1980). The Cu IUD causes a significant decrease in alkaline phosphatase and amylase of the cervical mucus with a maximum drop six months after insertion (Kandil et al. 1979). Acid phosphatase, on the other hand, shows a significant drop during the first three months followed by a sudden rise above control values (Figure 4). Copper content shows a significant increase starting from the first until the twelfth month with a maximum rise at the sixth month. However there is a relative decrease starting from the ninth month corresponding to the relative rise in amylase and alkaline phosphatase activities (Kandil et al. 1979).

On the other hand, inert IUDs such as the Lippes Loop cause a rise in alkaline phosphatase and a decrease in acid phosphatase levels, showing a maximal change after six months. Amylase shows a steady slow rise following a significant rise from the third to the twelfth month (Kandil et al. 1979).

The significance of these enzymatic changes in the cervical mucus is not clearly known. However, the depression of amylase activity may interfere with the availability of monosaccharides necessary for sperm survival and capacitation. Alkaline phosphatase, involved in energy metabolism of spermatozoa, may be implicated in the mechanism of action of copper devices.

The decreased activity of alkaline phosphatase and carbonic anhydrase in uterine secretions with copper may play an important role in the prevention of implantation (Moyer and Shaw 1980). There are increased amounts of neutral proteases, for

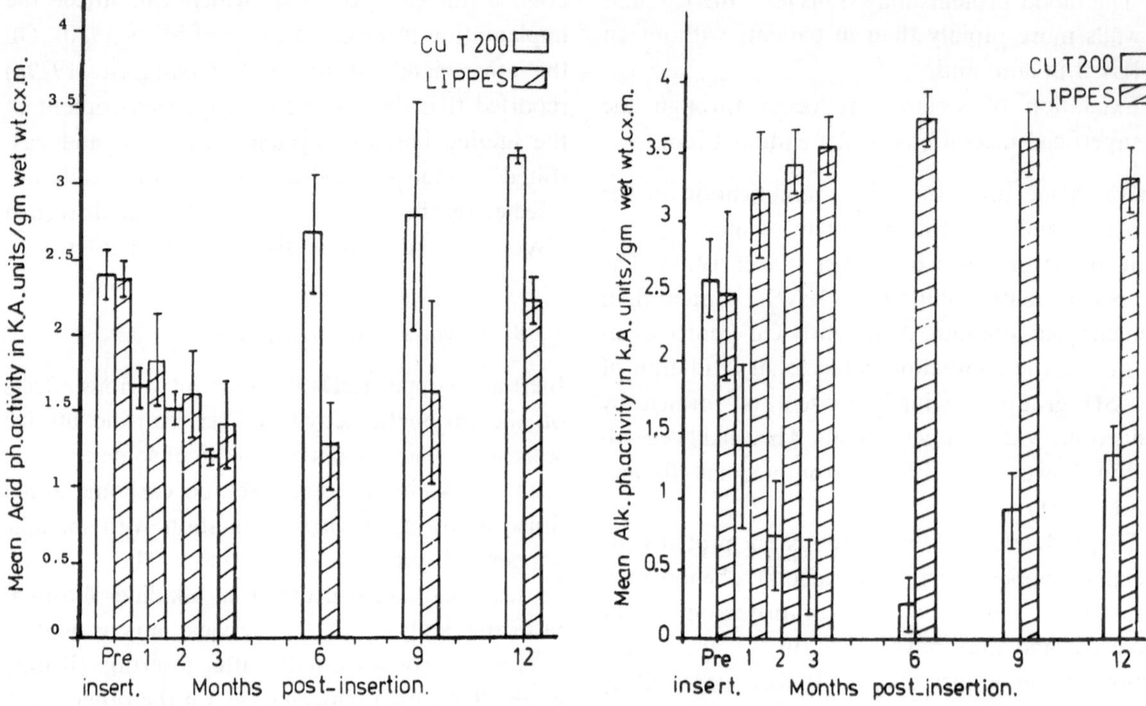

Figure 4. Acid and alkaline phosphatase activities in cervical mucus before and after insertion of inert and Cu T200 devices (Kandil et al. 1979).

example collagenase, elastase, plasminogen activators, and other trypsinlike enzymes, in response to IUD-stimulated inflammatory reaction (Moyer and Shaw 1980). These may represent one of the most important groups of chemical substances released and associated with antifertility action of the IUDs. The neutral proteases, elaborated from the macrophages adhering to the surface of the IUD, may have a profound effect on the preimplantation blastocyst and the implantation process.

The role of leukocytes in the contraceptive action of IUDs has been discussed in a previous section. Levels of the enzyme β-galactosidase were determined as it is a good measure of the quantities of leukocyte products although it plays no part in any toxicity process. Elstein and Sparks (1977) measured the β-galactosidase activity of the minimum concentration of leukocytic extracts that is lethal to the embryo, noting that it is less than the levels found in uterine secretions with an IUD in situ. This supports the role of foreign body reaction in the mechanism of action of the IUD.

VII. IMMUNOLOGICAL MECHANISM

Implantation of the blastocyst, with its genetically foreign cells invading the uterine epithelia, entails a sensitive form of immunologic tolerance. It is most likely that it is at this critical stage that the IUD has its contraceptive effect. Studies of the immunologic mechanisms in conception and pregnancy have been published (Edwards 1970), but further research is needed to evaluate the biochemical changes in the uterus in the presence of an IUD, the role of the immunoglobulins (Ig's) in the implantation and development of the blastocyst, and the action of the chemical mediators of the inflammatory process (Halub et al. 1971). The suggestion of the possible immunologic involvement in IUD function is supported by the poorer success of IUDs in nulliparous women (Viel and Lucero 1970). This could very well correlate with the increased incidence of preformed cytotoxic antibodies against lymphosytes in parous women (Patel and Terasaki 1969).

The circulating IgG and IgM levels increase in the presence of an IUD (Halub et al. 1971). The usual sequence of Ig alterations in antigen challenge, that is the IgM showing an earlier increase than the IgG, is seen from the data on Cu IUD patients. There is also a somewhat gradual increase in both immunoglobulins as long as the IUD is in place. Higher levels were observed at longer than twenty months exposure to the IUD as compared with patients with less than three months exposure. This data fits a model for a chronic immune reaction to the intrauterine exposure to the IUD (Halub et al. 1971).

The IUD-initiated inflammation is characterized by an increase in vascular permeability and the transport of IgG into the interstitial and intraluminal spaces (Halub et al. 1971). It is present also along the basement membrane of the endometrium (Tourville et al. 1970).

Nonantigenic chronic inflammation can induce the production of antibodies to endogenous cellular components, for example antilymphocytic globulin (ALG), which is IgG. A severe form of this autoimmunity to endogenous lymphocytes has been described in a subject who demonstrated persistent lymphocytopenogenic lymphocytotoxins (Schwartz 1969).

The increased level of circulating immunoglobulins and immunoglobulins in uterine secretion may have an important role in antifertility mechanisms of the IUD. Their possible modes of action are:

1. When the blastocyst interacts with the endometrial surface with the cellular elements characteristic of the inflammatory process, the immunologic tolerance may be lost and the blastocyst will be unable to implant or to resist phagocytic attack. It will disintegrate or will fail to develop (Halub et al. 1971).
2. Both IgG and IgM are possibly involved in the foreign body reactions to the IUD, perhaps causing a lymphocytotoxic or leukocytic chemotactic effect. This is supported by the fact that after the increase in vascular permeability in skin, a protease is found which converts the exuded IgG molecule to a chemotactic factor which causes the migration of polymorphonuclear leukocytes to the site of the inflammatory lesion (Yoshinage et al. 1970).

VIII. MECHANISM OF ACTION OF PROGESTERONE-RELEASING INTRAUTERINE DEVICES

As with inert and copper devices, the mechanism of action of progesterone-releasing devices is not fully understood, but the effect of a progesterone-releasing IUD on the uterine and oviductal environment, and the possible systemic effect has been investigated recently.

In one clinical study the action of the progesterone-releasing IUD was not only local but to a certain extent also systemic (Chapter 5). The endometrium metabolized large amounts of progesterone, 100–500 μg/day. The conversion of progesterone to its metabolites by the endometrial tissue takes place rapidly. The amount of hormone delivered by a 65μg/day progesterone IUD does not exceed the capacity of the endometrial tissue (Moyer and Shaw 1980). Progesterone and its metabolites appear in the uterine and peripheral vein plasma when a high-dose (80 μg/day) progesterone IUD is inserted into the uterine cavity of a baboon.

The application of progesterone-containing IUDs (Progestasert) alters the morphology of the endometrium drastically (Figure 5). These changes, irregular or arrested endometrial shedding, are similar to those of chronic nonspecific inflammation (Chapter 5). There is accumulation of secretory granules in the apex of the endometrial secretory cells because of increased rate of synthesis or a decreased rate of discharge of the granules from the cells. Both ciliated and secretory cells possess a relatively large number of lysosomal aggregates (Figure 6) which are typical of the first trimester of pregnancy (Chapter 5). The endometrial glands become smaller and are decreased in number (Hagenfeldt and Landgren 1975).

There are significant variations in the metabolism of the endometrial tissues and the enzyme levels. Activity of the alkaline phosphatase enzyme is decreased but the activity of acid phosphatase is only slightly increased. The β-glucuronidase activity of the normal endometrium, localized mainly in the glandular epithelium, increases with estrogen stimulation and decreases in users of Progestasert IUDs in contrast to users of inert and copper IUDs, indicating minimal leukocytic infiltration and foreign body reaction (Moyer and Shaw 1980).

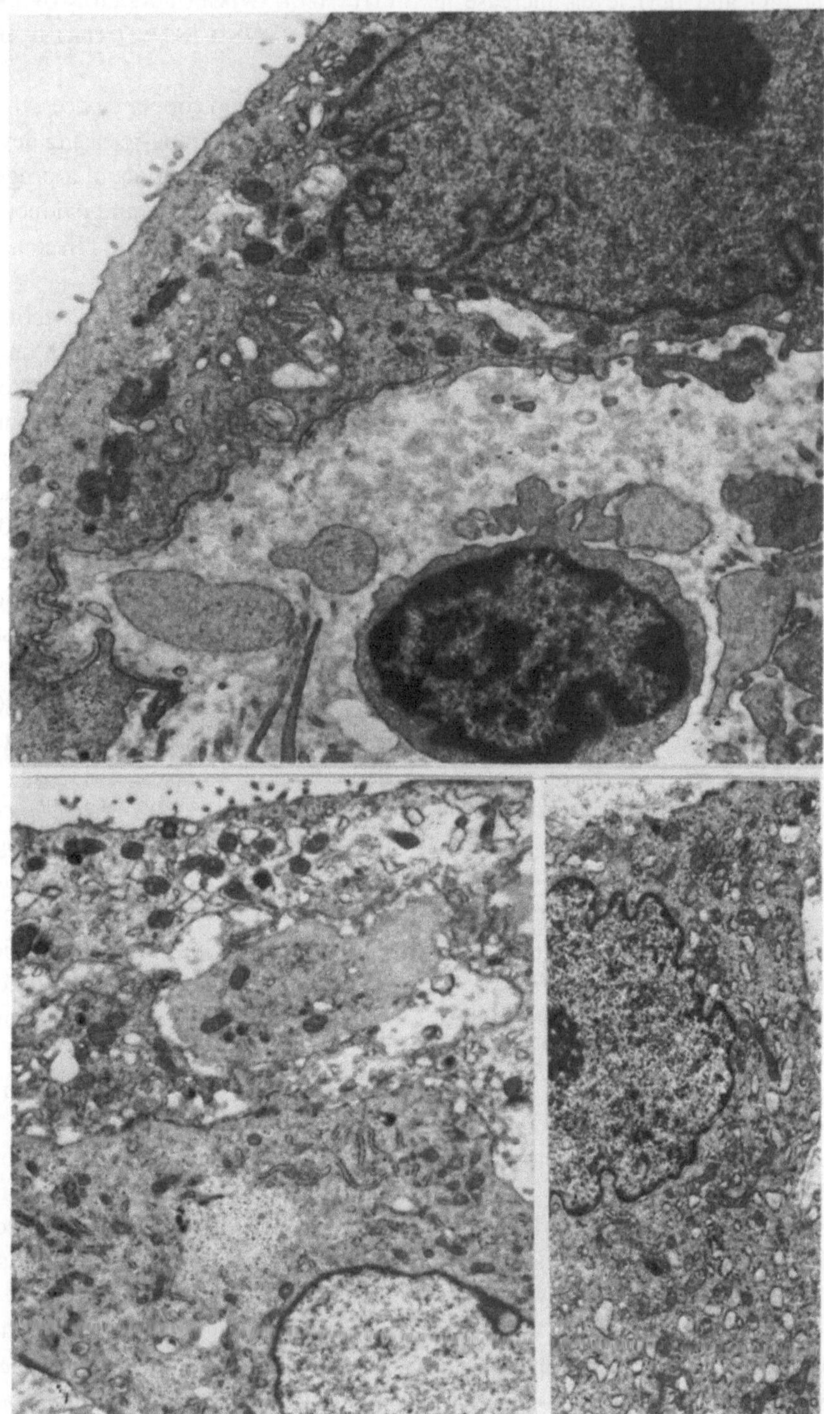

Figure 5. Transmission electron micrographs of a surface epithelial cell of endometrium. *Top:* note the decrease in height and disappearance of microvilli (× 12,000). *Lower left:* note decrease in microvilli, dilatation of endoplasmic reticulum, and glycogen in stromal decidual cell (× 9,000). *Lower right:* decidual cell frequency in the stroma of endometrium (× 10,000) (From Gonzalez - Angulo et al. 1979).

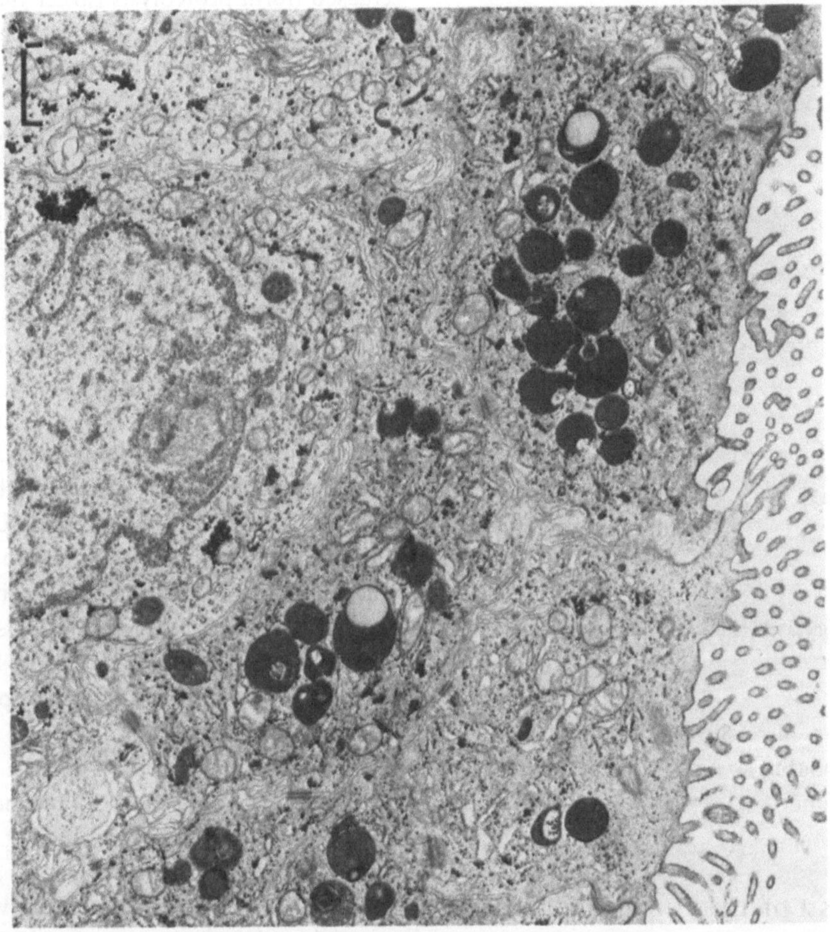

Figure 6. Transmission electron micrograph of secretory cells from oviduct with progesterone IUD in situ for twelve months. Dark inclusions are lysosomal aggregates typical of first trimester of pregnancy (× 9,000) (From Spornitz et al. 1979).

The total amount of protein in the endometrial tissues (protein/mg DNA) slightly increases 3-6 months after the insertion of the Progestasert IUD (Hagenfeldt and Landgren 1975). There is a significant decrease in oxygen uptake and glucose utilization, and an inhibition of the peptidase activity in the endometrium with the progesterone-releasing IUD (Moyer and Shaw 1980).

There are decreases in fucose, sialic acid, zinc, and calcium concentrations in the endometrial tissues of women wearing progesterone IUDs during the proliferative phase. At the same time there is an increase in the concentrations of sodium and potassium.

The effect of Progestasert devices on sperm transport and activity has been investigated in animals. The metabolism and capacitation of human and rabbit spermatozoa are affected by the progesterone IUD (Rosado et al. 1974).

Several physiological mechanisms have been attributed to the contraceptive action of progesterone-releasing IUDs (Figure 7; see also Chapter 5):

1. The number of endometrial granulocytes is drastically decreased compared with the untreated endometrium, particularly in the tissue adjacent to the IUD.
2. The formation of the nucleolar channel system is completely suppressed.
3. The formation of glycogen and the subsequent discharge of glycogen are diminished.
4. The number of ciliated cells in the surface epithelium and in the glandular epithelium is decreased.
5. Basal giant mitochondria are not formed in the endometrial gland cells.

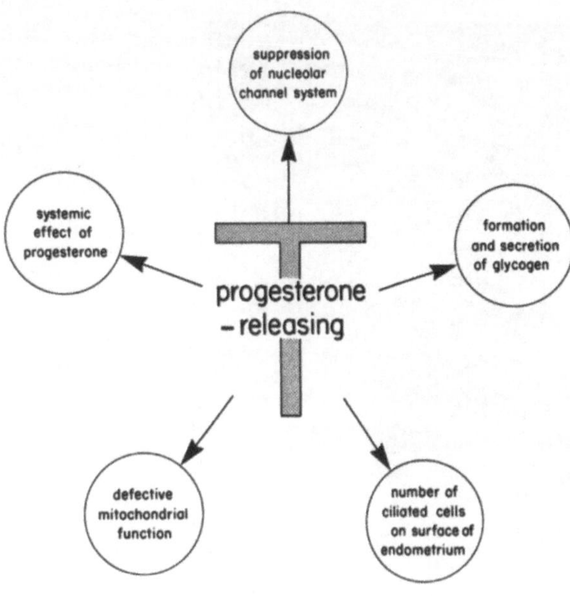

Figure 7. Physiological mechanisms of the progesterone-releasing IUD.

6. The oviducts also show some morphological changes, probably as a result of systemic effects of progesterone.

IX. MECHANISM OF UTERINE BLEEDING INDUCED BY INTRAUTERINE DEVICES

The problem of abnormal uterine bleeding following IUD insertion continues to be one of the major setbacks to this method of contraception. Device-induced uterine bleeding following insertion is not, in some women, accompanied by altered coagulability of the blood or by increased capillary fragility (Perkash et al. 1968). The empirical use of vitamins K, C and calcium for the treatment of bleeding following insertion of an IUD has not been successful.

Attempts have been made to correlate the frequency and the severity of clinical uterine bleeding with the morphologic changes in the endometrium. There is no significant correlation between clinical bleeding and histologic changes, however an increased number of mononuclear cells appears to be associated with a history of abnormal uterine bleeding (Moyer and Mishell 1971). Except in instances of severe bleeding, it is likely that the increased bleeding associated with an IUD results from increased fibrin proteolysis rather than from erosion of superficial blood vessels or other morphologic abnormalities (Figure 8; Shaw 1979).

The insertion of inert or copper IUDs causes an increased fibrinolytic activity (Shaw 1979; Bonnar and Sheppard 1979; Rybo 1979). The fibrinolytic activity is confined mainly to the superficial layer of the endometrium in contact with the device (Larsson et al. 1979). This fibrinolytic activity seems to be a combined effect of two plasminogen activators, namely the urokinaselike activator (Casslen and Astedt 1979) and the tissue blood activator.

Extensive fibrinolytic activity was present also in the endothelium of stromal capillaries and venules exposed by erosion of surface epithelium of endometrium associated with inert IUDs (Figure 9; Bonnar and Sheppard 1979). There is a remarkable difference in the fibrinolytic activity of the endometrium adjacent to inert IUDs and to progesterone-releasing devices (Figure 10). Fibrinolytic activity is evident in areas of epithelial erosion below the Lippes Loop and in areas of intact surface epithelium away from the device. In contrast, there is greatly reduced fibrinolytic activity in the case of progesterone-releasing IUDs (Bonnar and Sheppard 1979; Larsson et al. 1979; Rybo 1979). Inert IUDs are associated with more menstrual blood loss than copper IUDs (Figure 11). Progestasert IUDs produce the least menstrual blood loss. Increased fibrinolytic activity is the most accepted explanation for the increased menstrual blood loss in IUD users (Rybo 1979; Shaw 1979).

The other type of bleeding disturbance in IUD users is the intermenstrual bleeding (IMB) which occurs more frequently during the first cycles but gradually declines. The amount of blood lost through IMB is very small, and does not significantly contribute to a negative iron balance. The causes of IMB are still obscure, but it may be due to mechanical damage to the endometrium (Rybo 1979).

IX.A. Mast cells

There is an increase in the mast cell count as well as the histamine content of the uterus following introduction of an IUD in the rat (Mathur and Chaudhury 1968). However little is known about mast cells in the human uterus following IUD insertion

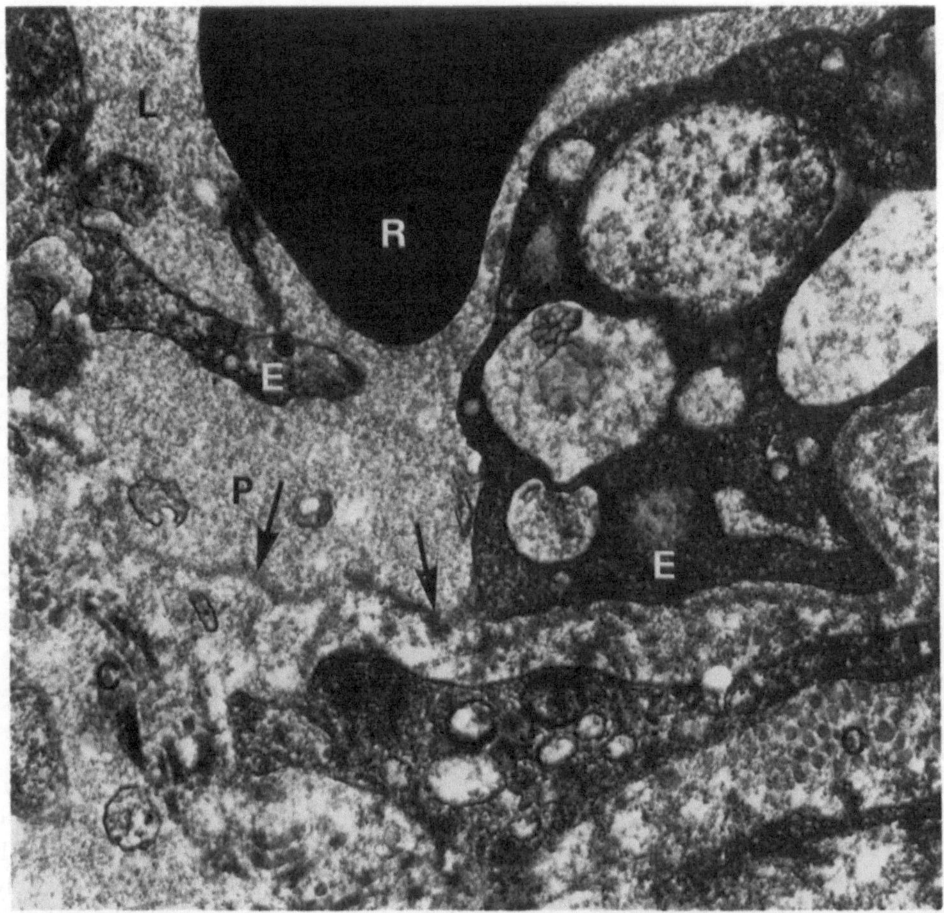

Figure 8. Electron micrograph of human endometrial vessel with IUD in situ. Note the gap separating two endothelial cells(E). The basal lamina (arrows) is discontinuous in the region of the gap. Plasma(P) is exposed to basal lamina and collagen(C), known stimulators of coagulation. *However, no hemostatic products (fibrinol platelets) are present.* A red cell(R) in vessel lumen(L) is approaching the vessel defect. Erythrocytes escape into the interstitium and eventuallly into the uterine cavity through such gaps. Finding exposed endometrium also suggests altered coagulation in this tissue (× 39,500) (Shaw 1979).

(Mehra et al. 1973). Mast cells are a rich source of heparin, histamine and 5-hydroxytryptamine. It is suggested that abnormal bleeding following insertion of an IUD may be related to mast cell changes in the endometrium, but the IUD as such does not cause a rise in the mast cell count, which appears to be increased only when the sample is obtained at the time of bleeding (Mehra et al. 1973). Based on the fact that the increased mast cell count could reflect an increase in histamine and capillary permeability, there was administration of a long-acting antihistaminic drug to women who were bleeding following IUD insertion; this resulted in a reduction in uterine bleeding (Bedi et al. 1968).

A therapeutic trial comparing the efficacy of antihistaminics in reducing bleeding and correlating the results with endometrial mast cell count in the same subject would indicate whether the antihistaminics control the bleeding by a specific action on the mast cells. Further studies are needed to correlate endometrial mast cell counts with protamine titrations in cases of dysfunctional uterine bleeding following IUD insertion. The therapeutic response to antihistaminic drugs, such as protamine sulphate and toluidine blue, should also be evaluated.

X. CONCLUDING REMARKS

The mechanism of action of the IUD is not known.

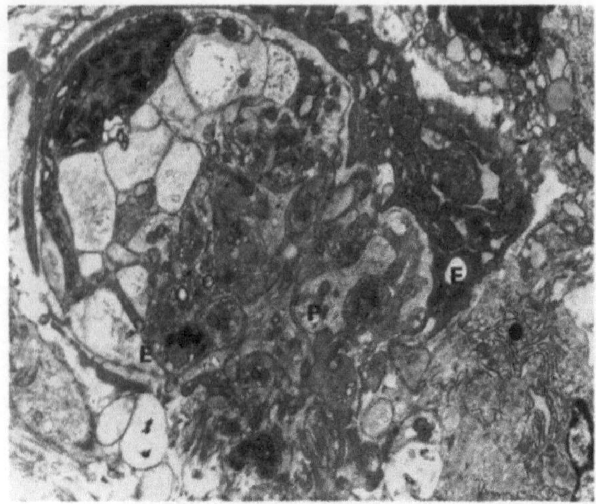

Figure 9. Transmission electron micrograph of stromal capillary in endometrium adjacent to a Lippes Loop D. Platelets (P) fill gap in endometrium (E) of vessel (× 7,000) (Sheppard and Bonnar 1979).

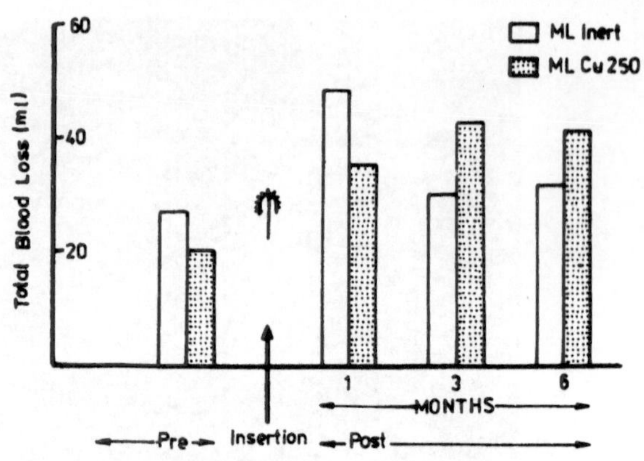

Figure 11. Menstrual blood loss in users of ML Cu-250 and ML inert IUDs (Aref et al. 1979).

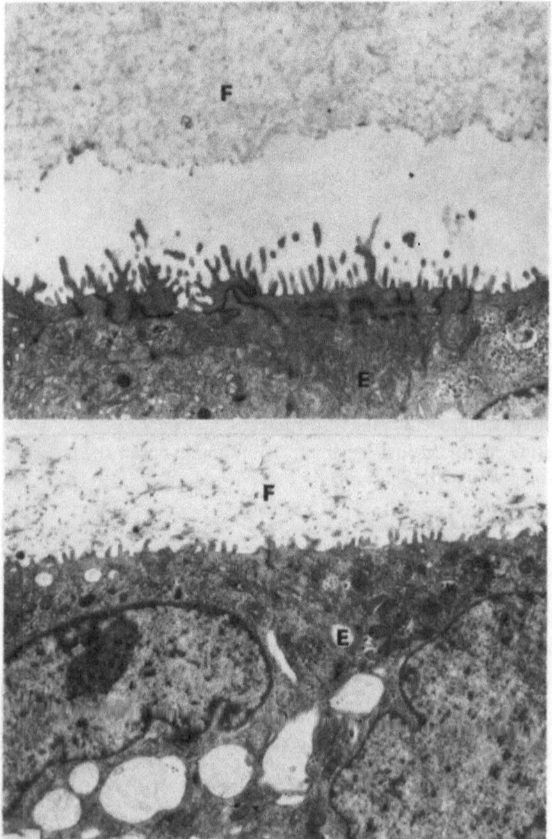

Figure 10. Electron micrograph of the endometrium adjacent to an inert IUD (*top*) and to a Progestasert IUD (*bottom*). *Top:* note a clear zone of lysis between the fibrin film (F) and the epithelium (E), 5 min incubation (× 7500). *Bottom:* note the absence of lysis. The fibrin film (F) remains totally in contact with the surface epithelium(E), 15 min incubation (× 7500) (From Sheppard and Bonnar 1979).

The suggested possible antifertility mechanism and possible failure causes are summarized in Figure 12, Figure 13 and Table 1. Inert IUDs possibly produce their antifertility effect mainly through the associated endometrial foreign body reaction. The copper IUD can produce even more severe foreign body reactions but its antifertility effect is enhanced by the local effect of copper ions on the biochemical component of the endometrium, sperm transport and survival, and blastocyst-endometrial interaction. The enzymatic changes and the immunological response to the IUD may also play an important role in the mechanism of action of both inert and copper devices.

The mechanism of action of the Progestasert IUD and its effect on the morphology of the endometrium is different from that of the other devices (see Figure 7). It is not associated with endometrial foreign body reactions and the IUD's systemic effect is doubtful.

The cause of IUD-induced bleeding is the increase in the fibrinolytic activity of the endometrium. The Progestasert IUDs are not associated with an increase in the fibrinolytic activity and, hence, they produce less menstrual bleeding than the other devices.

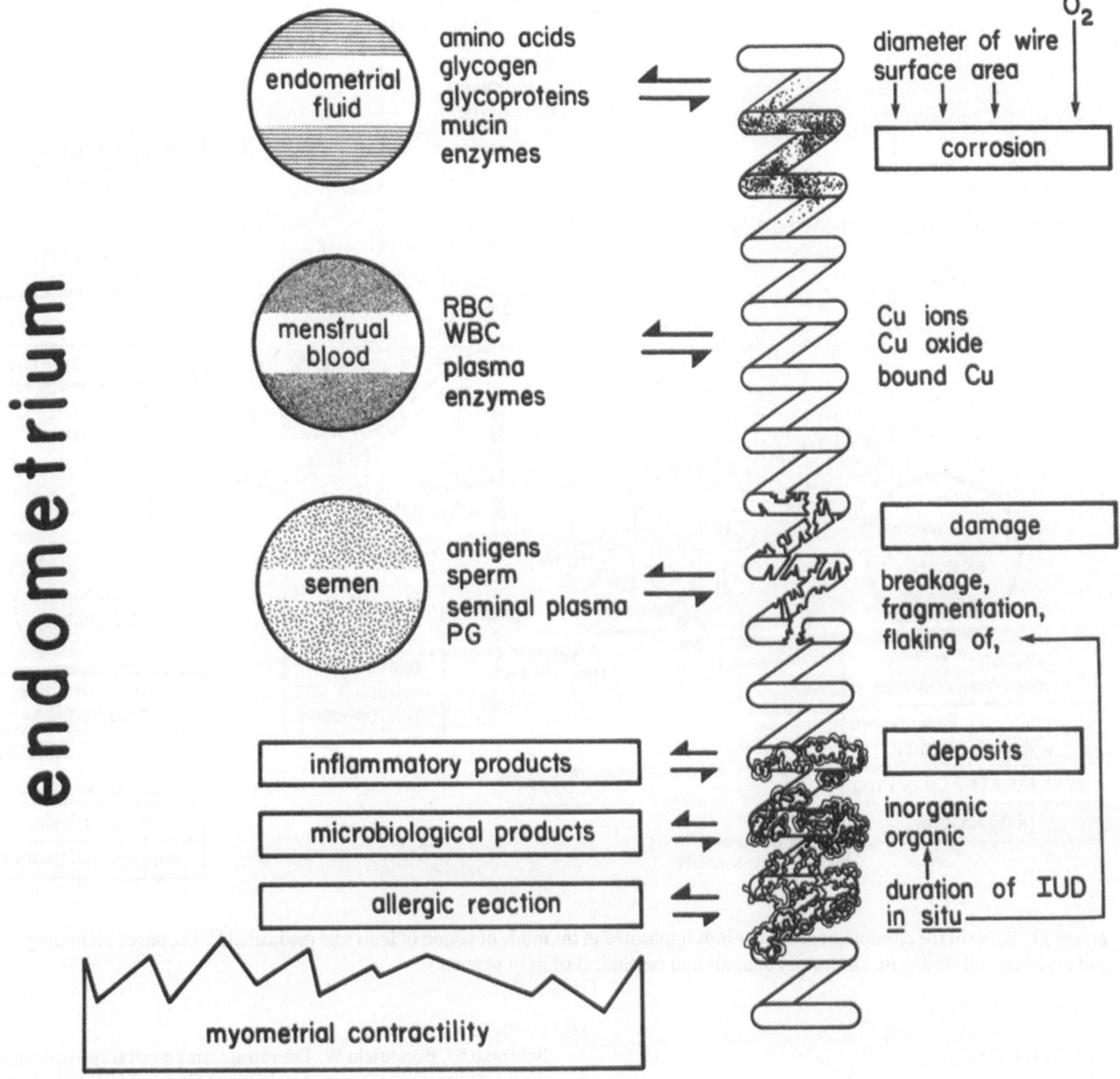

Figure 12. Factors affecting IUD failure: corrosion of copper, damage and deposition of inorganic and organic material, position in uterine lumen.

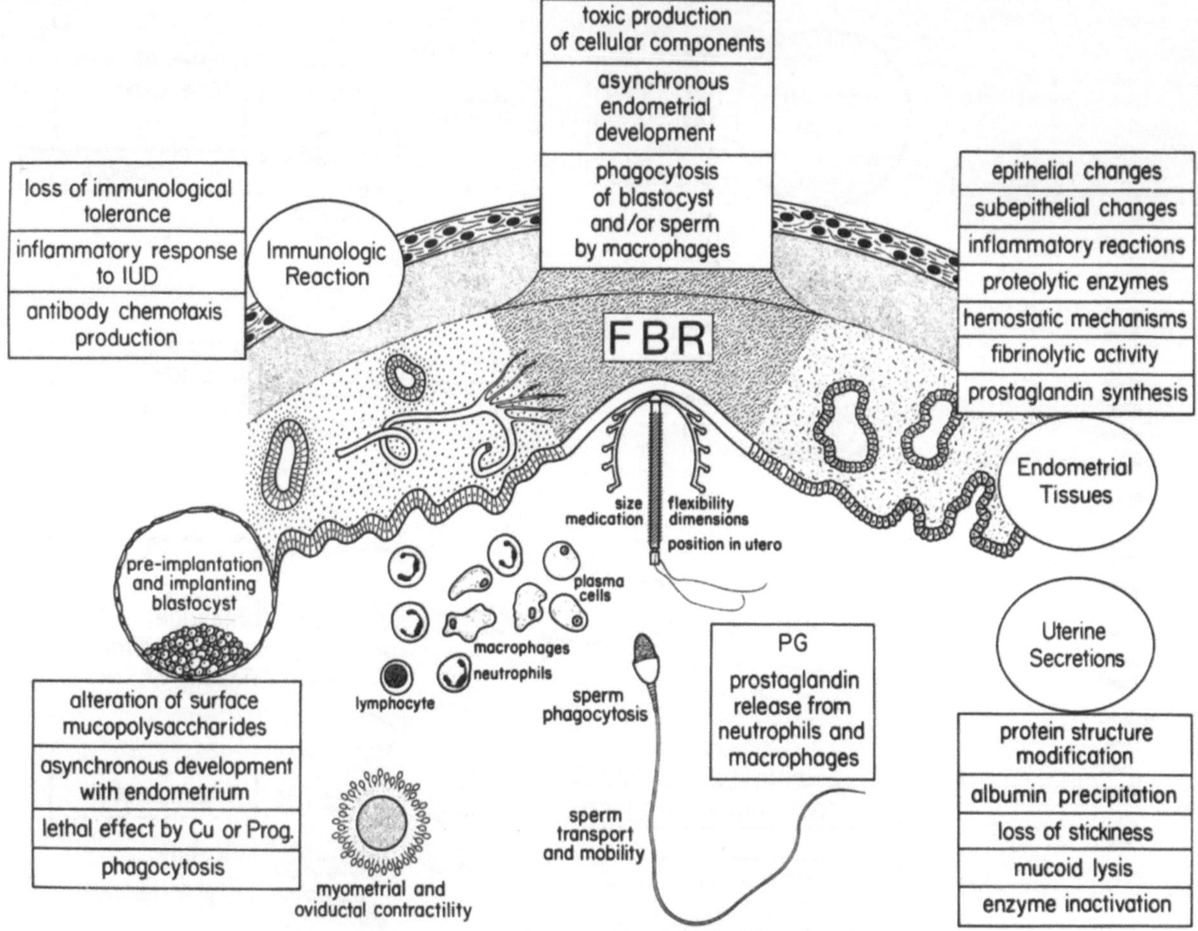

Figure 13. Some of the physiological mechanisms implicated in the mode of action of inert and medicated IUDs, based on findings and experimental studies on laboratory animals and on clinical trials in women.

REFERENCES

Abdalla MI, Ibrahim II, Makhlouf AM, Aboul Dahab T: Effect of Lippes Loop and copper T200 on pituitary-ovarian function. Presented at the symposium: Medicated IUDs and polymeric delivery systems, Amsterdam, 1979.

Adedevoh BK, Dada OA: Effect of intrauterine copper on the uptake of estradiol-C^{14} by rat tissues. Fertil Steril 24: 54-59, 1973.

Aref I, Hefnawi F, Kandil O, Yacout M, Said E: Effect of ML Cu-250 IUD on menstrual blood loss and sperm migration. Presented at the symposium: medicated IUDs and polymeric delivery systems, Amsterdam, 1979.

Barkoff J Jr: Urticaria secondary to copper intrauterine device. Int J Dermatol 15: 594-595, 1976.

Batar I, Taylor RN, Lampe L: Can the inert IUDs be further improved? Lippes Loop D, Intrauterine membranes and Ypsilon-Y. Presented at the symposium: medicated IUDs and polymeric delivery systems, Amsterdam, 1979.

Bedi P, Devi PK, Chaudhury RR: Preliminary report of a trial of a long-acting antihistaminic, buclizine hydrochloride in patients with bleeding after insertion of an intrauterine device. Br J Med Res 56: 884, 1968.

Behrman SJ, Burchfield W: The intrauterine contraceptive device and myometrial activity. Am J Obstet Gynecol 100: 194, 1968.

Behrman SJ, Archie JT, O'Brian OP: Myometrial activity and the IUCD II: propagation waves. Am J Obstet Gynecol 104: 123, 1969.

Beling CG, Cederqvist LL, Fuchs F: Demonstration of gonadotrophin during the second half of the cycle in women using intrauterine contraception. Am J Obstet Gynecol 125: 855, 1976.

Bengtsson LP, Moawad AH: The effect of the Lippes Loop on human myometrial activity. Am J Obstet Gynecol 98: 957, 1967.

Bhalla RC, Casida LE: Effect of intrauterine devices on pituitary gonadotrophins, ovulation and pseudopregnancy in rabbits. Biol Reprod 2: 58, 1970a.

Bhalla RC, Casida LE: Effect of intrauterine devices in sheep as affected by duration of progesterone influence and by the age of the corpus luteum. Biol Reprod 3: 214, 1970b.

Bhalla RC, Memon GN, Woody CO, Casida LE: Effect of bilateral intrauterine devices on some pituitary and ovarian characteristics near the time of ovulation in holstein heifers. J Anim Sci 28: 48, 1969.

Bonnar J, Sheppard BL: Fibrinolytic activity in the endometrium with inert and medicated IUDs. Presented at the symposium: Medicated IUDs and polymeric delivery systems, Amsterdam, 1979.

Casslen B, Astedt B: IUD and endometrial bleeding: biochemical aspects. Presented at the symposium: Medicated IUDs and polymeric delivery systems, Amsterdam, 1979.

Chakrabarti S, Dube DK, Roy SC: Effects of enetine and cyclohexamide on mitochondrial protein synthesis in different systems. Biochem J 128: 461-462, 1972.

Chang CC, Tatum JH, Kincl FA: The effect of intrauterine copper and other materials on implantation in rats and hamsters. Fertil Steril 21: 274, 1970.

Dada OA, Adedevoh BK: The effect of intrauterine contraceptive devices on the estrogen-induced incorporation of (^{3}H-5) uridine into RNA by the rat uterus. Acta Endocrinol 81: 165-169, 1976.

Doyle LL, Clewe TH: Preliminary studies of the effect of hormone-releasing intrauterine devices. Am J Obstet Gynecol 101: 544, 1968.

Eckstein P: Mechanisms of action of intrauterine contraceptive devices in women and other mammals. Br Med Bull 26: 52, 1970.

Edwards RG: Immunology of conception and pregnancy. Br Med Bull 26: 72, 1970.

El Sahwi S, Moyer DL: Antifertility effect of the intrauterine foreign body. Contraception 2:1, 1970.

El Sahwi S, Moyer DL: The leukocytic response to an intrauterine foreign body in the rabbit. Fertil Steril 22: 398, 1971.

El Sahwi S, Moyer DL: In vivo study of the embryotoxic activity of leukocytes. Contraception 16: 437, 1977.

Elstein M, Sparks RA: Intrauterine contraception volume one Annual research reviews I, St. Albans, Vermont, Eden Medical Research, 1977.

Faucher GL, Ellegood JO, Mahesh VB, Greenblatt RB: Urinary estrogens and pregnanediol before and after insertion of an intrauterine contraceptive device. Am J Obstet Gynecol 104: 502, 1969.

Flickinger CJ: Decreased formation of Golgi bodies in amebae in the presence of RNA and protein synthesis inhibitors. J Cell Biol 49: 221-226, 1971.

Flowers CE, Wilborn WH: New observations of physiology of menstruations. Am J Obstet Gynecol 51: 16, 1977.

Gonzalez-Angulo A, Aznar-Ramos R, Revilla-Monsalve MC: Ultrastructure changes in endometrium of women exposed to progesterone-releasing intrauterine contraceptive devices for more than five years. Presented at the symposium, Medicated IUDs and Polymeric Delivery Systems, Amsterdam, 1979.

Gordon S, Unkeless J, Cohn ZA: The macrophage as secretory cell. In: Immune recognition, Rosenthal TS (ed), New York, Academic Press, 1975, p 589-614.

Gosh M, Roy SK, Kar AB: Effect of a copper intrauterine contraceptive device and nylon suture on the estradiol 17 β-6,7-H^3 and progesterone 1,2-H^3 in the rat uterus. Contraception 11: 45-51, 1975.

Greenwald GS: Interruption of pregnancy in the rat by a uterine suture. J Reprod Fertil 9: 9, 1965.

Hagenfeldt K: The modes of action of medicated intrauterine devices. J Reprod Fertil [Suppl] 25: 117-132, 1976.

Hagenfeldt K, Landgren B: Contraception by intrauterine release of progesterone: effects on endometrial trace elements, enzymes and steroids. J Steroid Biochem 6: 895, 1975.

Hagenfeldt K, Johannisson E, Brenner P: Intrauterine contraception with the copper-T device in: effect upon endometrial mophology. Contraception 6: 207, 1972.

Hall HH, Sedlis A, Chabon I, Stone ML: Effect of intrauterine stainless steel ring on endometrial structure and function. Am J Obstet Gynecol 93: 1031, 1965.

Halub WR, Reyner FC, Forman GH: Increased level of serum immunoglobulins G and M in women using intrauterine contraceptive devices. Am J Obstet Gynecol 110: 362, 1971.

Hawk HW: Some effects of intrauterine devices on reproductive function in the ewe. Fertil Steril 20: 1, 1969.

Hawk HW: Rapid disruption of sperm transport mechanism by intrauterine devices in the ewe. J Reprod Fertil 23: 139, 1970.

Hersh EM, Bodey GP: Leukocytic mechanisms in inflammation. Annu Rev Med 21: 105, 1970.

Hurley JV: Substances promoting leukocyte emigration. Ann NY Acad Sci 116: 918, 1964.

Janakiraman K, Agarwal SP, Buch NC: Interference with pituitary luteinizing hormone activity by intrauterine devices in goats. Indian J Exp Biol 7: 202, 1969.

Jessen DA, Lane RE, Greene RR: Intrauterine foreign body: a clinical and histopathologic study on the use of the Graefenberg ring. Am J Obstet Gynecol 85: 1023, 1963.

Kandil O, Hefnawi F, Mahmoud M, Islam A, Askalani AH, Zaki K: Changes in some enzymatic activities of cervical mucus in users of Cu-T200 and Lippes Loop. Presented at the symposium: Medicated IUDs and polymeric delivery systems, Amsterdam, 1979.

Kar AB, Engineer AD, Goel R, Kamboj VP, Dasgupta PR, Chowhury SR: Effect of an intrauterine contraceptive device on biochemical composition of uterine fluid. Am J Obstet Gynecol 101: 966, 1968.

Khanna NM, Iyer RN, Kar B, Mundle M: Antifertility effect of emetine dimer. J Sci Indust Res 21: 84-90, 1962.

Koch VJ, Vogel M: Effect of ML Cu-250 on endometrium and sperm migration. Presented at the symposium: Medicated IUDs and polymeric delivery systems, Amsterdam, 1979.

Landesman R, Coutinho EM, Saxena B: Detection of human chorionic gonadotropin in blood of regularly bleeding women using copper intrauterine contraceptive devices. Fertil Steril 27: 9, 1976.

Larsson B, Liedholm P, Sjöberg N-O, Astedt B: Variations in fibrinolytic activity of the endometrium by different IUDs. Presented at the symposium: Medicated IUDs and polymeric delivery systems, Amsterdam, 1979.

Lietman PS: Mitochondrial protein synthesis: inhibition by emetine hydrochloride. Mol Pharamacol 7: 122, 1970.

Lifchez AS, Scommegna A: Diffusion of progestogens through Silastic rubber implants. Fertil Steril 21: 425, 1970.

Lindblom B, Larsson B, Hamberger L: Influence of copper on human oviductal motility. Presented at the symposium: Medicated IUDs and polymeric delivery systems, Amsterdam, 1979.

Little JR, Brecher G, Bradley TR, Rose S: Determination of lymphocyte turnover by continuous infusion of H^3 thymidine. Blood 19: 236, 1962.

Lövgren T, Pettersson K, Lundberg B, Punnonen R: Effect of Cu^{++} ions on the binding of estrogen to the human myometrial estrogen binding protein. Contraception 18 (2): 181, 1978.

McLennan CE, Rydell AH: Extent of endometrial shedding during normal menstruation. Obstet Gynecol 26: 605, 1965.

Malkani PK, Sujan S: Sperm migration in the female reproductive tract in the presence of intrauterine devices. Am J Obstet Gynecol 88: 963, 1964.

Margulies LC: Intrauterine contraception: a new approach. Obstet Gynecol 24: 515, 1964.

Marston JH, Kelly WA, Eckstein P: Effect of an intrauterine device on gamete transport and fertilization in the rhesus monkey. J Reprod Fertil 19: 149, 1969.

Martinez-Manautou J, Maqueo M, Aznar R: Endometrial morphology in women exposed to uterine systems releasing progesterone. Am J Obstet Gynecol 121: 175, 1975.

Mastroianni L Jr, Suzuki S, Manabe Y, Watson F: Further observations on the influence of the intrauterine device on ovum and sperm distribution in the monkey. Am J Obstet Gynecol 99: 649, 1967.

Mathur VS, Chaudhury RR: The effect of an intrauterine plastic device on the mast cell count in the rat uterus. J Reprod Fertil 15: 135, 1968.

Mehra U, Devi PK, Chakravarti RN, Chaudhury RR: The relationship between endometrial mast cell count and bleeding in women following insertion of an intrauterine device. Am J Obstet Gynecol 117: 852, 1973.

Mehta S, Pawar V, Joshi J, Kora S, Rajani V, Virkar KD, Raikar RS, Sheth AR: Serum prolactin levels in women using copper IUDs. Contraception 15: 327-334, 1977.

Middleton JC, Kennedy M: The biological actions of endouterine copper. Contraception 11: 209-225, 1975.

Mishell DR Jr, Bell JH, Good RG, Moyer DL: The intrauterine device: a bacteriologic study of the endometrial cavity. Am J Obstet Gynecol 96: 119, 1966.

Mizumoto H, Hohman W, Moyer D: Effects of intrauterine device on nuclear deoxyribonucleic acid metabolism in rabbit blastocysts: an autoradiographic study. Fertil Steril 27: 449, 1976.

Moore PJ, Rosenquist TH: The effect of an intrauterine device on myometrial glycogen in the hamster. Fertil Steril 32: 115, 1979a.

Moore PJ, Rosenquist TH: Some effects of an intrauterine device on glucosaminoglycans of the hamster uterus. Fertil Steril 32: 120, 1979b.

Morgenstern LL, Orgebin-Christ MC, Clewe TH, Bonney WA, Noyes RW: Observations on spermatozoa in the human uterus and oviducts in the chronic presence of intrauterine devices. Am J Obstet Gynecol 96: 114, 1966.

Moyer DL, Mishell DR Jr: Reactions of the human endometrium to the intrauterine foreign body II: long-term effects on the endometrial histology and cytology. Am J Obstet Gynecol 111: 66, 1971.

Moyer DL, Shaw ST: Mode of action of intrauterine devices. In: Human reproduction, Hafez ESE (ed), 1980.

Moyer DL, Rimdusit S, Mishell DR Jr: Sperm distribution and degradation in the human female reproductive tract. Obstet Gynecol 35: 831, 1970a.

Moyer DL, Mishell DR Jr, Bell J: Reactions of human endometrium to the intrauterine device I: correlation of the endometrial histology with the bacterial environment of the uterus following short-term insertion of the IUD. Am J Obstet Gynecol 106: 799, 1970b.

Moyer DL, Thompson RS, Berger I: Anti-implantation action of a medicated intrauterine delivery system (MIDS). Contraception 16: 39, 1977.

Nogales-Ortiz PJ, Nogales FF: The normal menstrual cycle: chronology and mechanism of endometrial desquamation. Obstet Gynecol 5: 259, 1978.

Noyes RW, Dickmann Z, Doyle LL, Gates AH: Ovum transfers, synchronous and asynchronous, in the study of implantation. In: Delayed implantation, Enders AC (ed), Chicago, University of Chicago Press, 1963.

Noyes RW, Dickmann Z, Clewe TH, Bonney WA: Pronuclear ovum from a patient using an intrauterine contraceptive device. Science 147: 744, 1965.

Nutting E, Mueller M: The effect of a copper intrauterine device during the early stages of pregnancy in the rabbit. Fertil Steril 26: 838, 1975.

Nygren KG, Johansson EDB: Premature onset of menstrual bleeding during ovulatory cycles in women with an intrauterine contraceptive device. Am J Obstet Gynecol 117: 971, 1973.

Oster GK: Reaction of metallic copper with biological substrates. Nature 234: 153, 1971.

Oster GK: Chemical reactions of the copper intrauterine device. Fertil Steril 23: 18, 1972.

Oster GK, Salgo MP: The copper intrauterine device and its mode of action. N Engl J Med 293: 9, 1974.

Oster G, Salgo MP: The copper intrauterine device and its mode of action. N Engl J Med 293: 432-438, 1975.

Parr EL: Intrauterine foreign bodies: a toxic effect of leukocyte extracts on rat morulae in vitro. Biol Reprod 1: 1, 1969.

Patel T, Terasaki PI: Significance of the positive crossmatch test in kidney transplantation. N Engl J Med 280: 735, 1969.

Perkash A, Bedi P, Chaudhure RR: Screening for bleeding tendency in patients with bleeding after insertion of an intrauterine device. Am J Obstet Gynecol 101: 766, 1968.

Polidoro JP, Black DL: The failure of the copper IUD to inhibit fertilization in the rabbit. J Reprod Fertil 23: 151, 1970.

Polidoro JP, Culver RM, Thomas S, Hahn DW: Mechanism of anti-implantation by copper IUD in the rabbit: transport and recovery of ova. Contraception 10: 481-490, 1974.

Potts M, Pearson RM: A light and electron microscopic study of cells in contact with intrauterine contraceptive devices. J Obst Gyn Br Comm 74: 129, 1967.

Rosado A, Hicks JJ, Aznar R, Mercado E: Intrauterine contraception with the progesterone-T device. Contraception 9: 40, 1974.

Rybo G: IUD and endometrial bleeding: qualitative and quantitative aspects. Presented at the symposium: medicated IUDs and polymeric delivery systems, Amsterdam, 1979.

Sagiroglu N, Sagiroglu E: The cytology of intrauterine contraceptive devices. Acta Cytol 14: 58, 1970a.

Sagiroglu N, Sagiroglu E: Biologic mode of action of the Lippes Loop in intrauterine contraception. Am J Obstet Gynecol 106: 506, 1970b.

Sammour MB, Iskander SG, Rifai SF: Combined histologic and cytologic study of intrauterine contraception. Am J Obstet Gynecol 98: 946, 1967.

Schwartz RS: Lymphocytopenogenic lymphocytotoxins. N Engl J Med 281: 324, 1969.

Sedlis A, Reyniak JV: Endometrial leukocytes in patients using intrauterine contraceptive devices. Am J Obstet Gynecol 108: 120, 1970.

Sedlis A, Kandemir E, Stone ML: Intrauterine pH of women using stainless steel contraceptive devices. Obstet Gynecol 30: 114, 1967.

Seshadri B, Gibor Y, Scommegna A: Antifertility effects of intrauterine progesterone in the rabbit. Am J Obstet Gynecol 109: 536-541, 1971.

Sharman A: Reproductive physiology of the postpartum period, Edinburgh, Livingstone, 1966.

Sharpe RM, Wrixon W, Hobson BM, Corker CS, McLean HA, Short RV: Absence of HCG-like activity in the blood of women fitted with intrauterine contraceptive devices. J Clin Endocrinol Metab 45: 496, 1977.

Shaw, ST: Studies on pathophysiology of IUD-induced endometrial bleeding. Presented at the symposium: medicated IUDs and polymeric delivery systems, Amsterdam, 1979.

Sheppard BL, Bonnar J: Response of endometrial blood vessels to inert and medicated IUDs as shown by scanning and transmission electron microscopy. Presented at the symposium: Medicated IUDs and polymeric delivery systems, Amsterdam, 1979.

Shorter RG, Huizenga KA, ReMine SG, Spencer RJ: Effects of preliminary incubation of lymphocytes with serum on their cytotoxicity for colonic epithelial cells. Gastroenterology 58: 843, 1970.

Spector WG, Gyan GB: New evidence for the existence of long lived macrophages. Nature 221: 860, 1969.

Spornitz UM, Ludwig KS, Mall-Haefeli M, Werner-Zodrow D, Uettwiller A: Effect of a progesterone containing IUD on the morphology of endometrium and oviduct. Presented at the symposium, Medicated IUDs and Polymeric Delivery Systems, Amsterdam, 1979.

Stormshak F, Lehmann RP, Hawk HW: Effect of intrauterine plastic spirals and HCG on the corpus luteum of the ewe. J Reprod Fertil 14: 373, 1967.

Tietze C: Studies in family planning. The Population Council, 55: 1, 1970.

Tourville DR, Ogra SS, Lippes J, Tomasi TB: The human female reproductive tract: immunohistological localization of gamma A, gamma G, gamma M, secretory 'piece', and lactoferring. Am J Obstet Gynecol 108: 1102, 1970.

Vickery BH, Erickson GI, Bennett JP, Mueller NS, Haleblian JK: Antifertility effects in the rabbit by continuous low release of progestin from an intrauterine device. Biol Reprod 3: 154-162, 1970.

Viel B, Lucero S: An analysis of 3 years' experience with intrauterine devices among women in the western area of the city of Santiago, July 1, 1964 to June 30, 1967. Am J Obstet Gynecol 106: 765, 1970.

Vorys N, de Neef JC, Boutselis JG, Dettman FG, Scott WP, Stevens VC, Besch PK: Intrauterine contraception. In: Proceedings of the second international conference, Segal SJ, Southam AL, Shafer KD (eds), Excerpta medica foundation international congress series 86, Amsterdam 1965 p 147ff.

Wagner H: Copper release of different IUD models demonstrated by a biological test system. Presented at the symposium: Medicated IUDs and polymeric delivery systems, Amsterdam, 1979a.

Wagner H: Action of copper on the surface of copper IUDs and human endometrium. Presented at the symposium: Medicated IUDs and polymeric delivery systems, Amsterdam, 1979.

Warren JE Jr, Hawk HW: Effect of an intrauterine device on sperm transport and uterine motility in sheep and rabbits. J Reprod Fertil 26: 419, 1971.

Wynn RM: Intrauterine devices: effects on ultrastructure of human endometrium. Science 156: 1508, 1967.

Yoshinaga M, Mayuni M, Yamamoto S, Hayashi H: Immunoglobulin G as possible precursor of chemotactic factor. Nature 225: 1138, 1970.

Zipper JA, Medel M, Prager R: Suppression of fertility by intrauterine copper and zinc in rabbits. Am J Obstet Gynecol 105: 529, 1969a.

Zipper JA, Tatum HJ, Pastene L, Medel M, Rivera M: Metallic copper as an intrauterine contraceptive adjunct to the 'T' device. Am J Obstet Gynecol 105: 1274, 1969b.

Zipper JA, Tatum HJ, Medel M, Pastene L, Rivera M: Contraception through the use of intrauterine metals I: copper as an adjunct to the 'T' device. Am J Obstet Gynecol 109: 771, 1971.

8. THE ROLE OF PROSTAGLANDINS IN THE MECHANISM OF ACTION AND THE SIDE EFFECTS IUDs

M. TOPPOZADA and E.S.E. HAFEZ

The actual contraceptive mechanism of action of IUDs in women is not definitely established. Many theories have been suggested but the fine mediating factors in each hypothesis still remain unknown. In view of the potent activity of prostaglandins these substances appeared to fit as a possible link between the presence of an intrauterine foreign body and the target response which blocks conception (Chaudhury 1971). The position is even more vague with respect to the complications of IUDs but recent evidence is in support of a possible role for prostaglandins in this connection as well (Damarawy and Toppozada 1976).

I. MECHANISM OF ACTION

I.A. Increased prostaglandins (endometrial) in the presence of IUDs

I.A. 1. Animal data

A large number of publications have documented that the intrauterine presence of a contraceptive device in laboratory and farm animals leads to release of significant amounts of prostaglandins which may contribute to the contraceptive action. Studies in rats, guinea pigs, hamsters and sheep showed a marked increase of prostaglandin-F (PGF) concentrations in the endometrium or utero-ovarian venous blood obtained from uterine horns containing IUDs over those found in control horns (Poyser et al. 1971; Spilman and Duby 1972; Saksena and Harper 1974; and Saksena et al. 1974). The elevated PGF levels were particularly obvious in the endometrium which was in contact with the IUD, in comparison with other areas of the uterus (Spilman and Duby 1972). Also, there is some evidence in support of an increased release of PGE_2 like material from the rat uterine horns bearing IUDs (Chaudhury 1973).

I.A. 2. Human data

In the human female the situation may differ to a considerable degree from that in subprimate animal species since the factors which control cycle events and conception are quite different. The effect of IUDs on endometrial prostaglandin levels in the human has received little attention in the past and only two recent studies attempted to measure such concentrations before and after insertion of the devices. In the first study $PGF_{2\alpha}$ and its 15 keto, 13,14-dihydro metabolite were measured by gas chromatography and mass spectrometry. The results indicated that IUD insertion did not induce any increase in either compound (Green and Hagenfeldt 1975). The other publication, however, reported on the endometrial concentrations of both E and F types using radioimmunoassay and showed a significant increase in the E but not the F types following IUD insertion (Hillier and Kasonde 1976). It has also been claimed earlier that uterine fluid from women fitted with IUDs exhibits increased pharmacological activity suggestive of the presence of prostaglandins (S.K. Batta, personal communication, 1971).

Tissue measurements of prostaglandin concentrations is a doubtful issue which suffers from certain limitations. These compounds are known to be rapidly released within seconds from tissues subjected to trauma such as the procedure of sampling. Thus the reported tissue levels may only represent an 'artificial' prostaglandin formation during tissue removal. This drawback has been minimized by immediate immersion of the endometrial samples in liquid nitrogen or in solutions containing enzyme inhibitors, to avoid such unphysiological biosynthesis. However, the investigators had confidence at least in the relative concentrations since all the samples (before and after insertion of IUDs) were processed in exactly the same manner.

It has been suggested that the macrophages on the surfaces of IUDs can serve as a potent source for the increased prostaglandin production. These macrophages constitute the predominant cell type adherent to IUDs and can produce large amounts of prostaglandins (Sagiroglu and Sagiroglu 1970; Myatt et al 1975). The macrophages adherent to the surface of extracted IUDs (plain and copper-bearing) were cultivated and PGE_2 and $PGF_{2\alpha}$ were measured by radioimmunoassay in culture fluids collected at 24 hr. The prostaglandin production correlated with the total number of cells on the IUD; the production of the F type predominated over the E variety in most instances (Myatt et al. 1975). The relative overproduction of $PGF_{2\alpha}$ as compared to PGE_2 may be a reflection of the presence of copper which favours the biosynthesis of the former (Maddox 1973).

A definite variation in the number of leukocytes attached to IUDs throughout the menstrual cycle has been reported, with a significantly greater number of cells on inert as compared to copper-bearing devices which was consistent at all phases of the cycle (Myatt et al. 1977). The latter finding was explained either on the basis of device size or due to the cytotoxic action of copper. The leukocytes on IUDs produced PGE_2 and $PGF_{2\alpha}$ which followed a rising pattern with a peak of $PGF_{2\alpha}$ immediately prior to the next period, a pattern which simulates the endometrial release of prostaglandins in the normal cycle (Figure 1).

I.A.3. Medicated IUDs

Endometrial samples obtained in humans following the insertion of copper-bearing IUDs also showed the increase in PGE levels observed with inert devices (Hillier and Kasonde 1976). The copper ion has been shown to modify the enzymatic conversion of arachidonic acid in a specific way towards a stimulated PGF and an inhibited PGE production (Maddox 1973). Such an effect may have a beneficial role on the incidence of side-effects with copper-bearing devices.

The effect of progesterone on endometrial prostaglandin release in response to the presence of an IUD has not yet been investigated. The synthesis of $PGF_{2\alpha}$ by human endometrium in tissue culture was inhibited by progesterone but the effect on the

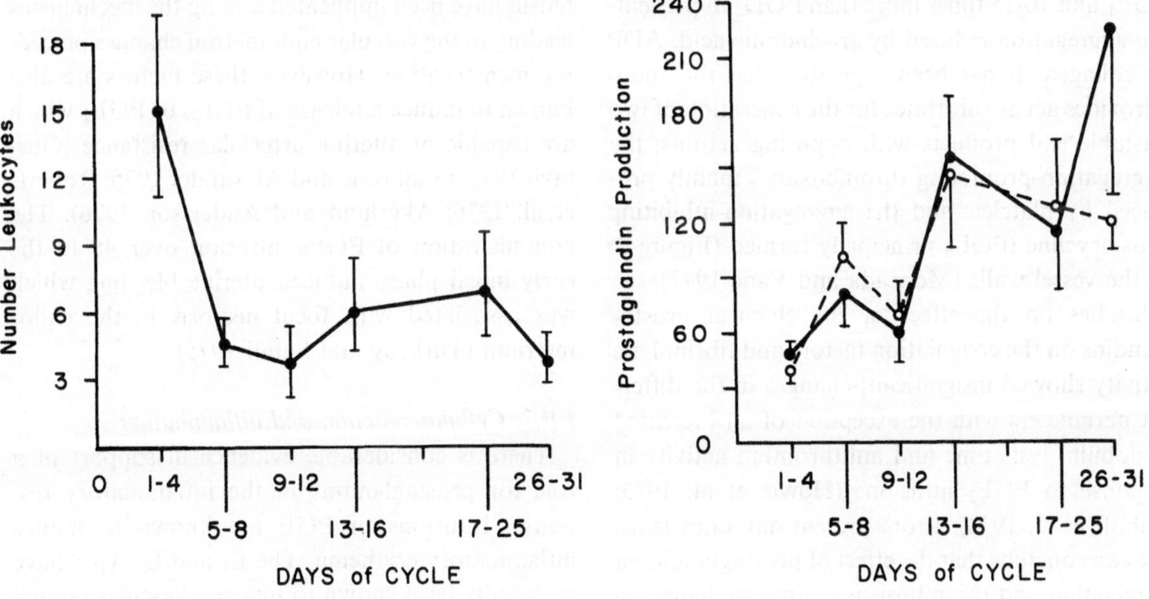

Figure 1. Left: number of leukocytes X 10^7 adherent to IUDs removed at various cycle phases. Right: mean production rates of PGE_2 (broken line) and $PGF_{2\alpha}$ (continuous line) by leukocytes adherent to IUDs (ng/10^7) (from Myatt et al. 1977).

release of the E type has not been studied (Cane and Villee 1975). On the other hand, exogenous administration of progestogens was reported to make the myometrium relatively insensitive to prostaglandins (Toppozada et al. 1976; Shaala et al. 1977). In this context the effects and biological responses of the uterus in the presence of Progestasert require further evaluation.

I.B. Prostaglandins (Biological actions) of released in relation to IUDs

I.B. 1. Vascular effects

Of the classical prostaglandins PGE_1 was found to be an inhibitor of platelet aggregation while PGE_2 had an initial weak inhibitory effect on the first phase of aggregation followed by a stimulatory action on the second phase induced by adenosine diphosphate – ADP (Kloeze 1967; Shio and Ramwell 1972). Prostaglandin$_{2\alpha}$ neither promoted nor inhibited aggregation. The endoperoxide intermediates (PGG_2 and PGH_2) as well as the thromboxanes (A_2 and B_2) are powerful aggregating agents on human platelets. Prostacycline (PGX or PGI_2) on the other hand was found to be a very powerful inhibitor of platelet aggregation to an extent which was 20-30 times more potent than PGE_1 and 10-15 times more than PGD_2 in preventing aggregation induced by arachidonic acid, ADP or collagen. It has been suggested that the endoperoxides act as substrates for the generation of two unstable end products with opposing actions; the aggregation-promoting thromboxanes mainly produced by platelets and the aggregation-inhibiting prostacycline (PGI_2) principally formed (Figure 2) in the vessel walls (Moncada and Vane 1977).

Studies on the effect of the classical prostaglandins on the coagulation factors and fibrinolytic activity showed insignificant changes in the different parameters with the exception of an increased euglobulin lysis time and antithrombin activity in response to PGE_2 infusions (Howie et al. 1973; Duboff et al. 1974). From present-day knowledge one can conclude that the effect of prostaglandin on coagulation and thrombosis is mainly mediated via their influence on platelet function and only to a minor extent by affecting the factors responsible for fibrin formation and fibrinolysis.

In most peripheral vascular beds, the prostaglandins of the A and E types usually induce vasodilatation. The B_2 variety has a potent vasoconstrictor property while $F_{2\alpha}$ has a qualitatively similar but weaker effect (Kadowitz 1972; Greenberg et al. 1974). The recently discovered prostaglandins (I_2 and D_2) have the capacity of relaxing some vascular smooth muscles, while the endoperoxide intermediates (PGG_2 and PGH_2) have the opposite effect.

Intrauterine instillation of low doses of $PGF_{2\alpha}$ approximating physiological levels induced a dramatic fall in endometrial blood flow in the subhuman primate (Einer-Jensen 1973). Whether this response is secondary to myometrial contraction or due to a direct vascular constriction remains to be definitely clarified. However, it appears that $PGF_{2\alpha}$ has a little influence on uterine vascular resistance (Brody and Kadowitz 1974). The E and A series on the other hand cause potent relaxation of uterine vessels and depress the sensitivity of uterine vascular muscles to adrenergic constrictor stimuli (Clark et al. 1978). Inhibitors of prostaglandin synthesis have been shown to reduce uterine PGE concentrations with a consequent rise in uterine vascular resistance.

Lysosomal stress and release of vasoactive substances such as oxytocin, vasopressin and angiotensin have been implicated among the mechanisms leading to the vascular endometrial changes preceding menstruation. However, these factors are also known to induce a release of $PGF_{2\alpha}$ or PGE_2 which are capable of altering arteriolar resistance (Gustavii 1972; Gimbrone and Alexander 1975; Roberts et al. 1976; Akerlund and Andersson 1976). The administration of $PGF_{2\alpha}$ infusion over 48 in the early luteal phase induced uterine bleeding which was associated with focal necrosis in the endometrium (Turksoy and Safaii 1975).

I.B.2. Cellular reaction and inflammation

There is considerable evidence in support of a role for prostaglandins in the inflammatory response. Infusions of PGE are known to induce inflammatory erythema. The E_1 and E_2 types have repeatedly been shown to increase vascular permeability while the F group was without effect. (Crunkhorn and Willis 1969). A dual mechanism has been suggested for the PGE_1-induced vascular

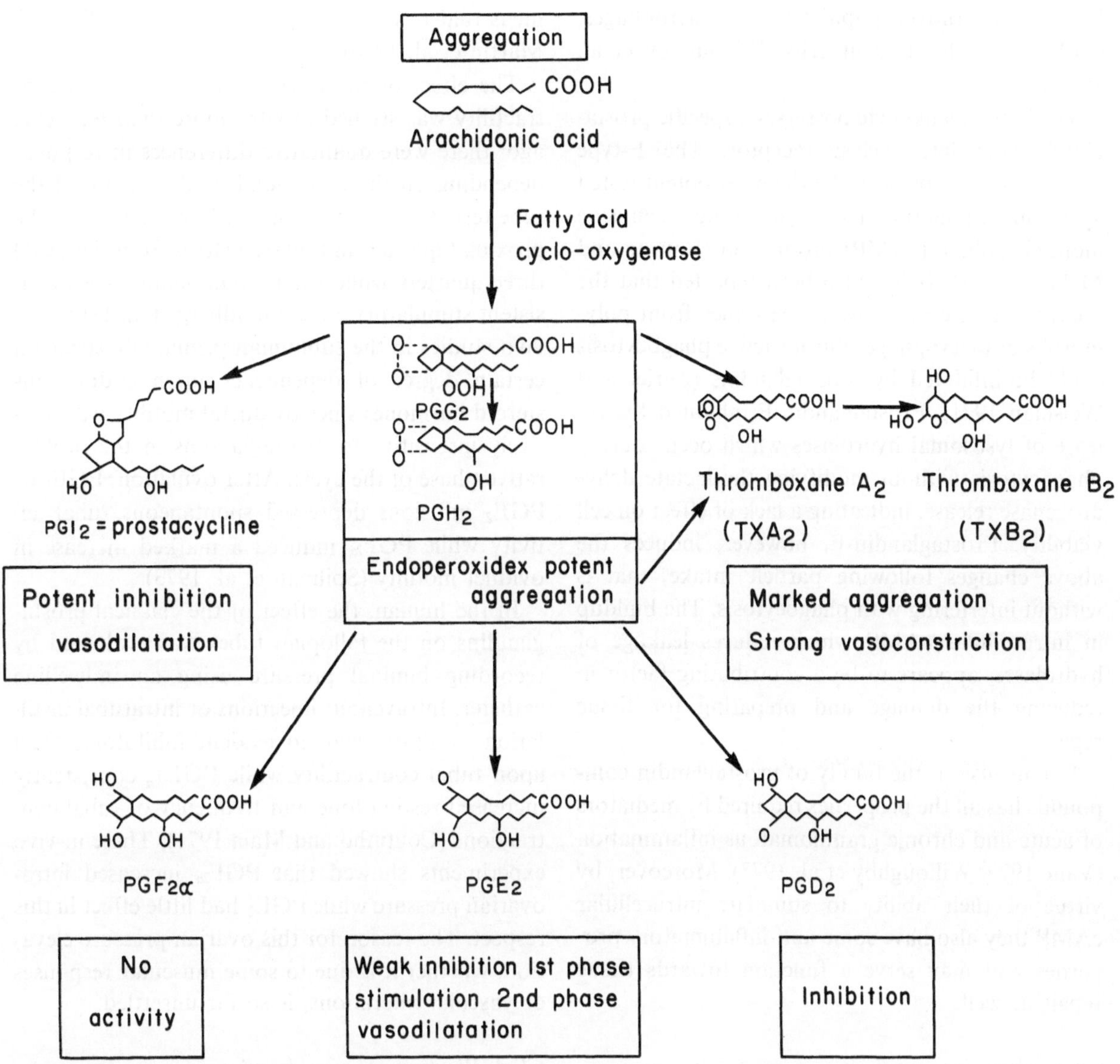

Figure 2. Pathways of prostaglandin and thromboxane biosynthesis and their effects on platelets and blood vessels.

permeability which includes a direct action and an indirect mechanism through histamine release (Willoughby et al. 1973). Prostaglandins of the E type potentiate vascular leakage induced by other mediators such as bradykinin or histamine and may oppose the effect of endoperoxides in this respect (Vane 1976). Prostaglandin-$F_{2\alpha}$ showed an antagonistic effect to the vascular permeability increased by PGE_1 and PGE_2 (Crunkhorn and Willis 1971).

An important function of certain prostaglandins in relation to the mechanism of action of IUDs is their ability to cause leukocyte emigration (Kaley and Weiner 1972). This is particularly evident in response to members of the PGE group and also with $PCF_{1\alpha}$ while PGF_2 was ineffective in this respect. The active agents caused a typical picture of nonimmune inflammation with early dominance of polymorphs that was then replaced by a wave of mononuclear cells.

Subsequent to the migration of leukocytes to the site of inflammation, which is coincident with the raised levels of prostaglandins, there are alternative pathways to the source of inflammatory response ranging from resolution to the development of a chronic type of reaction. The latter is characterized by a high-turnover population of macrophages, epithelioid cells or giant cells (Willoughby et al. 1973).

The human leukocyte possesses a specific prostaglandin/adenylate cyclase receptor. The E-type prostaglandins appear to be the most potent tested agent in stimulating leukocyte cyclic adenosine monophosphate (cAMP) production (Bourne and Melmon 1971). It has also been reported that the selective release of lysosomal enzymes from polymorphs or macrophages during active phagocytosis could be inhibited by prostaglandins (Zurier and Weisman 1971). Prostaglandin-E inhibited the release of lysosomal hydrolases which occur during phagocytosis without modifying the lactate dehydrogenase release, indicating a lack of effect on cell viability. Prostaglandin-E, however, induces the above changes following particle intake, that is without interfering with phagocytosis. The buildup in intracellular cAMP which reduces leakage of hydrolases, appears to be a contributing factor in reducing the damage and preparing for tissue repair.

In conclusion, the family of prostaglandin compounds has all the properties required by mediators of acute and chronic granulomatous inflammation (Vane 1972; Willoughby et al. 1973). Moreover, by virtue of their ability to stimulate intracellular cAMP they also have some anti-inflammatory properties and may serve a function towards tissue repair as well.

I.B.3. Muscular responses

With only few exceptions, the classical prostaglandins (E_2 and $F_{2\alpha}$) have been shown to be very potent myometrial stimulants under in-vivo conditions in the nonpregnant state, but with varying degrees of sensitivity probably related to the endocrine phase of the cycle. A midcycle phase of relative insensitivity to prostaglandins has been reported (Toppozada et al 1975,1977; Martin et al. 1978) while intake of combined oral contraceptives results in a significant reduction in the uterine response to prostaglandins at all phases of the cycle (Toppozada et al. 1976; Shaala et al. 1977). The two main exceptions in the quality of uterine response are related to a definite inhibition observed following local intrauterine instillation of PGE_2 around ovulation time (Figure 3) and during active menstrual bleeding (Toppozada et al. 1975, 1977; Martin et al. 1978).

The effect of the E and F types on tubal contractility was studied in vitro more than ten years ago; there were qualitative differences in response depending on the compound used and site of the tube tested. The E type induced contraction of the proximal quarter and relaxed strips from the distal three-quarters while the F compounds had a consistent stimulatory effect (Sandberg et al. 1965). In-vivo studies in the subhuman primate illustrated a certain degree of dependence upon endogenous steroid hormones since oviductal motility was relatively insensitive to prostaglandins in the proliferative phase of the cycle. After ovulation, PGE_1 or PGE_2 infusions depressed spontaneous tubal activity while $PGF_{2\alpha}$ induced a marked increase in oviduct motility (Spilman et al. 1973).

In the human, the effect of the classical prostaglandins on the fallopian tubes was evaluated by recording luminal pressure using an indwelling catheter. Intravenous injections or intratubal instillation of PGE_2 had an evident inhibitory effect upon tubal contractility while $PGF_{2\alpha}$ consistently increased resting tone and frequency of tubal contractions (Coutinho and Maia 1971). These in-vivo experiments showed that $PGF_{2\alpha}$ increased intraovarian pressure while PGE_2 had little effect in this respect. The reason for this ovarian pressure elevation, whether it is due to some muscular responses or vascular alterations, is so far unsettled.

I.B.4. Biochemical considerations

The different prostaglandins possess diverse biochemical actions and are capable of inducing chemical alterations in various tissues. These biologically potent compounds either stimulate or inhibit the formation of other humoral agents or modify the tissue response to known stimuli. The mode of action of prostaglandins in this respect varies to a considerable degree from one situation to another.

The interaction of prostaglandins with catecholamines, pituitary-ovarian hormones and many other humoral agents has well been documented. The effect on adenylate cyclase and other enzyme systems as well as the conspicuous effects on cAMP and GMP indicate a possible role for prostaglandins in the control of intracellular functions. Also, it has been shown that some prostaglandins can alter

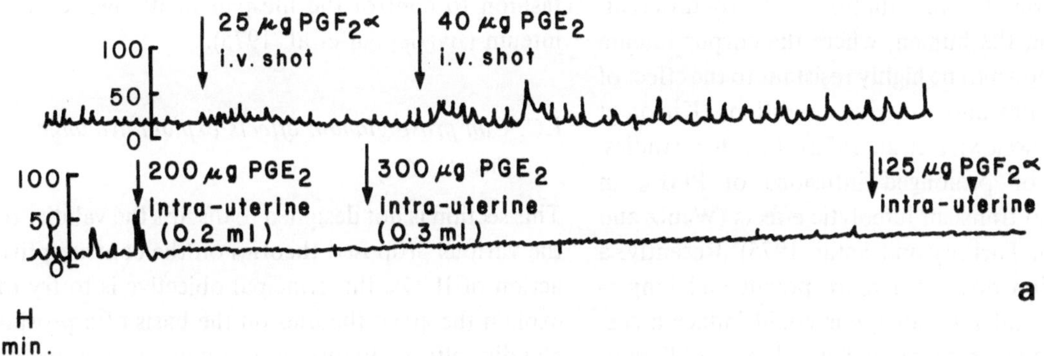

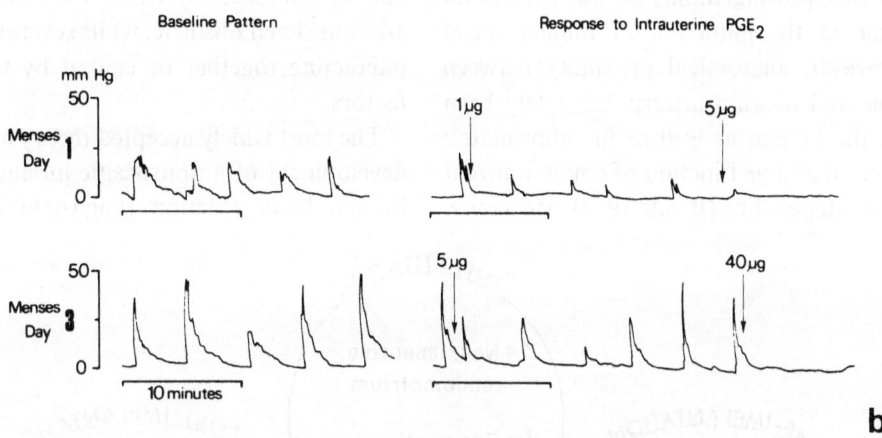

Figure 3. Inhibition of nonpregnant uterine activity by local instillation of PGE_2. a: at a midcycle (from Toppozada et al. 1975). b: at menstruation (from Martin et al. 1978).

cellular nucleic acid and protein synthesis. Moreover, some prostaglandin types were reported to modify the function of membranes by displacing membrane-bound calcium.

I.B.5. Endocrine changes

There is ample evidence in support of the theory that $PGF_{2\alpha}$ is probably the factor which controls the lifespan of the corpus luteum in subprimate animal species. The source of this luteolytic substance is believed to be the adjacent uterine horn which releases the prostaglandin into the uterine vein in response to estrogens, uterine distension and presence of foreign bodies. A countercurrent mechanism has been suggested to explain the mode of transfer of prostaglandin from the uterine vein to the closely related ovarian artery (McCracken 1971).

In the primate, the situation is clearly different, especially in the human, where the corpus luteum has been shown to be highly resistant to the effect of prostaglandins under in-vivo conditions (Kirton et al. 1970; Jewelewicz et al. 1972). In a few studies, high-dose or prolonged infusions of $PGF_{2\alpha}$ in humans had transient luteolytic effects (Wentz and Jones 1973; Turksoy and Safaii 1975). Recently, a high infusion dose of a more potent and longer-acting prostaglandin analogue could induce a sustained luteolytic response in few volunteers (Toppozada et al. 1978). Based upon these data, and the lack of an apparent route for transfer of uterine prostaglandins to ovarian tissue in the human, it was argued that prostaglandins do not possess an essential role in the induction of human luteal demise. However, anatomical proximity between uterine veins and ovarian arteries has lately been reported in the human as well as in subprimates; this may serve the same function of countercurrent transfer of prostaglandins (Bendz 1977). Moreover, it has been suggested that prostaglandins locally produced by the ovary may function in a feedback fashion to control the lifespan of its own corpus luteum (Bygdeman et al. 1975).

I.C. Can prostaglandin effects explain available theories ?

This section is not designed to discuss the validity of the various proposed theories on the contraceptive action of IUDs; the principal objective is to try to explain the given theories on the basis of a prostaglandin effect. Figure 4 summarizes the major theories suggested over the past two decades. It also shows if any of these mechanisms can be mediated by a prostaglandin action or the observed inflammatory cell reaction. Many of the included theories are considered obsolete, while several others may be interacting together or caused by the same basic factors.

The most widely accepted theory at present is the development of a nonspecific inflammatory cell or foreign body reaction (Sagiroglu and Sagiroglu

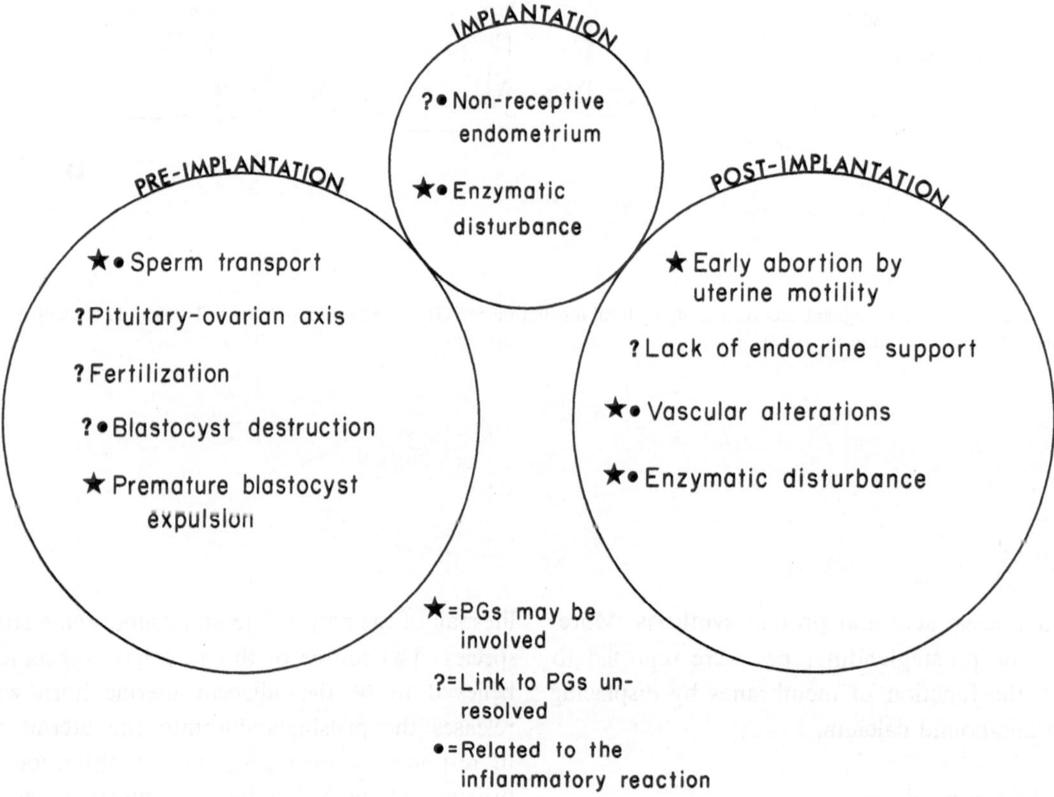

Figure 4. Proposed theories for the mechanism of action of IUDs. Possible involvement of prostaglandins or of the inflammatory cell reaction are indicated.

1970; El Sahwi and Moyer 1971; Moyer and Mishell 1971; Gawad et al 1977). Both prostaglandins and the inflammatory response are capable, each on their own, of producing biological effects of contraceptive significance. What makes the situation even more complex and perplexing is the fact that either prostaglandins or the migrating leukocytes can be the primary mediators, since prostaglandins are chemotactic inducing migration of white blood cells, and the leukocytes on IUDs can release prostaglandins (Kaley and Weiner 1972; Myatt et al. 1975, 1977). Thus a vicious circle is established, but which of these constitutes the initial stimulus remains so far unresolved. The different prostaglandins that may contribute to the mechanism of action of IUDs and their modes of achieving this goal are illustrated in Figure 5.

I.D. Does prostaglandin inhibition interfere with the efficacy of IUDs ?

The question whether prostaglandin inhibition interferes with the efficacy of IUDs is difficult to answer at present. If administration of prostaglandin antagonists or inhibitors of their biosynthesis results in an increased failure rate (pregnancies) in users of IUDs then this would constitute substantial evidence in favour of an obligatory role for prostaglandins in the mechanism of action of IUDs. Such an experimental approach is only feasible in animal studies. In fact only two investigations in subprimates have tackled this problem, with contradictory conclusions. The first study was conducted in rabbits and showed that the anti-implantation effect of an IUD could be reversed by an inhibitor of prostaglandin (Saksena and Harper 1974). Such an experiment is a very delicate one requiring precise timing and dosage to avoid the antifertility effects of the anti-prostaglandin (Indomethacin) itself.

The second study used rats as the experimental animal and polyphloretin phosphate as the prostaglandin antagonist (Chaudhury et al. 1977). The latter compound has a different mechanism of prostaglandin inhibition; it acts as a mild competitive antagonist to prostaglandins at the receptor site. This drug could not prevent the antifertility effect of the intrauterine foreign body, leading the

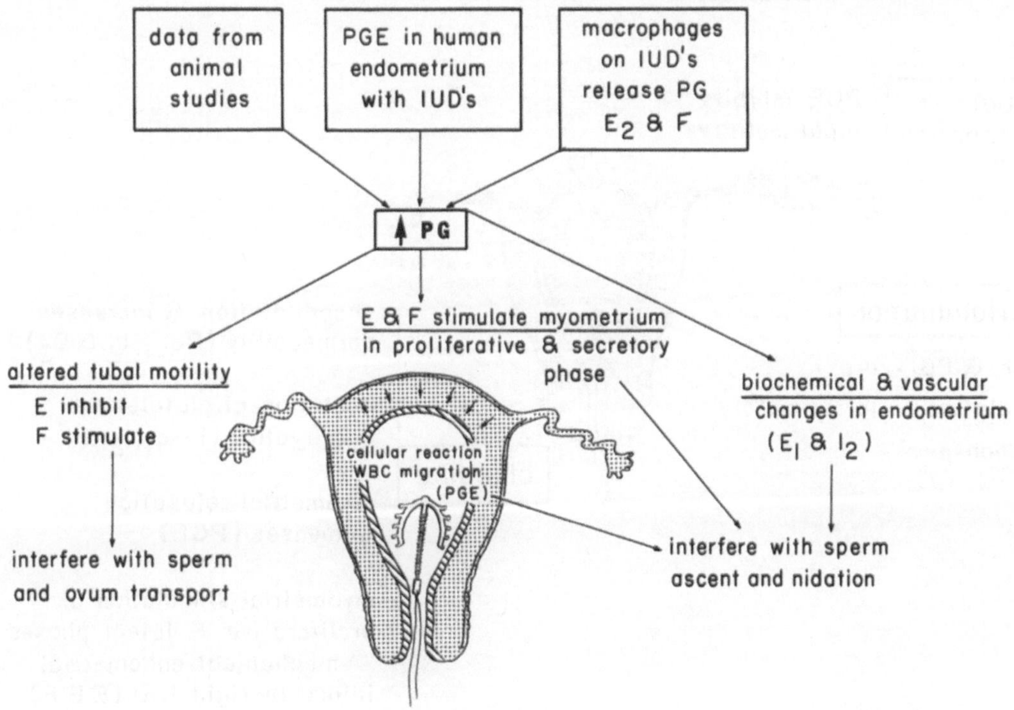

Figure 5. The role of prostaglandins in the mechanism of action of IUDs. The compound most probably involved is indicated in relation to the different mechanisms.

authors to conclude that IUDs do not act by releasing prostaglandins. It appears therefore that this issue still remains unsettled and further investigations, especially in subhuman primates, are required before a final judgement of the role of prostaglandins can be established.

II. SIDE-EFFECTS

II.A. Bleeding

Irregular, unpredictable and excessive uterine bleeding (Figure 6) is the most annoying side-effect of IUD use and is the most prevalent reason for requests for removals (discontinuation). The vascular properties of certain prostaglandins make these substances fit as possible mediators to the abnormal blood loss with IUDs. This is particularly true with respect to PGE_1, PGD_2 and PGI_2 (prostacycline), which inhibit platelet aggregation and induce uterine vasodilatation. These members can thus be termed the prohemorrhagic prostaglandins in contradistinction to the antihemorrhagic derivatives such as PGB_2, $PGF_{2\alpha}$, PGG_2, PGH_2 and the thromboxanes.

Besides vascular factors, muscular (myometrial) responses can also operate to produce or exaggerate IUD-induced uterine bleeding. The inhibition of uterine activity has been observed only during menses in response to lacal instillation of PGE_2 (Martin et al. 1978) may contribute to an increased menstrual blood loss. Moreover, myometrial stimulation by PGF compounds at any phase or PGE types at the proliferative and luteal phases of the cycle may cause endometrial injury as a result of mechanical irritation against the rigid IUD.

It should be emphasized here that our knowledge regarding the above factors is quite deficient and a great deal still needs to be done in this area

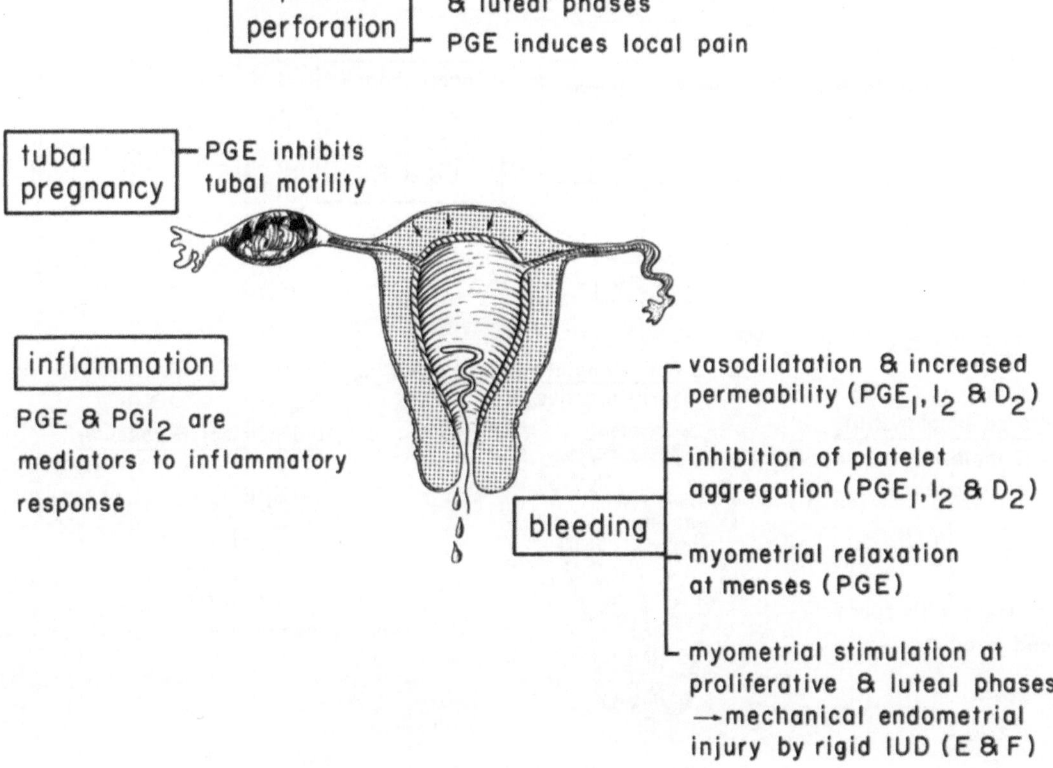

Figure 6. The role of prostaglandins in the side effects of IUDs. The most likely compound involved in each side effect is indicated.

before a definite link can be established and a proper therapeutic approach can be designed. For instance, there is lack of evidence to show that women with abnormal bleeding due to IUDs have abnormal production rates of prostaglandins. No one has so far attempted to measure prostaglandin concentrations in excessive bleeders to compare them with those IUD users with normal menstrual blood loss. In this context, prostaglandins of the E type appear to be more eligible as mediators than the F variety due to their vasodilator property and effect on platelets. The role of prostacycline and thromboxanes may well be prominent in this respect but this is only speculative. Also, the myometrial response to prostacycline, PGD_2, and the endoperoxides and thromboxanes has not yet been investigated in humans.

The effect of local copper or progesterone (in medicated IUDs) in reducing blood loss may , at least in part, be mediated through their influence on prostaglandin synthetase activity. The copper ion has been shown to modify the enzymatic conversion of arachidonic acid in a specific way towards a stimulated F and inhibited E production (Maddox 1973). Also progesterone was reported to inhibit $PGF_{2\alpha}$ release from the endometrium in tissue culture but the effect on PGE_2 has not been evaluated (Cane and Villee 1975).

The first striking evidence to support the hypothesis of prostaglandin involvement in abnormal bleeding due to IUDs appeared in January 1976 when prostaglandin synthesis inhibitors were successfully used to control this type of bleeding (Damarawy and Toppozada 1976). The authors based their approach on the theoretical assumption that excessive PGE production may be an active factor in this respect (Table 1). Soon after this initial publication, an increased endometrial PGE production in response to IUDs, but not specifically in bleeders, was reported (Hillier and Kasonde 1976). Also, other clinical reports soon confirmed the fact that nonsteroidal anti-inflammatory drugs (NSAID), probably through prostaglandin synthetase inhibition, could check excessive bleeding due to IUDs or in cases of dysfunctional uterine bleeding (Anderson et al. 1976; Guillebaud et al. 1978). The latter studies were more precise as they relied on objective measurement of menstrual blood loss while the original investigation was principally a subjective evaluation (Figure 7).

The administration of NSAID in IUD users induced a highly significant reduction in mean total blood loss regardless of whether the therapy started before or coincided with the first day of menses (Guillebaud et al. 1978). The effect on the duration of bleeding appeared to be less conspicuous than on the amount of blood loss. Also, the clinical value of these agents on intermenstrual spotting could not be demonstrated. Those data, along with the original study of Damarawy and Toppozada (1976), established the basis for future research aiming at improvement of the clinical performance of IUDs.

The best agent to use, with minimal side effects and optimum schedule of administration, remains unsettled. However, chronic local release or systemic therapy of NSAID throughout the cycle as a control measure of excessive blood loss in IUD users suffers fom three possible major hazards. These are interference with the contraceptive action of IUDs, teratogenic potential if a pregnancy oc-

Table 1. Result of Indomethacin treatment as compared with placebo in patients with IUDs.

Treatment groups	*Total. no.*	*Satisfactory outcome*	*Failure*	*Percentage success*
Indomethacin group:				
1. Menorrhagia	30[a]	27	2	90
2. Prophylactic against menorrhagia	20	19	1	95
Placebo group (control)	25	6	19[b]	24

[a] One case was lost in the follow-up.

[b] Bleeding on ten of these cases was later controlled by Indomethacin. The other nine cases did not receive Indomethacin and continued to bleed for 7-10 days.

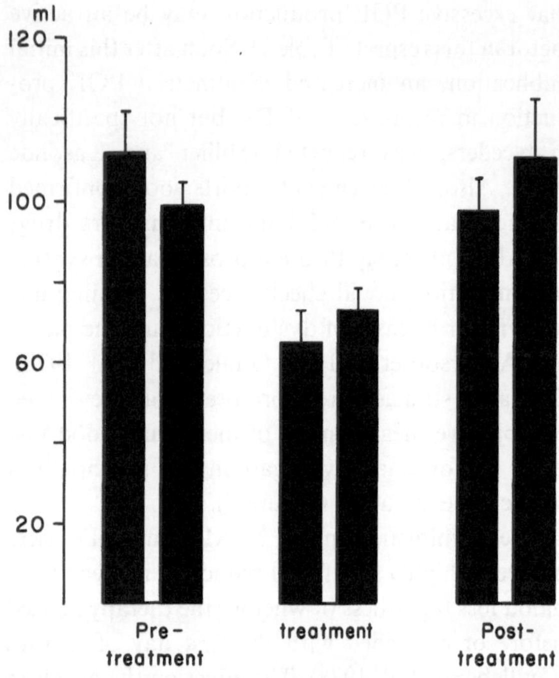

Figure 7. Effect of treatment with mefenamic acid for two cycles on mean total menstrual blood loss in 15 women with IUDs and heavy menstrual blood loss (80 ml or more) as compared to pre-treatment and post-treatment cycles (from Guillebaud et al. 1978).

curs, and the side effects that may occur as a result of prolonged administration of these potent agents. Therefore, the suggested approach for control by NSAID of excessive menstrual blood loss in women with IUDs should be restricted to an intermittent intake starting with the onset of bleeding.

The mechanism of NSAID in reducing excessive blood loss in women with IUDs is not fully understood. It was presumed that these agents act by interfering with prostaglandin synthetase activity but the exact pathway inhibited is not known since our knowledge in this area is still in the stage of infancy. However it has been shown that NSAID inhibited PGE_2 and $PGF_{2\alpha}$ which may serve as a possible mechanism (Maddox 1973).

II.B. Pain and missed loop

Pelvic pain (Figure 6) is one of the common reasons for discontinuation of use of IUDs. The pain may be uterine or extrauterine, continuous or menses-related and colicky or dull-aching in nature. Two major factors contribute to IUD-associated pain; these are abnormal or excessive uterine contractility and pelvic inflammatory disease.

Abnormal or modified uterine activity is known to occur following insertion of IUDs (Bengtsson and Moawad 1976). Most of the earlier studies were directed toward an evaluation of whether altered motility is involved in the mechanism of action of IUDs. Recently, however, a correlation between the IUD-induced dysmenorrheic pain, increased uterine activity and prostaglandin concentrations appeared as a logical assumption in view of the potent spasmogenic properties of these compounds and their probable crucial role as mediators in primary dysmenorrhea (Pickles et al. 1965; Halbert et al. 1975; Lundstrom et al. 1976). Prostaglandin synthetase inhibitors have been shown to reduce the plasma concentrations of $PGF_{2\alpha}$ and its 15-keto, 13,14-dihydro metabolite significantly in dysmenorrheic subjects and were also reported to induce dramatic pain relief in severe cases (Lundstrom et al. 1976). Also, administration fo relatively low doses of prostaglandins, either systemically or locally is known to cause appreciable uterine cramps like those of primary or IUD-induced dysmenorrhea (Lundstrom et al. 1976). In view of the above considerations, prostaglandin synthetase inhibitors are currently being evaluated by the WHO for their effect on pain and uterine contractions (Rowe 1977). In rats, intra-uterine foreign bodies stimulated uterine contractility which could be inhibited by prostaglandin biosynthesis inhibitors (Chaudhury 1975). In humans with IUDs there are several aspects which still require confirmation, such as an increased uterine activity and prostaglandin production in IUD users complaining of pain. Also, if suppressed contractility and decreased prostaglandin release concomitant with pain relief induced by prostaglandin sunthesis inhibitors can be demonstrated in such cases, it would constitute substantial evidence in support of a role for prostaglandins in IUD-induced pain (Figure 8).

Missed loop includes spontaneous expulsions, uterine perforations and malpositioning or elevation of the IUD inside the uiterine cavity (Figure 6). It appears logical to believe that abnormal or excessive uterine activity may be crucial predisposing factors in the establishment of these conditions.

These functional myometrial disturbances may

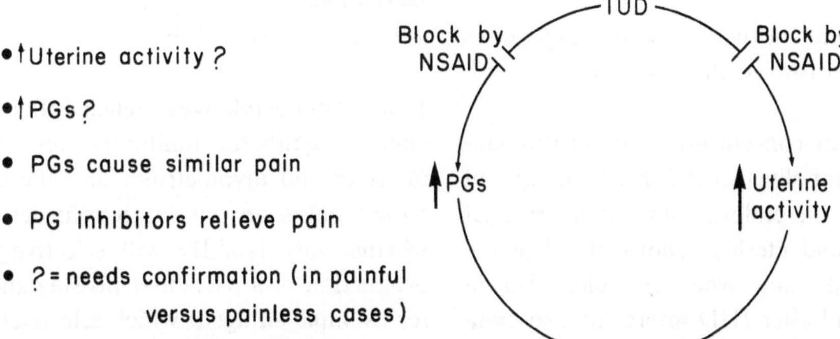

Figure 8. Evidence for the role of prostaglandins mediators in IUD-induced pain, also valid for primary dysmenorrhea.

be induced by excessive or abnormal release rates of different prostaglandin compounds. Moreover, abnormal relaxation of the cervix should also be considered in connection with IUD expulsions particularly if prostaglandins of the E type possess an inhibitory influence on the nonpregnant isthmus as they do on the pregnant myometrium (Embrey and Morrison 1968).

II.C. Pelvic inflammation

It is becoming gradually recognized that pelvic inflammatory disease is one of the complications of IUDs and comes as the third major cause after pain and bleeding in the list of reasons for removals. It is not known whether this inflammation is a primary IUD complication or only represents an IUD induced flare-up of previously existing dormant infection. In the former situation prostaglandins can serve as valid mediators. It is established that this group of lipids have potent inflammatory effects; they are released in the inflammatory exudate and can attract inflammatory cells; NSAIDs act by inhibiting prostaglandin production (Vane 1976). It is also probably true that excess prostaglandin of the E type may be involved in exacerbation of a pre-existing chronic pelvic inflammatory disease in view of their causing pelvic congestion (vasodilatation) and stimulating uterine activity.

II.D. Pregnancy; intrauterine or extrauterine

If prostaglandins possess an essential role in the mechanism of action of IUDs then a deficient release would be the cause of accidental unwanted pregnancies. This assumption may be true both for intrauterine and extrauterine pregnancies. However there is some evidence showing that there is an increased risk of ectopic pregnancy among IUD users. This has been explained on the basis that IUDs afford a much higher rate of protection against intra-uterine relative to extrauterine implantation. In this context, PGE compounds, which are released in excess by IUDs, are known to inhibit tubal motility and may thus contribute to the occurrence of ectopic gestation (Coutinho and Maia 1971).

III. FUTURE DEVELOPMENTS

The role of prostaglandins and thromboxanes in the mechanism of action of IUDs and their side effects is still not definitely established. However, available data suggest prostaglandin involvement in these mechanisms. Confirmation of such assumptions and further in-depth analysis of the delicate and complex intermediary steps would permit active measures to correct aberrations thus improving efficacy rates and reducing side-effects and complications.

III.A. Basic studies on the role of prostaglandins and thromboxanes

Future development on the role of prostaglandins should be directed toward the following:

1. Measurement of concentrations of prostaglandins and their metabolites, of endoperoxides and of thromboxanes in the endometrium, in uterine jet wash specimens and uterine venous blood in the subhuman primate and when feasible, also in women before and after IUD insertion; also comparison of the analytical data of users having side effects with those of asymptomatic users, e.g. excessive bleeders versus normal bleeders.

2. Studies on the effect of prostaglandins endoperoxides and thromboxanes on endometrial, myometrial and uterine vascular tissues. There is need to study the binding capacity of these compounds to the above uterine components and the humoral factors controlling the binding. Also, histological, cytological and histochemical changes induced by local instillation of the various compounds should be investigated to find out whether such administration can reproduce the observed changes with IUds (heavy bleeders and normal bleeders). It is also of interest to evaluate the effect of various prostaglandins and thromboxanes on endometrial blood flow concomitant with a recording of uterine activity. Since prostacycline (PGI_2) is a potent inhibitor of platelet aggregation, a powerful pro-inflammatory substance and an efficient dilator of microcirculation, its role in the inflammatory reaction and excessive bleeding induced by IUDs should be carefully evaluated.

3. Studies on the prostaglandin synthetase enzyme activity of the endometrium at the different phases of the menstrual cycle prior to and in the presence of IUDs: these would help to achieve a better understanding of the various pathways of prostaglandin production and their controlling factors. The enzyme activity is different in different tissues. and is subject to modification by humoral factors. What governs the pathway of arachidonic acid into a specific direction to form a certain prostaglandin or thromboxane is presently unknown.

III.B. Effect of prostaglandin synthesis inhibitors

Development with regard to the effect of prostaglandin synthesis inhibitors should include:

1. Study of the relative potencies of different prostaglandin synthesis inhibitors on human endometrium and myometrium and the effect of hormonal status on this inhibition; determination of whether any NSAID will selectively inhibit the production of a particular prostaglandin pathway, for example an agent which selectively inhibits the synthesis of PGE_1, PGD_2, and PGI_2 (all inhibitors of platelet aggregation and vasodilators) would be very useful to control excessive blood loss. Also, the effect of different NSAIDs on the prostaglandin binding capacity of endometrium should be investigated.

2. Histological, electronmicroscopic and histochemical effects of locally administered prostaglandin synthesis inhibitors on the endometrium in normal and abnormal menstrual blood loss.

3. Based upon the theory that prostaglandins mediate the contraceptive action of IUDs, there is a need to explore whether long-term local or systemic administration of prostaglandin synthetase inhibitors would interfere with the efficacy of IUDs. Subhuman primate studies are the most suitable for this purpose. Also, the question of teratogenic influence that may result from such treatment needs to be answered; this is of significance in cases of IUD failures.

4. Comparative clinical evaluation of different prostaglandin synthesis inhibitors for the control of blood loss in IUD users in order to select the most effective agent with least side effects and also to determine the most suitable route of drug delivery: for the present time, one is only permitted to use these drugs on an intermittent basis at menstruation until the issue of possible failures and teratogenicity are resolved.

5. If chronic local release of NSAID is considered

safe, then in-vitro and in-vivo studies should be conducted to find out the best type of delivery system, duration of action and release rate. Also, acute and chronic local and systemic toxicity evaluation should be an essential prerequisite.

REFERENCES

Akerlund M, Andersson KE: Vasopressin response and terbutalin inhibition of the human uterus. Obstet Gynecol 48: 528, 1976.

Anderson ABM, Haynes PJ, Guillebaud J. Turnbull AC.Reduction of menstrual blood loss by prostaglandin synthetase inhibitors. Lancet 1: 774, 1976.

Bendz A: The anatomical basis for a possible counter-current exchange mechanism in the human adnexa. Prostaglandins 13: 355, 1977.

Bengtsson L.P Moawad AH The effect of the Lippes loop on human myometrial activity. Am J Obstet Gynecol 98: 957, 1967.

Bourne HR, Melmon KL Adenyl cyclase in human leucocytes: evidence for activation by separate beta-adrenergic and prostaglandin receptors. J. Pharmacol Exp Ther 178: 1–7, 1971.

Brody MJ Kadowitz PJ: Prostaglandins as modulators of the autonomic nervous system. Fed Proc 33:46, 1974.

Bygdeman M, Toppozada M, Wiqvist N. The prostaglandins. In: Progress in infertility, Behrman SJ, Kistner RW (eds), Boston, Little, Brown, 1975, pp 963-983

Cane EM Villee CA. The synthesis of prostaglandin-F by human endometrium in organ culture. Prostaglandins 9: 281, 1975.

ChaudburyG. Intra-uterine device: possible role of prostaglandins. Lancet 1: 48, 1971.

Chaudbury G. Release of prostaglandins by the IUCD. Prostaglandins 3: 773-784, 1973.

Chaudbury G. Influence of indomethacin, an inhibitor of prostaglandin synthesis, on IUD mediated increase in motility and hypertrophy of the rat uterine horn. In : Analysis of intrauterine contraception, Hefnawi F, Segal S (eds), New York, American Elsevier, 1976, p 471 ff.

Chaudhury MR, Mathur VS, Chaudhury RR, Isrankun P: Study to elucidate the mechanism of action of intrauterine device in rat:(abstract). Asian Cong Obstet Gynecol 1: 264, 1977.

Clark KE, Ryan MJ, Brody MJ: Effect of prostaglandins on vascular resistance and adrenergic vasoconstrictor responses in the canine uterus. Prostaglandins 12: 71, 1978.

Coutinho EM, Maia HS: The contractile response of the human uterus, Fallopian tubes, and ovary prostaglandins in vivo. Fertil Steril 22: 539-543, 1971.

Crunkhorn P, Willis AL: Actions and interactions of prostaglandins administrations intradermally in rat and in man. Br J Pharmacol 36: 216, 1969.

Crunkhorn P, Willis AL: Interaction between prostaglandin-E and F given intradermally in the rat. Br J Pharmacol 41: 507-512, 1971.

Damarawy H, Toppozada M: Control of bleeding due to IUDs by a prostaglandin biosynthesis inhibitor. IRCS med Science 4: 5, 1976.

Duboff GS, Penner JA, Rohwedder J: Effect of prostaglandins E_1 and E_2 and $F_{2\alpha}$ on human blood coagulation. Nature 251: 430-434, 1974.

Einer-Jensen N: Decreased endometrial blood flow and plasma progesterone level after instillation of 19 mg $PGF_{6\alpha}$ into the lumen of the uteri of Rhesus monkey. Prostaglandins 4: 517-522 1973.

ElSahwi S, Moyer DL: The leucocytic response to an intrauterine foreign body in the rabbit. Fertil Steril 22: 298, 1971.

Embrey MP, Morrison DL: The effect of prostaglandins on human pregnant myometrium in vitro. J. Obst Gyn Br Cwlth 75: 829, 1968.

Gawad AA, Toppozada HK, ElSawi M, Saleh F, ElSahwi S: Study of the uterine environment in association with intrauterine contraceptive devices. Contraception 16: 469-485, 1977.

Gimbrone MA, Alexander RW: Angiotensin II; stimulation of prostaglandin production in cultured human vascular endothelium. Science 189: 219-220, 1975.

Green K, Hagenfeldt K: Prostaglandins in the human endometrium: gas-chromatographic/massspectrometric quantitation before and after IUD insertion. Am J Obstet Gynec 122: 611-613,1975.

Greenberg S, Wilson WK, Howard L: Mechanism of the vasoconstrictor action of prostaglandin. B. J Pharmacol Exp Ther 190: 59-69, 1974.

Guillebaud J, Anderson ABM, Turnbull AC: Reduction by mefenamic acid of increased menstrual blood associated with intra-uterine contraception. Br J Obstet Gynaecol 85: 53, 1978.

Gustavii B: Labour: a delayed menstruation. Lancet 1: 1149-1150, 1972.

Halbert DR, Demers LM, Fontana J, Jones DED: Prostaglandin levels in endometrial jet wash specimens in patients with dysmenorrhea before and after indomethacin therapy. Prostaglandins 10: 1047, 1975.

Hillier K, Kasonde JM: Prostaglandin E and F concentrations in human endometrium after insertion of intra-uterine contraceptive device. Lancet 1: 15-16, 1976.

Howie PW, Calder AA, Forbes CD, Prentice CRM: Effects of intravenous prostaglandin-E_2 on platelet function, coagulation and fibrinolysis. J Clin Pathol 26: 354-358, 1973.

Jewelewicz R, Cantor B, Dyrenfurth, Warren MP, Van der Wiele R: Intravenous infusion of prostaglandin-$F_{2\alpha}$ in the mid-luteal phase of the normal human menstrual cycle. Prostaglandins 1: 443-1972.

Kadowitz PJ: Effects of prostaglandins E_1 and E_2 and A_2 on vascular resistance and responses to noradrenaline nerve stimulation and angiotensin in the dog hind limb. Br J Pharmacol 46: 395-400, 1972.

Kalley C, Weiner R: Effect of prostaglandin-E_1 on leucocyte migration. Nature (New Biol) 234: 114-115, 1972.

Kirton KT, Pharris BB, Forbes AD: Luteolytic effects of prostaglandin $F_{2\alpha}$ in primates. Proc Soc Exp Biol Med 133: 314, 1970.

Kloeze J: Influence of prostaglandins on platelet adhesiveness and platelet aggregation. In : Prostaglandins: proceedings of Nobel symposium II, Bergstrom S, Samuelsson B (eds), Stockholm, Almquist & Wiksell, 1967 p 241ff.

Lundstrom V, Green K, Wiqvist N: Prostaglandins, indomethacin and dysmenorrhea. Prostaglandins 11: 893, 1976.

McCracken J: Prostaglandins and corpus luteum regression.

Ann NY Acad Sci 180: 456, 1971.

Maddox IS: The role of copper in prostaglandin synthesis. Biochim Biophys Acta 306: 74-81, 1973.

Martin JN Jr, Bygdeman M, Eneroth P: The influence of locally administered prostaglandin E_2 and $F_{2\alpha}$ on uterine motility in the intact non-pregnant human uterus. Acta Obstet Gynecol Scand 57: 141-147, 1978.

Moncada S, Vane JR: In: Biochemical aspects of prostaglandins and thromboxanes (Kharasch N, Fried J, (eds), Academic Press, 1971 p 155 ff.

Moyer DL, Mishell DR Jr: Reactions of human endometrium to the intrauterine foreign body. Am J Obstet Gynecol 111: 66-80, 1971.

Myatt L, Bray MA, Gordon D, and Morley J: Macrophages on intrauterine contraceptive devices produce prostaglandins. Nature 257: 227-228, 1975.

Myatt L, Chaudhury G, Gordon D, Elder M: Prostaglandin production by leucocytes attached to intrauterine devices. Contraception 15: 589, 1977.

Pickles VR, Hall WJ, Best FA, Smith GN: Prostaglandin in endometrium and menstrual fluid from normal and dysmenorrhoeic subjects. J Obst Gyn Br Cwlth 72: 185-192, 1965.

Poyser NL, Horton EW, Thompson CL, Los M: Identification of $PGE_{2\alpha}$ released by distention of guinea-pig uterus in vitro. Nature (London) 230: 526-529, 1971.

Roberts JS, McCracken JA, Gavagan JE, Soloff MS: Oxytocin-stimulated release of prostaglandin-$F_{2\alpha}$ from ovine endometrium in vitro: correlation with estrus cycle and oxytocin receptor binding. Endocrinology 99; 1107-1114, 1976.

Rowe P: Medicated intrauterine devices : review. In : WHO symposium on advances in fertiliy regulation, Diczfalusy E (ed), Moscow, 1976, p 381 ff.

Sagiroglu N, Sagiroglu E: Biologic mode of action of the Lippes Loop in intra-uterine contraception. Am J Obstet Gynecol 106: 506-515, 1970.

Saksena SK, Harper MJI: Prostaglandin-mediated action of intrauterine devices I: F-prostaglandins in the uterine horns of pregnant rabbits with unilateral intrauterine devices. Fertil Steril 25: 121-126, 1974.

Saksena SK, Lau LF, Casttracane V: Prostaglandin-mediated action of IUDs (II): F-prostaglandins (PGF) in the uterine horn of pregnant rats and hamsters with intrauterine devices. Prostaglandins 5: 97-106, 1974.

Sandberg F, Ingelman Sundberg A, Ryden G: The effect of prostaglandin $F_{1\alpha}$, $f_{2\alpha}$, $f_{2\beta}$ on the human uterus and fallopian tubes in vitro. Acta Obstet Gynecol Scand 44: 585-594, 1965.

Shaala S, Khowessah M, El-Damarawy H, ElSahwi S, Osman M, Toppozada M: Reduced uterine response to $PGF_{2\alpha}$ under oral contraceptives. Prostaglandins 14: 523-533, 1977.

Shio H, Ramwell P: Effect of prostaglandin-E_2 and aspirin on the secondary aggregation of human platelets. Nature New Biol 236: 45-46, 1972.

Spilman CH, Duby RT: Prostaglandin-mediated luteolytic effect of intra-uterine device in sheep. Prostaglandins 2: 159-168, 1972.

Spilman CH, Forbes AD, Norland JF: Oviduct motility during the Rhesus monkey menstrual cycle: effect of prostaglandins, Biol. Reprod 9: 68, 1973.

Toppozada M, Gaafar A, Shaala S, Osman M: The relaxant property of local prostaglandin-E_2 on the non-pregnant uterus, a cyclic triphase response. Prostaglandins 9: 475, 1975.

Toppozada M, Khowessah M, Shaala S, Said S, Osman M: Uterine response to prostaglandins-E_2 under oral contraceptives. Contraception. 13: 749-761, 1976.

Toppozada M, Khowessah M, Shaala S, Osman M, Rahman HA: Aberrant uterine response to prostaglandin E_{-2} as possible etiologic factor in functional infertility. Fertil Steril 28: 434-439, 1977.

Toppozada M, Khabil T, El-Sokkary H: Role of prostaglandins in the control of human pituitary ovarian function. Asia Oceania Congr. Endocrinol 6(1): 143-151,1978.

Turksoy RN, Safaii MS: Immediate effect of prostaglandin-$F_{2\alpha}$ during the luteal phase of the menstrual cycle. Fertil Steril 26: 634-637, 1975.

Vane JR: Prostaglandins and the aspirin-like drugs. Hosp Pract 7: 61-71, 1972.

Vane JR: Prostaglandins as mediators of inflammation. In: Advances in prostaglandin and thromboxane research II. Samuelsson B, Paoletti R (eds), New York, Raven, 1976, p 791-801.

Wentz A, Jones GS: Transient luteolytic effect of prostaglandin-$F_{2\alpha}$ in the human. Obstet Gynecol 42: 172, 1973.

Willoughby DA, Geroud JP, Di Rosa M, Velo GP: The control of the inflammatory response with special reference to the Prostaglandins. In: Prostaglandins and cyclic AMP, Kahm RH, Lands WEM (eds), New York, Academic Press, 1973, p 187-206.

Zurier RB, Weisman G: Inhibition by prostaglandin-E_1 of lysosomal enzyme discharge from human polymorphs. Arthritis Rheum 14: 191-192, 1971.

9. PITUITARY-OVARIAN FUNCTION IN IUD USERS

M.I. Abdalla, I.I. Ibrahim, M.I. Osman and M.A. Bayad

It is notable that remarkable progress in the technology of intrauterine contraception has taken place in the last fifteen years. Research activities in this direction were stimulated by reports that linked the administration of contraceptive steroids with a higher incidence of systemic complications in women users. It was estimated in 1974 that more than fifteen million women around the world were using the IUD (Speidel and Ravenholt 1974). This number is on the increase every year, paralleled with further achievements in studies performed to minimize the complications and side effects of appliances used for intrauterine contraception.

The pain and bleeding frequently associated with the use of intrauterine appliances are the most common reasons for their removal. Both complications can be correlated in one way or another with changes in the pituitary-ovarian function. Distension of the uterine horns in experimental animals by beads or other foreign bodies was shown to induce premature regression of the corpus luteum (Bland and Donovan 1966). Pain, as a stressful event, was shown to cause insufficient function of the corpus luteum and a short luteal phase of the menstrual cycle in some women (Johansson et al. 1971). Various etiological factors have been suggested to explain the mechanisms of abnormal bleeding with IUDs, among them are inflammatory (Willson et al. 1964), mechanical (Davis and Israel 1964; Kamal et al. 1971) and endocrine factors (Lippes 1962; Vorys et al. 1964; Johansson and Nygren 1975).

Furthermore, the mechanism of contraceptive action of the intrauterine device is still poorly understood. Although local endometrial changes are believed to be the main mode of contraceptive efficacy, some investigators have pointed to the possibility of associated ovarian or pituitary change (Ancla and Brux 1969; Faucher et al. 1969; Cuadros and Tovar 1972). In this respect most of the studies were conducted on experimental animals; the few studies in humans involved only a small number of patients and cycles. The results were characterized by marked species variations in animals as well as a difference in response between animals and humans.

I. ANIMAL STUDIES

Although the contraceptive end result of IUDs in animals is uniform in all species, the associated endocrine response varies according to species studied. The reported data, as far as the pituitary-ovarian function is concerned, focusses on one of three modes of reaction as a result of the presence of the intrauterine appliance.

I.A. Impairment of corpus luteum function

The IUD can impair the luteal function in rabbits, guinea pigs, cattle, sheep and pigs. An earlier regression of the corpus luteum was observed in the sheep with the intrauterine appliance placed in the horn adjacent to the ovary containing the corpus luteum than when it was placed in the opposite horn (Ginther et al. 1966). Premature menstrual bleeding was demonstrated in baboons fitted with Margulies Spirals, subsequent to shortening of the interval between the midcycle estradiol peak and the onset of menses (Breed et al. 1972). Shorter estrous cycles were also observed in cows (Yamauchi and Nakahara 1958), goats (Gadgil et al. 1968) and water buffalo heifers (Janakiraman et al. 1970). These animals appear to be dependent on a release of prostaglandins from the uterus to interfere with the lifespan of the corpus luteum. In support of this concept is the demonstration of higher concentrations of prostaglandins in the uteri of mice wearing IUDs (Lau et al. 1974).

In contrast with the above observations, no change in cycle length was demonstrated in other species, for example in Kan Krej cows and Surti buffalo (Buch and Shukla 1966) and in pigs (Ferrits and Hawk 1966).

I.B. Interference with ovulation

There is evidence of delayed ovulation in rabbits fitted with IUDs, subsequent to late or diminished release of luteinizing hormone (Janakiraman and Casida 1968). Partial failure of ovulation in Holstein heifers was reported by Hawk et al. (1964), while complete blockage of ovulation in Surti buffalo heifers in the presence of IUDs was demonstrated by Buch et al. (1964).

I.C. Interference with pituitary gonadotropic activity

Studies reflecting the integrity of the pituitary gonadotropin secretion in animals fitted with intrauterine appliances are inconsistent. While some investigators reported changes in follicle-stimulating hormone (FSH) and luteinizing hormone (LH) secretion patterns, others failed to confirm such findings in different species. Janakiraman and Casida (1968) reported that LH activity 11 h after mating was higher in rabbits fitted with IUDs than in controls. On the other hand, in a study on Holstein heifers 26 h after detection of ovulation, Bhalla et al. (1969) showed no difference in the relative FSH and LH activity between the IUD-treated group and the controls. However they reported that the weights of the anterior pituitary in the IUD-treated group were significantly greater than in the controls. In rats, IUDs were found to have no effect on pituitary LH and FSH and failed to affect significantly the ovarian weight and the number of corpora lutea (Labhsetwar 1970).

To reach a conclusion from the data collected from animal studies is difficult. The evidence prevailing is that IUDs can affect the pituitary-ovarian interrelation either by interfering with the process of ovulation or by hampering the normal and natural growth of corpora lutea. The mechanism whereby these effects are produced remains to be substantiated by more evidence.

II. HUMAN STUDIES

Exploration of the pituitary-ovarian interrelation in women wearing different types of intrauterine contraceptive devices was the subject of few studies in the last fifteen years. This is attributed to the overwhelming reports on the local action and endometrial changes subsequent to IUD insertion, which was the main concern of most of the investigative efforts.

II.A. Cycle length in IUD users

Essentially, ample evidence was submitted during the Second International Conference on IUDs in 1964 proving that IUD users do have ovulatory menstrual cycle. However, reports appeared in the late sixties providing evidence that IUD wearers have shorter corpus luteum life span. Sammour et al. (1967) and Faucher et al. (1969) suggested that intrauterine contraceptive devices may interfere in one way or another with the life span of the corpus luteum. Their studies were based on the finding of shorter luteal phases in over 70% of a small group of women wearing Lippes Loops. They evaluated their cases by vaginal cytological changes as well as decrease in urinary estrogens and pregnanediol in the second half of the menstrual cycle. These results were confirmed by Haukkamaa et al. (1974) who reported a higher incidence of anovulatory cycles or cycles with insufficient function of the corpus luteum in a small group of women wearing Copper T, based on urinary pregnanediol assays. However, the majority of the Copper T cycles studied were the cycle of insertion of the IUD.

II.B. Pituitary gonadotropins and ovarian steroids in IUD users

Pursuing this line of investigative research, Nygren and Johansson (1973) estimated the day-to-day ovarian steroid levels in thirteen women fitted with Cu-T200 IUDs. They followed their cases for three years with occasional monthly studies. The results were synchronized according to the first day of menses; they demonstrated an average 2.5 days advancement in the onset of menstrual bleeding compared with the cycles preceding the IUD insertion, in spite of normal levels of serum estradiol and progesterone in those days. The general pattern of these two hormones during the menstrual cycle, in their study, did not change after Cu- T200 insertion. Martin and Brown (1973) gave data similar to the above findings in ten women wearing the Lippes Loop, Gräfenberg Ring and Inhiband intrauterine appliances. The menstrual bleeding in their study was premature in relation to the estrogen and pregnanediol values obtained by urinary assays. Brenner and Mishell (1975) confirmed the normal secretion pattern of progesterone and estradiol in women using the IUD.

The secretion pattern of pituitary gonadotropins and ovarian steroids was estimated in two groups of women using Lippes Loop and Cu- T200 devices (Abdalla et al. 1978a, 1978b, 1979). The women chosen in their study had the appliances fitted for more than one year, were regularly menstruating, and were of similar ages and comparable parity. The cycles were synchronized according to the LH peak (which was regarded as day 0 of the menstrual cycle, preceding ovulation by 24 h) and the results compared with a control group of the same specifications, not fitted with IUDs and not using any hormonal contraceptives. Each cycle was classified into seven intervals according to the LH peak: day −9 to −15, −2 to −8, −1, 0, +1, +2 to +8, and +9 to +15.

Statistical analysis of FSH data revealed no significant differences between the mean values of the three groups at days −1, 0 and +1. Nonsignificant differences were present in the Cu group at days −9 to −15 and in the Lippes group at days −2 to −8 and +2 to +8. A significant decreased level was present in the remaining intervals in both Cu and Lippes groups (Figure 1).

Statistical analysis of LH data revealed decreased values at days −9 to −15 in both Cu and Lippes groups, at days −2 to −8 in Cu only and days +2 to +8 in the Lippes group only (Figure 2).

Statistical analysis of estradiol data showed nonsignificant differences at days 0, −1, +1, +2 to +8 and +9 to +15 between the three groups. The estradiol level was lower in the Cu group and there

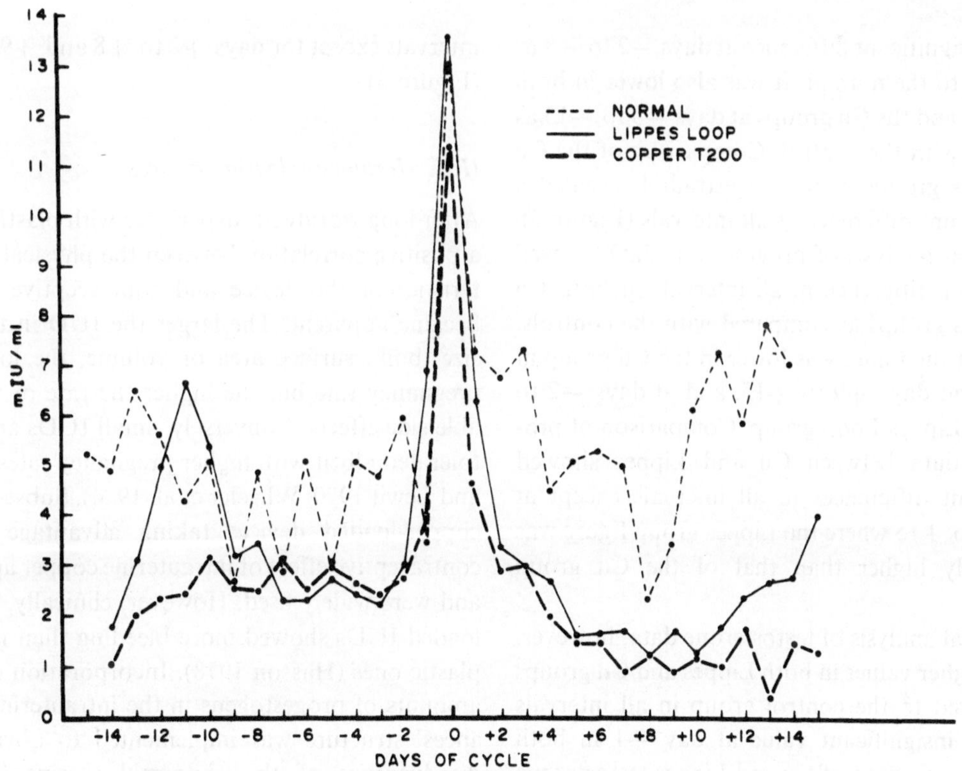

Figure 1. Serum levels of FSH in normal, Cu-T200 and Lippes Loop groups.

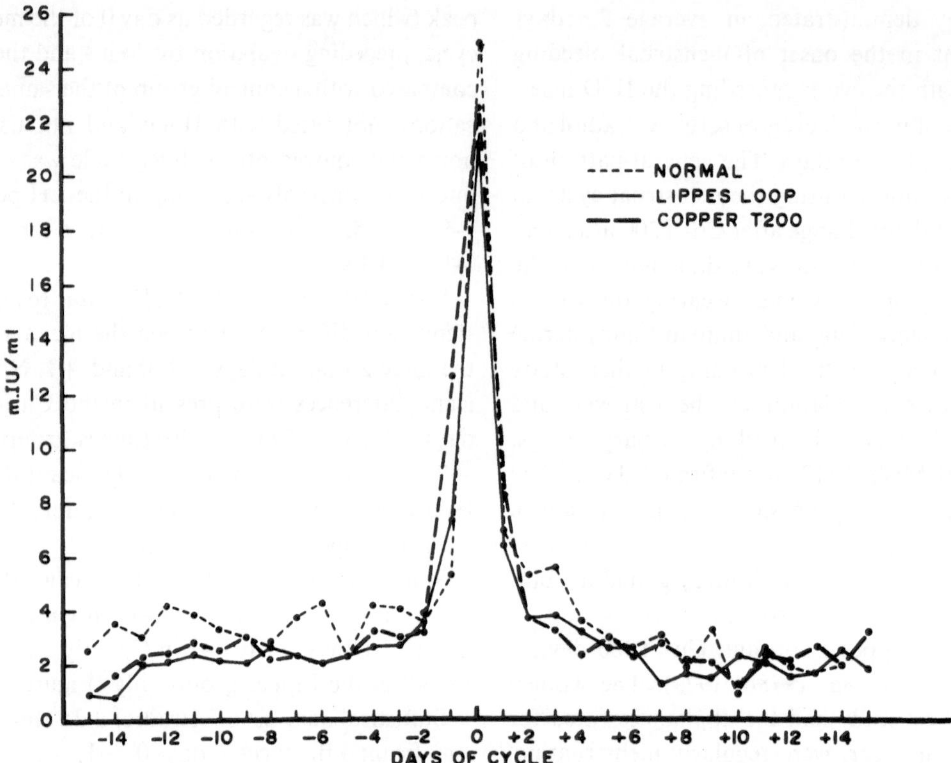

Figure 2. Serum levels of LH in normal, Cu-T200 and Lippes Loop groups.

was a nonsignificant difference at days −2 to −8 as compared to the normal. It was also lower in both the Lippes and the Cu groups at days −9 to −15 as compared with the control. Comparison of the Cu and Lippes groups' values of estradiol revealed a nonsignificant difference at all intervals (Figure 3).

Statistical analysis of progesterone data showed insignificant difference in all intervals in both Cu and Lippes groups as compared with the controls, except that the figure was lower in the Cu group at day −1 and days +9 to +15, and at days −2 to −8 in the Lippes Loop group. Comparison of progesterone data between Cu and Lippes showed insignificant differences in all intervals except at days +9 to +15 where the Lippes group figure was significantly higher than that of the Cu group (Figure 4).

Statistical analysis of testosterone data, however, showed higher values in both Lippes and Cu groups as compared to the control group in all intervals except an insignificant value at day +1 in both groups. Comparison of Cu and Lippes testosterone data revealed nonsignificant differences in all the intervals except for days +2 to +8 and +9 to +15 (Figure 5).

II.C. Hormone-releasing devices

After long worldwide experience with plastic IUDs, a positive correlation between the physical characteristics of the device and contraceptive efficacy became apparent. The larger the IUD in terms of size, bulk, surface area or volume, the lower the pregnancy rate but the higher the rate of undesirable side effects. Conversely, small IUDs are better tolerated albeit with higher pregnancy rates (Tietze and Lewit 1970; Wheeler et al. 1974). Subsequently, copper-loaded devices taking advantage of the contraceptive effect of intrauterine copper appeared and were widely used. However, clinically, copper-loaded IUDs showed more bleeding than identical plastic ones (Hasson 1978). Incorporation of small amounts of progestogens in the intrauterine appliances' structure was implemented to obviate the disadvantage of the abnormal uterine bleeding experienced with other devices and to preserve a high contraceptive efficacy.

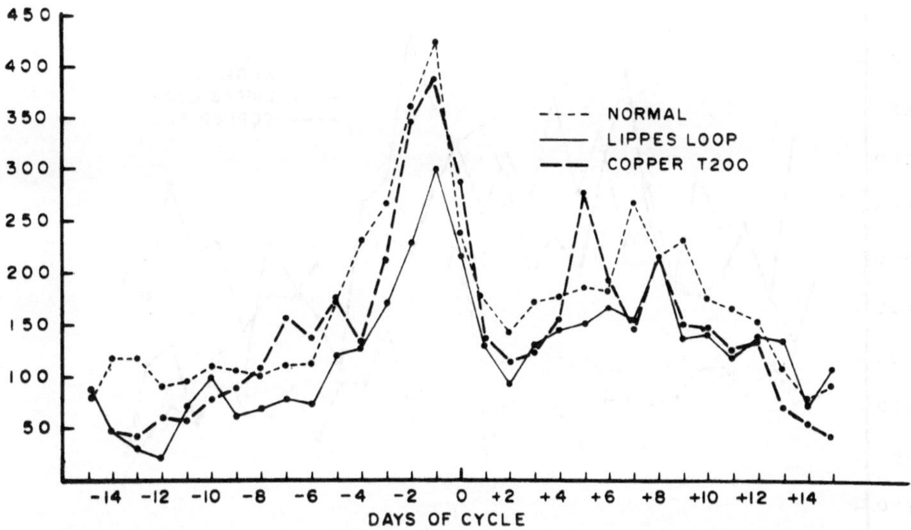

Figure 3. Serum levels of estradiol in normal, Cu- T200 and Lippes Loop groups.

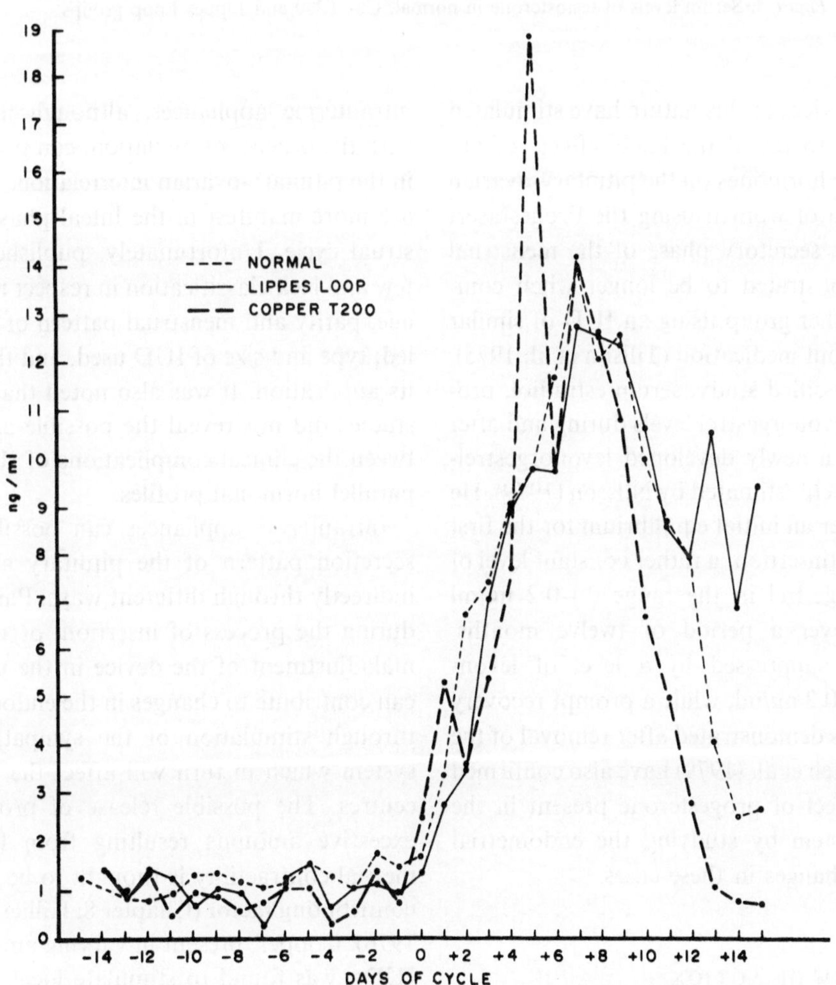

Figure 4. Serum levels of progesterone in normal, Cu- T200 and Lippes Loop groups.

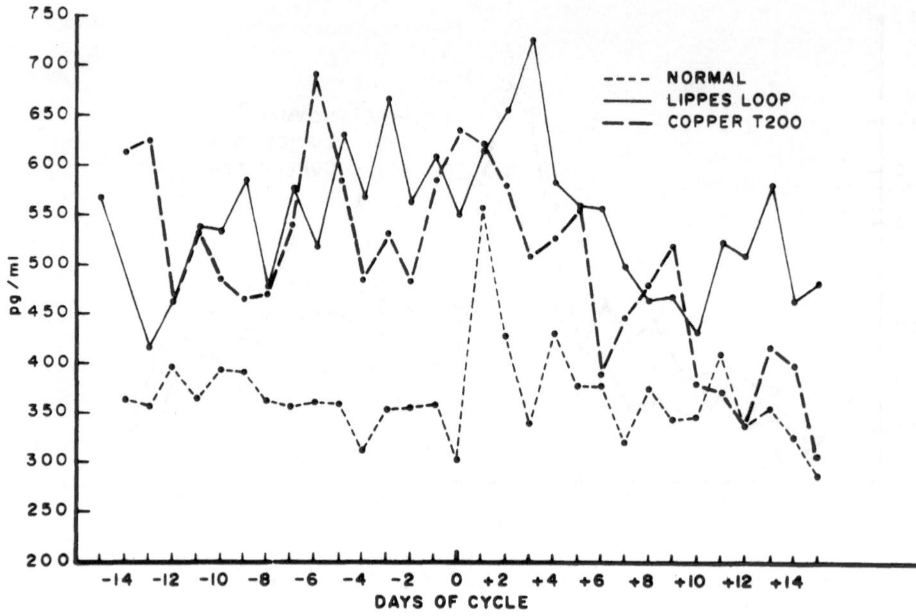

Figure 5. Serum levels of testosterone in normal, Cu- T200 and Lippes Loop groups.

Obviously, devices of this nature have stimulated research efforts to reveal the likely effects of absorbed synthetic hormones on the pituitary-ovarian axis. In a group of women using the Progestasert TM system, the secretory phase of the menstrual cycle was demonstrated to be longer when compared with another group using an IUD of similar design but without medication (Tillson et al. 1975).

In a more classified study, serum estradiol, progesterone and levonorgestrel levels during and after the removal of a newly developed levonorgestrel-releasing IUD were estimated by Nilsson (1979). He showed that after an initial equilibrium for the first twenty days postinsertion, a rather constant level of plasma levonorgestrel in the range 0.1-0.2 ng/ml was detected over a period of twelve months. Ovulation was suppressed by a level of levonorgestrel above 0.2 ng/ml, while a prompt recovery of ovulation was demonstrated after removal of the IUD. Mall-Haefeli et al. (1979) have also confirmed the systemic effect of progesterone present in the Progestasert system by studying the endometrial and oviductal changes in these cases.

III. MECHANISM OF ACTION

The impression gained from human studies is that intrauterine appliances, although not interfering with the process of ovulation, can produce changes in the pituitary-ovarian interrelation. These changes are more manifest in the luteal phase of the menstrual cycle. Unfortunately, published studies are few and lack classification in respect to the number, age, parity and menstrual pattern of subjects studied; type and size of IUD used, and the duration of its application. It was also noted that the reported studies did not reveal the possible association between the clinical complications of IUDs and their parallel hormonal profiles.

Intrauterine appliances can possibly affect the secretion pattern of the pituitary and the ovary indirectly through different ways. Pain, developing during the process of insertion, or resulting from maladjustment of the device in the uterine cavity, can contribute to changes in the endocrine function through stimulation of the sympathetic nervous system which in turn will affect the hypothalamic centres. The possible release of prostaglandin in excessive amounts resulting from forceful myometrial contractility is thought to be an additional contributing factor (Chapter 8; Hillier and Kasonde 1976). Copper, present in varying amounts in some IUDs, was found to stimulate local prostaglandin production (Oster and Salgo 1975). Abdalla et al. (1978c) demonstrated that intravenous prostaglandin-E_2 (Sulprostone) produced a significant reduction in pituitary and ovarian hormones in both the follicular and luteal phases of the menstrual cycle.

IV. CONCLUSIONS

The final conclusion to this issue has not even been approached yet. More research activity in this area is required because of the obvious clinical bearing of the subject. In helping to reach a conclusive view of the mechanism of action of IUDs, explanation of the most common complications of different appliances will be formulated. These complications, like bleeding and pain, are responsible for most IUD removals.

Medicated IUDs, especially hormone-releasing devices, have opened a new area of investigative research in contraceptive technology. The correlation between the likely impact of absorbed synthetic hormones on the pituitary-ovarian function and the improvement in clinical complications and contraceptive efficacy should be investigated.

REFERENCES

Abdalla MI, Ibrahim II, Aboul Dahab T, Marei A: Corpus luteum function in IUD users. Arab J Lab Med 4: 62, 1978a.

Abdalla MI, Ibrahim II, Aboul Dahab T, Makhlouf AM: Effect of Lippes Loop and copper T200 on pituitary gonadotropins. Arab J Lab Med 4: 288, 1978b.

Abdalla MI, Ibrahim II, Osman MI: Effect of prostaglandin-E_2 derivative (Sulprostone) on the pituitary-ovarian function in nonpregnant females. Presented at the International Sulprosterone Symposium Vienna, 1978c.

Abdalla MI, Ibrahim II, Makhlouf AM, Aboul Dahab T: Effect of Lippes Loop and copper T200 on pituitary-ovarian function. Presented at the symposium: Medicated IUDs and polymeric delivery systems, Amsterdam, 1979.

Ancla M, Brux JA: Ultrastructural studies on the endometrial lesions induced by intrauterine devices. J Reprod Med 3: 53, 1969.

Bhalla RC, Memon GN, Woody CO, Casida LE: Effect of bilateral intrauterine devices on some pituitary and ovarian characteristics near the time of ovulation in Holstein heifers. J Anim Sci 28: 48, 1969.

Bland KP, Donovan BT: In: Advances in reproductive physiology, Meharen A (ed), London, Logos, 1966.

Breed WG, Stephenson JM, Eckstein P, Peplow PV, Bett WR: J Reprod Fertil 28: 249, 1972.

Brenner P, Mishell DR Jr: Progesterone and estradiol pattern in women using an intrauterine contraceptive device. Obstet Gynecol 41: 456, 1975.

Buch NC, Shukla KP: Effect of intrauterine plastic devices on reproduction in Surti buffaloes and Kan Krej cows. Indian J Dairy Sci 19: 25, 1966.

Buch NC, Shukla KP, Hawk HW: Interference with ovulation by intrauterine plastic devices in Indian water buffaloes. Int Cong Anim Reprod AI 5 (2): 242, 1964.

Cuadros A, Tovar E: Histochemistry of uteri bearing copper intrauterine devices: light and electron microscopic study. Presented at the American Fertility Society Meeting, New York, 1972.

Davis HJ, Israel R: Uterine cavity measurements in relation to design of intrauterine contraceptive devices. In: Intrauterine contraception, Segal SJ, Southam AL, Shafer KD (eds), Amsterdam, Excerpta Medica, 1964, p 135-141.

Faucher GL, Ellegood JO, Mahesh VB, Greenblatt RB: Urinary estrogens and pregnanediol before and after insertion of an intrauterine contraceptive device. Am J Obstet Gynecol 104: 502, 1969.

Gadgil BA, Collins WE, Buch NC: Effects of intrauterine spirals on reproduction in goats. Indian J Exp Biol 6: 138, 1968.

Gerrits RG, Hawk HW: Effect of intrauterine devices on fertility in pigs: abstract. J Anim Sci 25: 1266, 1966.

Ginther OJ, Pope AL, Casida LE: Local effect of an intrauterine plastic coil on the corpus luteum of the ewe. J Anim Sci 25: 272, 1966.

Hasson HM: Copper IUDs. J Reprod Med 20 (3): 139, 1978.

Haukkamaa M, Luukkainen T, Timonen H: IUD on length of menstrual cycle. Ann Clin Res 6: 40, 1974.

Hillier K, Kasonde TM: Prostaglandin E and F concentrations in human endometrium after insertion of intrauterine contraceptive device. Lancet 1: 15, 1976.

Janakiraman K, Casida LE: Ovulation, corpora lutea development and pituitary LH activity in rabbits with intrauterine devices. J Reprod Fertil 15: 395, 1968.

Janakiraman K, Woody CO, Agarwal SP, Bhalla RC, Shukla KP, Gadgil BA, Buch NC, Casida LE: Interference with reproduction in water buffalo by intrauterine devices. J Reprod Fertil 22: 499, 1970.

Johansson EDB, Nygren KG: IUDs, ovarian function, and onset of menstrual bleeding. In: Proceedings of the third international conference on intrauterine contraception, Hefnawi F, Segal SJ (eds), Amsterdam, North-Holland Biomedical Press, 1975, p 335ff.

Johansson EDB, Wide L, Gemzell C: LH and progesterone in plasma and LH and oestrogens in urine during 42 normal menstrual cycles. Acta Endocrinol 68: 502, 1971.

Kamal I, Hefnawi F, Ghoneim M, Talaat M, Abdalla MI: Dimensional and architectural disproportion between the intrauterine device and the uterine cavity: a cause of bleeding. Fertil Steril 22 (8): 514, 1971.

Labhsetwar AP: Intrauterine device and pituitary FSH and LH in the rat. Fertil Steril 21 (2): 177, 1970.

Lau IF, Saxena SK, Chang MC: J Reprod Fertil 37: 429, 1974.

Lippes J: A study of intrauterine contraception: development of a plastic loop. In: Intrauterine contraceptive devices, Tietze C, Lewit S (eds), Amsterdam, Excerpta Medica, 1962, p 69ff.

Mall-Haefeli M, Werner-Zodrow I, Spornitz UM, Ludwig KS, Uettwiller A: The Progestasert system. Presented at the symposium: Medicated IUDs and polymeric delivery systems Amsterdam, 1979.

Martin PM, Brown, JB: J Clin Endocrinol Metab 36: 1125, 1973.

Nilsson CG: Clinical trial with a progestin-releasing IUD. Presented at the symposium: Medicated IUDs and polymeric delivery systems, Amsterdam, 1979.
Nygren KG, Johansson EDB: Premature onset of menstrual bleeding during ovulatory cycles in women with an intrauterine contraceptive device. Am J Obstet Gynecol 177: 971, 1973.
Oster G, Salgo MP: The copper intrauterine device and its mode of action. N Engl J Med 293: 432, 1975.
Sammour MB, Iskander SG, Rifai SF: Combined histologic and cytologic study of intrauterine contraception. Am J Obstet Gynecol 98: 946, 1967.
Speidel JJ, Ravenholt RT: In: Intrauterine devices: development, evaluation and program implementation, Wheeler RG, Duncan GW, Speidel JJ (eds), Academic press, New York, 1974.
Tietze C, Lewit S: Evaluation of IUDs: ninth progress report of the Cooperative Statistical Program. Stud Fam Plann 55: 1, 1970.
Tillson SA, Marian M, Hudson R, Wong B, Pharriss B, Aznar R, Martinez Manautau J: Gonadotropin and steroid hormone levels in women using the intrauterine hormone-releasing systems. Contraception 11: 179, 1975.
Vorys N, De Neef JC, Boutselis JG, Dettman FG, Scott WP, Stevens VC, Besch PK: Effect of intrauterine devices on the normal menstrual cycle. In: Proceedings of the second international conference on intrauterine contraception, New York, Population Council 1964.
Wheeler RG, Buschbom RL, Marshall RK: A rational basis for IUD design and development. In: Intrauterine devices: development, evaluation and programm implementation, Wheeler RG, Duncan GW, Speidel JJ (eds), New York, Academic Press, 1974, p 163-190.
Willson J, Bollinger CC, Ledger WJ: The effect of an intrauterine contraceptive device on bacterial flora of the endometrial cavity. Am J Obstet Gynecol 90 (6): 726, 1964.
Yamauchi M, Nakahara T: Effects of uterine distension on the estrous cycle of cattle. Jap J Anim Reprod 3: 121, 1958.

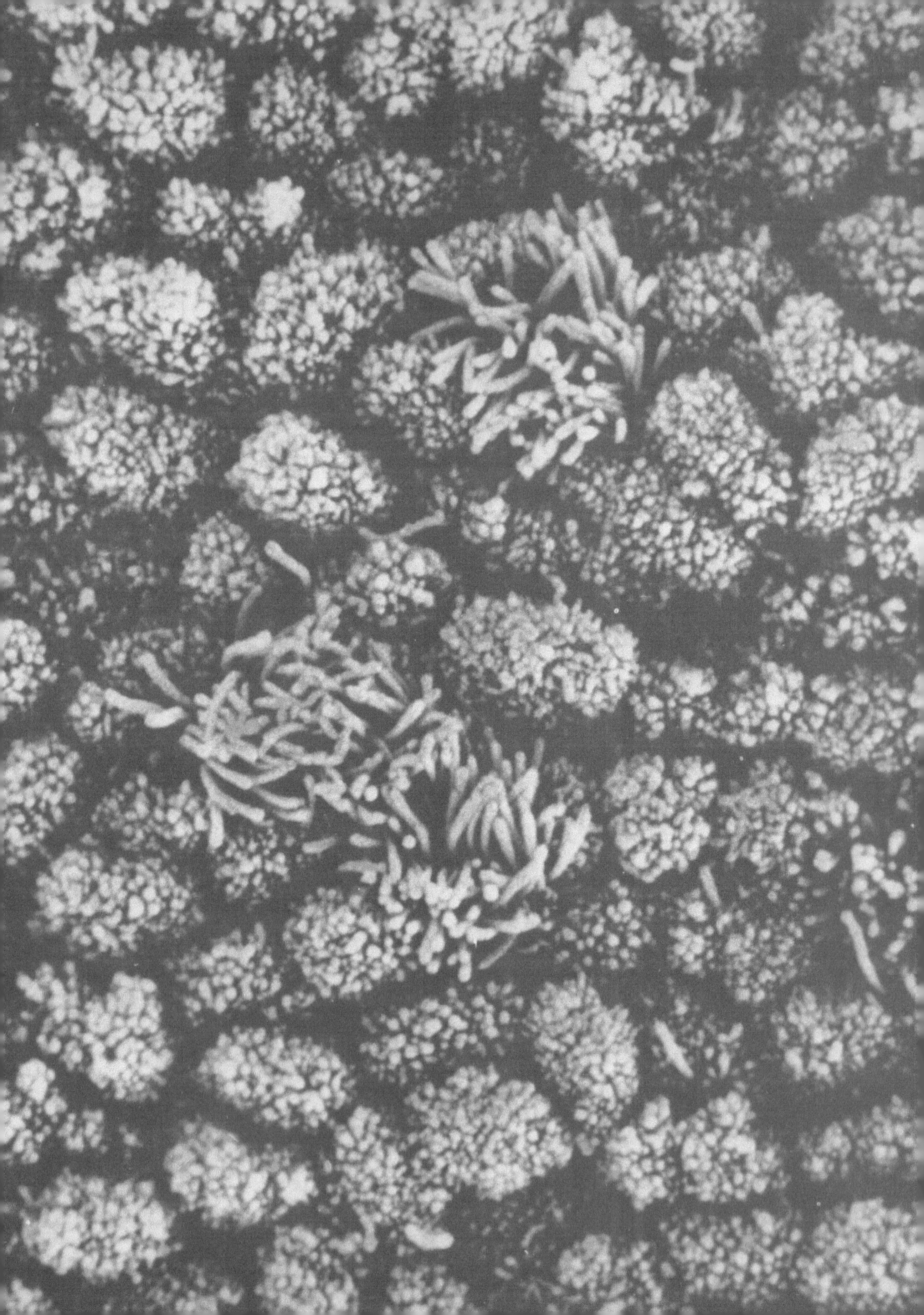

II. CLINICAL ASPECTS

10. COPPER IUDs: GENERAL CONSIDERATIONS

W.A.A. VAN OS, C.C.A. DE NOOYER and P.E.R. RHEMREV

Copper, as a trace element, has its role in the regulation of fertility. All human tissues contain copper, which is an essential component of certain enzymes and proteins. Gräfenberg was the first to introduce into the uterus a ring, partially made of copper, for regulation of fertility in the woman (see Figure 1). In this area, however, little was known about the 'inert' and 'active' intrauterine contraceptive devices (IUDs). After a long hiatus, plastic IUDs were developed, but their shapes and overall dimensions did not conform to the uterine cavity.

The studies of Tatum and Zipper (1968) and Zipper et al. (1968, 1969, 1970) revealed the low contraceptive effect of the inert T device, which configuration was based on the dimensions and functional integrity of the endometrial cavity. In the late sixties there was found a remarkable decrease in the number of implantations in the rabbit uterine horn fitted with copper wire with no reduction in the control horn. Based on such research a new concept in intrauterine contraception was introduced: the use of intrauterine pharmacologically-active substances in order to increase the effect of the inert IUD. In providing an inert T device with a copper wire of a surface area of 30 mm^2, the pregnancy rate is reduced from 18.3 to 4.9 per 100 users per year. Trials are presented in which a correlation is described between the surface area of copper on a T device and the contraceptive performance. A classic relationship is presented in Figure 2.

In an attempt to reduce the rates of pregnancy and expulsion, the effects of the Cu- T200 and 380A devices have been studied. The results of several clinical trials, completed in the early seventies, utilizing different models of the Cu-T, are summarized in Figure 3 (Zipper et al. 1971; Gibor et al. 1973; Roy et al. 1974; Timonen et al. 1974; Ti-

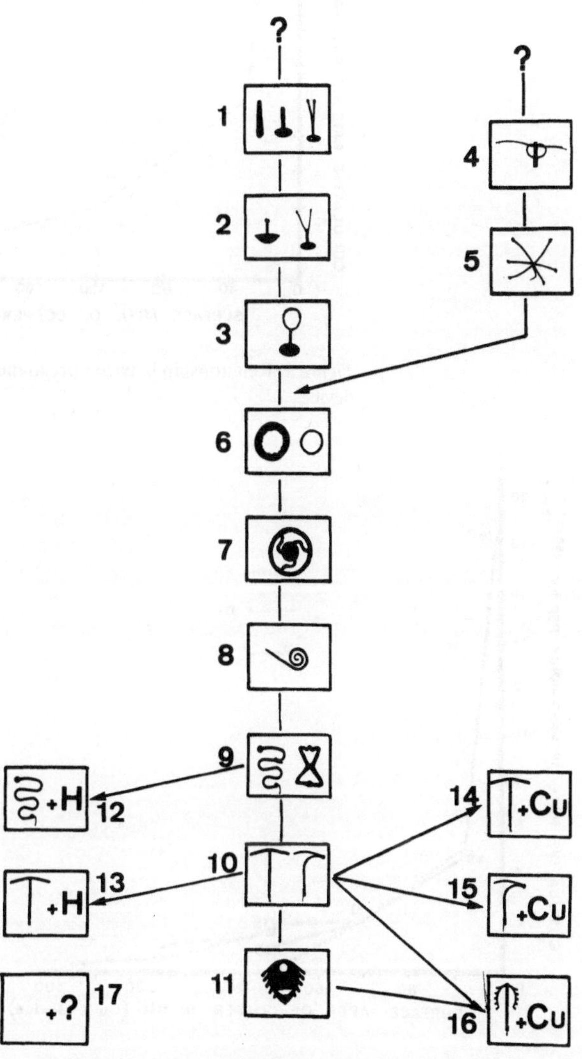

Figure 1. History of the IUD. 1, 2, 3: stem pessaries; 4: Richter's 'Seidenring'; 5, 6: Gräfenberg Ring; 7: Ota Ring; 8: Margulies Spiral; 9: Lippes Loop, Birnberg Bow; 10: T-device; 11: Dalkon Shield; 12: Lippes Loop progesterone IUD; 13: T-device with progesterone; 14: Cu-T device; 15: Cu-7 device; 16: combined Multiload copper IUD; 17: future IUD?

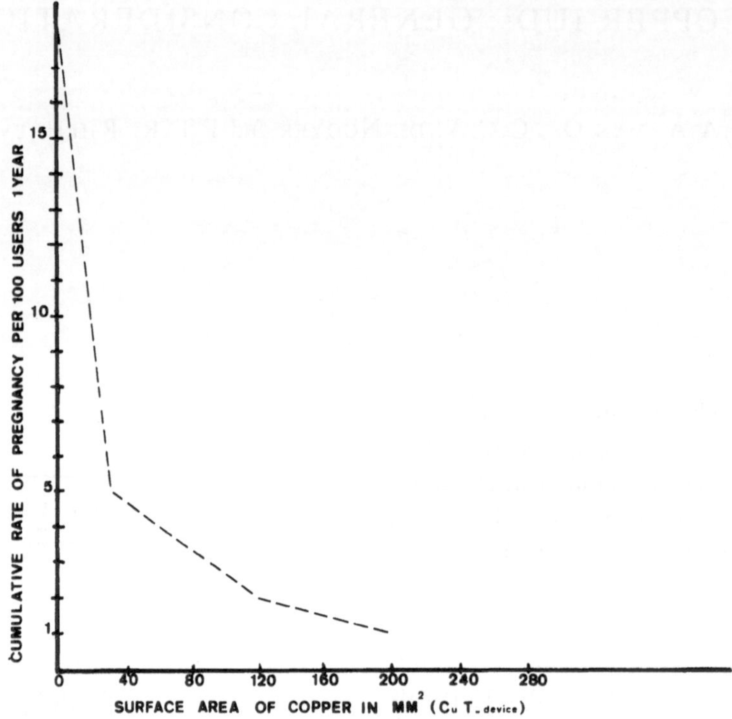

Figure 2. Relationship between pregnancy rate and surface area of copper on the T device.

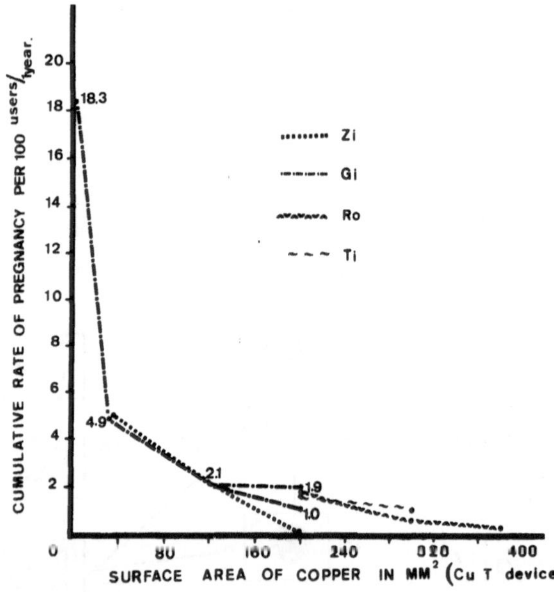

Figure 3. Relationship between pregnancy rate and surface area of copper on the T device in several clinical trials: Zi: Zipper et al. (1971); Gi: Gibor et al. (1973); Ro: Roy et al. (1974); Ti: Timonen (1974, 1976); Timonen et al. (1974).

monen 1976a, 1976b). The relation between pregnancy rate and surface area of copper is based on the performance of one type of IUD. Every IUD has its own relation depending on the shape. Data are influenced by the characteristics and cultural background of the groups of women involved. Trials are done in selected clinics, and results related to the technical skills of doctors. There is no correlation between pregnancy rate and surface area of copper and exposure time.

The consideration concerns the recent copper IUDs, the Copper-T, the Copper-7 and the combined Multiload Cu-250 and Cu-375 (van Os et al. 1977). The Multiload is a combination of the configuration of the Copper-T and the Dalkon Shield, after the central membrane has been removed. In order to improve theoretical effectiveness, a device with a surface area of 375 mm² has been developed, the Multiload Cu-375.

In this context the effects of copper include metallic copper as well as released copper ions.

I. MECHANISM OF ACTION OF THE COPPER IUD

The exact mechanism of action of the copper IUD is not precisely known. From animal experiments a number of theories have been evolved, which can explain the contraceptive effect, but each action can be different from species to species and is possibly dependent on variations in the shape of the IUD. Copper contributes to the contraceptive efficacy, but until now its exact effects have not been demonstrated. The most important theories on the mode of action of an IUD are summarized below.

I.A. Implantation

An anti-implantation or embryotoxic activity of polymorphonuclear leukocytes and macrophages is elicited by the IUD. Greenwald (1965) was the first to suggest a relation between the contraceptive action of an IUD and the presence of leukocytes in the endometrium. In the rabbit uterus a correlation exists between the number of leukocytes provoked by an IUD and the degree of fertility (El Sahwi and Moyer 1970), and the in-vitro development of rat and mouse embryos is prevented by polymorphonuclear leukocytes (Smith et al. 1974).

In-vitro and in-vivo studies confirm the embryotoxic activity of leukocytes (El Sahwi and Moyer 1977a, 1977b). No evidence is found in these experiments that phagocytes have a primary role in preventing the fertilized ovum from implanting.

I.B. Endometrial metabolism

In animals evidence exists for a link between the release of endometrium secretions and the blastocyst activity. A lack of stimulatory substances, or abnormal or noxious compounds produced by the endometrium in the vicinity of a copper IUD, can interfere with blastocyst activity and development or make implantation impossible. Effects are known on concentrations of zinc and enzymes, for example on alkaline phosphatase, β-gluceronidase and carbonic anhydrase (Chang and Tatum 1970); Hagenfeldt et al. 1972). The RNA level in human endometrium is negatively influenced by intrauterine copper relase (Hicks et al. 1975; Hernandez-Perez et al. 1976). Binding of a steroid to a receptor protein is inhibited by copper ions (Aitken and Harper 1978; Lövgren et al. 1978; Tamaya et al. 1976). Low circulating β-HCG levels in the luteal phase of fertile and sexually active copper IUD bearers have been demonstrated (Beling et al. 1976; Landesman et al. 1976), but also denied (Aubert et al. 1977; Klein and Mishell 1977; Sharpe et al. 1977). This controversy may be due to the assays used and their sensitivity (Saxena and Landesman 1978). A small amount of β-HCG is found in the serum of patients with malignant gynecological conditions and other neoplasms (Rutanen and Seppälä 1978; Braunstein et al. 1973). Material similar to HCG is detectable in normal human tissue (Yoshimoto et al. 1979).

I.C. Ovum transport

The transport of the fertilized ovum in the uterus is precisely timed and crucial for embryonic survival (Hunter 1977). Transport of the ovum through the tube and into the uterus can be influenced by the presence of a copper IUD. In-vitro copper affects smooth muscle activity; contraction frequencies are related to copper concentrations (Larsson et al. 1976).

I.D. Intrauterine copper

Copper, as a heavy metal, is toxic to the developing blastocyst and to sperm (Zielske et al. 1974). In the rabbit, entry of copper into blastocyst lysosomes results in cell death (Ambraham et al. 1974). The effects of a copper IUD in the sheep on embryonic survival and on intrauterine sperm cells were similar to those of a plastic IUD (Hawk et al. 1974). The postcoital test is not interfered with in copper IUD users, but copper ionization of the cervix in human volunteers is followed by a marked diminution of sperm count and depression in motility (Chattopadhyay et al. 1976). In-vitro incubation of cervical mucus with a copper device caused a reduction in sperm penetration (Rush and Elstein 1974). In clinical experiments no sperm was present in the fallopian tubes after artificial insemination of women using an IUD; this may indicate an influence on the intrauterine sperm transport (Tredway et al. 1975).

I.E. Prostaglandins

A copper IUD may influence the synthesis and concentrations of prostaglandins, resulting in altered contractility patterns of the uterus and oviduct. Prostaglandins E and F have different effects in vitro on isolated circular and longitudinal smooth muscle of the oviduct. The ratio between the concentrations of PGE and PGF is essential for the physiologic contractile function of the human fallopian tube (Lindblom et al. 1978). The concentration of $PGF_{2\alpha}$ in uterine flushings changes during the cycle, with highest values in the midsecretory phase of the cycle of normal women, an expression of endometrial prostaglandin metabolism (Maathuis 1978). Prostaglandins are involved in cell replication and platelet aggregation (Powles 1979).

Insertion of a foreign body into the guinea pig or sheep uterus results in the release of $PGF_{2\alpha}$ and increase of its level in uterine venous blood (Thompson 1973). In rabbit the anti-implantation effect of a unilateral IUD is reversed by prostaglandin inhibitors (Saksena and Harper 1974). Postinsertional changes in PGE and PGF concentrations in human endometrium are inconsistent; this is possibly due to the variability of the biopsy site (Hillier and Kasonde 1976; Scommegna et al. 1978). Both PGE and PGF can be isolated from macrophages adhering to the IUD (Abdel Gawad et al. 1977).

II. COPPER INTRAUTERINE DEVICES AND THE ENDOMETRIUM

Both medicated and inert IUDs are responsible for evoking an inflammatory response in the endometrium of their wearers. It is impossible to divide this mild inflammatory response on morphological grounds between a reaction to an inert IUD and an effect provoked by the addition of copper. Besides the influence of copper ions, the response of the endometrium is also related to:

- the compounds used in the IUD;
- the geometry of the IUD and the degree of endometrium compression;
- the endometrial area of surface covering;
- the immunological response of the user to a foreign body.

The infiltration of the endometrium by polymorphonuclear leukocytes and mononuclear cells is evoked by the presence of an inert IUD.

Studies of endometrium biopsies and specimens of endometrium after hysterectomy, with a Cu-T or Cu-7 in utero reveal a normal development of both the proliferative and secretory endometrium (Hagenfeldt et al. 1972; Chih Hsu et al. 1976). Compression, microerosions and microabscesses of the surface epithelium due to mechanical trauma of the copper IUD have been described (Chih Hsu et al. 1976). Polymorphonuclear leukocytes and mononuclear cells are present, primarily subepithelially and in relation to the implantation site. Intrauterine washings of uteri fitted with a Cu-T200 show an enormous cellular reaction. In association with this copper device relatively more polymorphs and fewer macrophages are counted than with the inert Lippes Loop (Abdel Gawad et al. 1977).

The presence of plasma cell infiltration of the endometrium is essential to a diagnosis of chronic endometritis. Some 30-50 percent of endometria of symptomatic women with an IUD show nonspecific chronic endometritis (Czernobilsky 1978). The development of a postinsertional plasma cell infiltrate is observed despite negative bacterial cultures (Moyer et al. 1970). Culture difficulties of certain species of micro-organisms or the very individual immunologic response to a foreign body may be responsible.

The ultrastructure of endometria of copper device wearers is not very different from that observed normally (Gonzalez-Angulo and Aznar-Ramos 1976). Mitochondrial changes are described in the vicinity of a Cu-T, and differences are found in the development of the nuclear channel system (Gonzalez-Angulo and Aznar-Ramos 1976; Wynn 1967). In epithelial cells of endometria in the presence of a copper IUD less frequent and smaller light areas are seen. As a long-term effect of copper ions an interference in the carbohydrate metabolism is postulated, but not proved (Nilsson et al. 1974). Of some interest also is the discovery of vascular defects in a study of endometria of copper IUD wearers (Hohman et al. 1977).

Vascular gaps, possibly caused by pressure of the device, are frequently noted in the superficial layer of the endometrium beneath an intact surface epithelium. Degeneration, separation and fragmentation of endothelial cells, followed by the formation of gaps filled with erythrocytes, can explain the intermenstrual spotting associated with an IUD on morphological grounds. But because the vascular gaps are located in the functional layer, and spiral vessels exhibit an intense vasoconstriction before the onset of menstruation, these gaps cannot explain enhanced menstrual blood loss.

III. COPPER EMISSION AND ABSORPTION

The antifertility effects of the copper IUD are only possible if copper atoms are dissolved in the uterine milieu and oxidized to oxides. An equilibrium is established depending on the surface area of metallic copper, the intrauterine pH, blood loss, the chemical characteristics of the compounds in the uterine fluid, and the metabolic activity of the endometrium (see Chapter 7). In female monkeys wearing copper IUDs higher copper levels than are present in controls are demonstrated in the endometrium, but analysis for copper in body organs and plasma reveals no effect of the device (Ranney et al. 1975; Moo-Young et al. 1973). After insertion of tracer elements ^{64}Cu and ^{67}Zn into rat uteria systemic absorption was demonstrated; however almost all of the copper disappeared within the feces (Okercke et al. 1972).

Different models of copper IUDs in man cause no measurable increase in serum copper concentrations (Hagenfeldt et al. 1972; Anteby et al. 1978). The loss of metallic copper is correlated with the surface area of the wire. In asymptomatic patients the release rate of copper from preweighed Cu-T200 devices averaged 44.0 μg/day, measured direct post-insertionally up to the fortieth month of use. The copper release rate from preweighed Cu-T devices with a surface area of 100, 200, 300 and 400 mm^2 is 26, 44, 75 and 74 μg/day during the first month of use (Timonen 1976). A higher release rate during the first sixty days is given by Hagenfeldt et al. (1972). Bleeding problems may explain this difference. The copper release rate during the first month of use from the Cu-T400 device is not significantly different from the release rate in the Cu-T300 devices. Wide standard deviations or a supersaturation of the uterine milieu can explain this fact. Furthermore one month of use gives too little information about the relation between release rate and exposure time. Theoretically a saturation of the uterine milieu is only attained in a steady-state situation. The continuous release of copper is confirmed in a clinical study in which copper concentrations are measured in the uterine fluid for four years after insertion; there was no reduction, indeed there was a significant increase, in the amount of copper loss (Larsson and Hamberger 1977). In contrast with this significant increase in copper loss are the findings of calcareous deposits on copper IUDs (Johnson et al. 1976; Gosden et al. 1977). The major constituent is calcium carbonate, which is known to be porous. Copper ions can be found in the asymmetric crusts. Like corrosion, the deposits are the results of an interaction between the copper IUD and the uterine milieu.

Pregnancy and expulsion rates were both significantly lower when a copper IUD was replaced after two years rather than using the same device continuously for three years (Newton et al. 1977). However no differences in pregnancy rates after one year and three years of continuation with the same device were found in a nonrandomized study (Silvin 1977).

Based on copper wires of 0.2 mm an exposure time of 3.5 years is advised for commercially available Cu-T200 and Cu-7 devices (Kosonen 1978). The Multiload Cu-250 carries sufficient copper to provide contraceptive effectiveness for several more years. Compared with the intact Multiload Cu-250, approximately 14 percent of the original amount of copper has been released after one year, 27 percent after two years and 40 percent after three years (Figure 4) in utero (Maes et al. 1978). Studies in the early seventies revealed no copper levels in endometria of users of copper devices by X-ray dispersive analysis (Chih Hsu et al. 1976; Gonzalez-Angulo and Aznar-Ramos 1976). Copper is identified in epithelial cells and biochemical analysis of subcellular structurers demonstrates the presence of copper in cytoplasm, nuclei and microsomes and endometrial cells (Hernandez-Perez et al. 1975).

IV. THE COPPER DEVICE AND THE ENDOCRINE PROFILE

Menstrual disorders in copper IUD users are not related to a systemic endocrine derangement but to local effects of the foreign body. Studies on peripheral plasma levels of LH, FSH, progesterone and estradiol during the menstrual cycle of IUD bearers

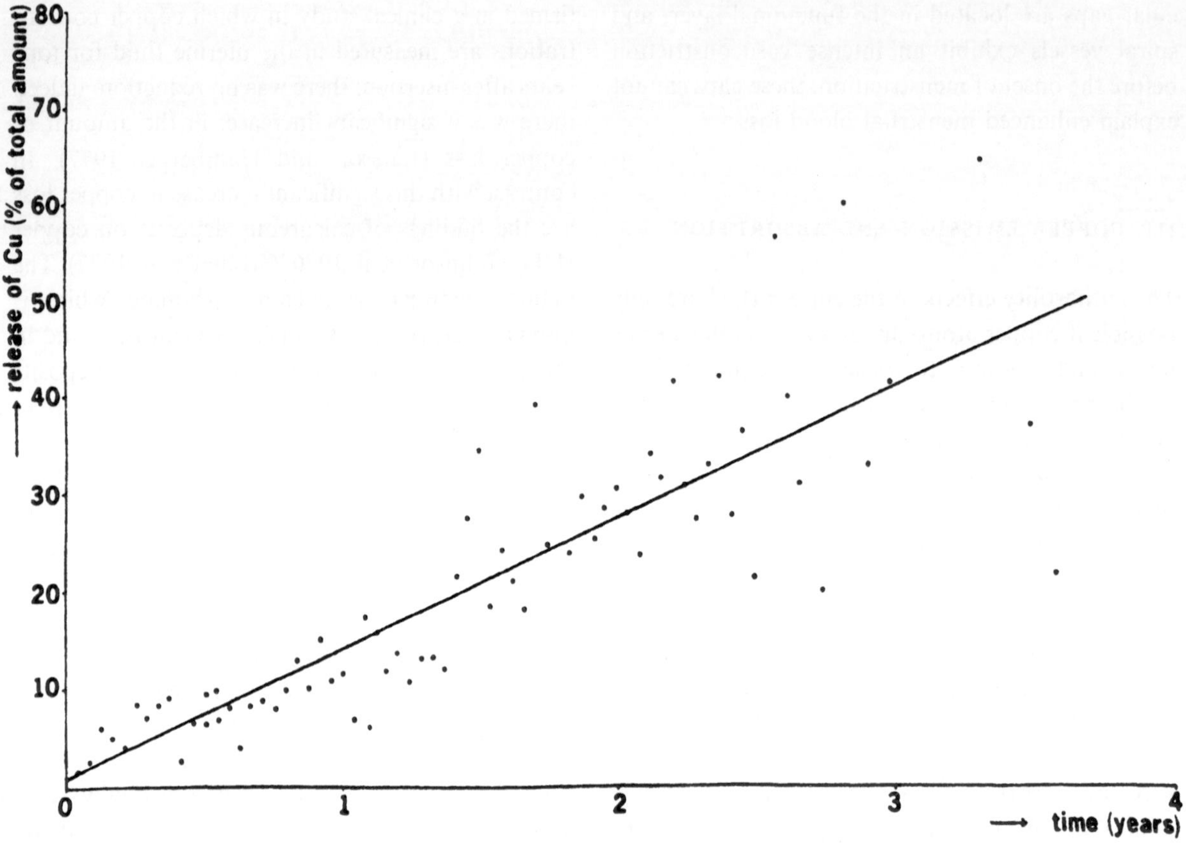

Figure 4. The relationship between the amount of copper lost from the Multiload Cu-250 and the length of time the device remained in utero (Maes et al. 1978).

do not demonstrate an influence of the copper device on follicular maturation, time of ovulation or corpus luteum function (Nygren and Johansson 1973; Brenner and Mishell 1975; Haukamaa et al. 1974); (see also Chapter 11).

The menstrual flow usually starts when levels of both estradiol and progesterone have not yet fallen to levels in control cycles. Bleeding does not necessarily imply endometrial desquamation (Nogaks Ortiz et al. 1978). Steroid hormones, lysosomes, prostaglandins and fibrinolytic activity are involved in the mechanism. Local changes within the endometrium in the vicinity of a copper IUD are the cause of the premature onset of the menstrual flow.

Changing concentrations of prostaglandings or their precursors, increase in the concentration of plasminogen activators, or blocking of the binding of estrogen or progesterone to their specific receptors can explain the menstrual disorders provoked by a copper IUD in utero (Hillier and Kasonde 1976; Kasonde and Bonnar 1976; Lövgren et al. 1978).

Serum prolactin levels in women using copper IUDs were higher compared with a control group, according to Mehta et al. (1977), however Spellacy et al. (1978) could not demonstrate any effect of copper IUD on prolactin levels.

V. TOXICOLOGICAL ASPECTS OF THE COPPER DEVICE

Little information is available on the acute and subacute toxicity of copper released from copper devices. The copper IUD does not seem to induce cancer of the endometrium or cervix.

The spatial relationship of the device to the uterine cavity is important with regard to both the antifertility effect and endometrial trauma. Replicas of human copper IUDs should be used in animals; insertion in the animal by the transvaginal route is often impossible, therefore surgical procedures are necessary.

The kinetics of intrauterine drug release and absorption, in combination with local body effects, are problems to consider, but an estimation of the acute toxicity of copper is actually impossible to make because of the way in which it is applied (McConnell 1974).

VI. CONCLUDING REMARKS

The mechanism of action of a copper device is not known, but it may be related to the inflammatory reaction or to the induction of the metabolic derangement in the intrauterine milieu.

An antifertility effect of copper is only possible if copper atoms are dissolved and oxidized to oxides, followed by an equilibrium.

The influence of copper on endometrial morphology is unknown.

After insertion of copper devices there is no measurable increase in serum copper concentration.

Neither deposits of calcium carbonate nor corrosion on the wire prevents the continuous release of copper.

Copper IUDs do not affect the cyclic endocrine profile. Menstrual disorders are an expression of the changed intrauterine milieu after insertion.

Toxicological studies are practically impossible because of the intrauterine application.

The incidence of cervical or endometrial carcinoma is not correlated with use of copper IUDs.

ACKNOWLEDGEMENT

The authors express their sincere thanks to Miss Elma van Ekeris for her editorial skills.

REFERENCES

Abdel Gawad A, et al.: Study of the uterine environment in association with intrauterine contraceptive devices. Contraception 16: 575, 1977.

Abraham R, et al.: Effects of intrauterine copper wire on blastocyst and uterine lysosomes of the rabbit: a cytochemical and ultrastructural study. J Reprod Fertil 36: 59, 1974.

Aitken RJ, Harper MJK: New methods for the regulation of implantation. Contraception 18: 181, 1978.

Anteby SD, et al.: The effect of intrauterine devices containing zinc and copper on their levels in serum. Fertil Steril 29: 30, 1978.

Aubert JM, et al.: Assessment of human chorionic gonadotropin levels during luteal phase in women using intrauterine contraception. Contraception 16: 557, 1977.

Beling CG, et al.: Demonstration of gonadotropins during the second half of the cycle in women using intrauterine contraception. Am J Obstet Gynecol 125: 855, 1976.

Braunstein GD, et al.: Ectopic production of human chorionic gonadotropin by neoplasms. Ann Intern Med 78: 39, 1973.

Brenner PF, Mishell DR Jr: Progesterone and estradiol patterns in women using an intrauterine contraceptive device. Obstet Gynecol 46: 456, 1975.

Chang CC, Tatum JH: A study of the antifertility effect of intrauterine copper. Contraception 1: 265, 1970.

Chattopadhyay SK, et al: Effects of copper ionisation of the cervix on sperm migration. Contraception 14: 331, 1976.

Chih Hsu FA, et al.: Endometrial morphology with copper-bearing intrauterine devices. Contraception 14: 243, 1976.

Czernobilsky B: Endometritis and infertility. Fertil Steril 30: 119, 1978.

El Sahwi S, Moyer DL: Antifertility effects on the intrauterine foreign body. Contraception 2: 1, 1970.

El Sahwi S, Moyer DL: Embryotoxic effects of homogenized polymorphs, macrophages, endometrial and liver cells in vitro. Contraception 16: 453, 1977a.

El Sahwi S, Moyer DL: In vivo action of the embryotoxic activity of leucocytes. Contraception 16: 453, 1977a.

Gibor Y, et al.: The association beteween the amount of copper and copper carrying IUDs and their contraceptive efficacy. Int J Reprod Med 11: 209, 1973.

Gonzalez-Angulo A, Aznar-Ramos R: Ultrastructural studies on the endometrium of women wearing T-Cu 200 intrauterine devices by means of transmission and scanning electron microscopy and X-ray dispersive analysis. Am J Obstet Gynecol 125: 170, 1976.

Gosden C, et al.: Intrauterine deposition of calcium on copper-bearing intrauterine contraceptive devices. Br Med J 1: 202, 1977.

Greenwald GB: Interruption of pregnancy in the rat by a uterine suture. J Reprod Fertil 9: 9, 1965.

Hagenfeldt K, et al.: Intrauterine contraception with the Copper-T device: effects upon endometrial morphology. Contraception 6: 207, 1972.

Haukamaa M, et al.: The effect of the Copper-T 200 IUD on the luteal phase plasma progesterone concentration in the normal menstrual cycle. Ann Clin Res 6: 40, 1974.

Hawk HW, et al.: Effects of a copper intrauterine contraceptive device on embryo survival, uterine spermicidal activity and endometrial vascular porosity in the ewe. Am J Obstet Gynecol 118: 480, 1974.

Hernandez-Perez O, et al.: Subcellular distribution of trace metals in the normal and in the copper-treated human secretory endometrium. Contraception 11: 451, 1975.

Hernandez-Perez O, et al.: RNA metabolism of the normal and copper-treated human endometrium. Contraception 14: 421, 1976.

Hicks JJ, et al.: Effects óf intrauterine copper on the nucleic acids, polysome patterns and glycoprotein composition of the human endometrium. Am J Obstet Gynecol 121: 931, 1975.

Hillier K, Kasonde JM: Prostaglandins E and F concentrations in human endometrium after insertion of intrauterine contraceptive device. Lancet 1: 15, 1976.

Hohman WR et al.: Vascular defects in human endometrium caused by intrauterine contraceptive devices. Contraception 16: 507, 1977.

Hunter RHF: Function and malfunction of the Fallopian tubes in relation to gametes, embryos and hormones. Eur J Obst Gyn Reprod Biol 7: 267, 1977.

Johnson AB, et al.: Calcareous deposits formed on IUDs in human exposures. Contraception 14: 507, 1976.

Kasonde JM, Bonnar J: Plasmicogen activators in the endometrium of women using intrauterine contraceptive devices. Br J Obstet Gynaecol 83: 315, 1976.

Klein TA, Mishell DR Jr: Absence of circulating chorionic gonadotropin in wearers of intrauterine contraceptive devices. Am J Obstet Gynecol 129: 626, 1977.

Kosonen A: Corrosion of copper in utero. Fertil Steril 30: 59, 1978.

Landesman R, et al.: Detection of human chorionic gonadotropin in blood of regularly bleeding women using copper intrauterine contraceptive devices. Fertil Steril 27: 1062, 1976.

Larsson B, Hamberger L: The concentration of copper in human uterine secretion during four years after insertion of a copper-containing IUD. Br Med J 22: 197, 1977.

Larsson B, et al.: The influence of copper on the in vitro motility of the human Fallopian tube. Am J Obstet Gynecol 125: 683, 1976.

Lindblom B, et al.: Differentiated contractile effects of prostaglandins E and F on the isolated circular and longitudinal smooth muscle of the human oviduct. Fertil Steril 30: 553, 1978.

Lövgren T, et al.: Effect of Cu^{++} ions on the binding of estrogen to the human myometrial estrogen-binding protein, 1978.

Maathuis JB: Cyclic changes in the concentration of prostaglandin-F_2 in human uterine flushings. Br J Obstet Gynaecol 85: 207, 1978.

McConnell RG: Special requirements for toxicological testing of metal-releasing intrauterine devices. Acta Endocrinol [Suppl] 185, 1974.

Maes RAA, et al.: Copper release from the Multiload Cu-250 IUD. IRCS Med Sciences 6: 507, 1978.

Mehta S, et al.: Serum prolactin levels in women using copper IUDs. Contraception 15: 327, 1977.

Moo-Young AJ, et al.: Copper levels in tissues of rhesus monkeys bearing intrauterine or intra-abdominal copper devices. Fertil Steril 24: 848, 1973.

Moyer DL, et al.: Reactions of human endometrium to the intrauterine device. Am J Obstet Gynecol 106: 799, 1970.

Newton J, et al.: Continuous intrauterine copper contraception for 3 years: comparison of replacement at 2 years with continuation. Br Med J 1: 197, 1977.

Nilsson O, et al.: Ultrastructural signs of an interference in the carbohydrate metabolism of human endometrium produced by the intrauterine Copper-T device. Acta Obstet Gynecol Scand 53: 139, 1974.

Nogaks-Ortiz F, et al.: The normal menstrual cycle: chronology and mechanism of endometrial desquamation. Obstet Gynecol 51: 259, 1978.

Nygren KG, Johansson EDB: Premature onset of menstrual bleeding during ovulatory cycles in women with intrauterine contraceptive devices. Am J Obstet Gynecol 117: 971, 1973.

Okercke R, et al.: Systemic absorption of intrauterine copper. Science 177: 358, 1972.

Os WAA van, et al.: Evaluation of the combined Multiload copper intrauterine device. World Cong Fertil Steril 9(28): 291, 1977.

Powles RJ: Prostaglandins and cancer. Cancer Topics 2: 4, 1979.

Ranney RE, et al.: Uterine copper distribution in monkeys implanted with copper-carrying intrauterine devices. Fertil Steril 26: 80, 1975.

Roy S, et al: Experience with three different models of the Copper-T intrauterine contraceptive device in nulliparous women. Am J Obstet Gynecol 119: 44, 1974.

Rush F, Elstein M: The effect of incubating a copper-releasing intrauterine device on sperm penetration and spinnbarkeit of cervical mucus. J Obst Gyn Br Comm 8: 483, 1974.

Rutanen EM, Seppälä, M: The HCG submit radioimmunoassay in non-trophoblastic gynecologic tumors. Cancer 41: 692, 1978.

Saksena SK, Harper MJK: Prostaglandin-medicated action of intrauterine devices: F-prostaglandins in the uterine horns of pregnant rabbits with unilateral intrauterine devices. Fertil Steril 25: 2, 1974.

Saxena BB, Landesman R: Does implantation occur in the presence of an IUD? Res Reprod 10: 3, 1978.

Scommegna A, et al.: Endometrial prostaglandin-F content of women wearing non-medicated or progestin-releasing intrauterine devices. Fertil Steril 29: 5, 1978.

Sharpe RM, et al.: Absence of HCG-like activity in the blood of women fitted with intrauterine contraceptive devices. J Clin Endocrinol Metab 45: 496, 1977.

Silvin J: Effect of calcium deposition on copper IUDs. Br Med J 6: 387, 1977.

Smith DM, et al.: Effect of polymorphonuclear leucocytes on the development of mouse embryos cultured from the two-cell stage to blastocysts. Biol Reprod 4: 74, 1974.

Spellacy WN, et al.: Plasma prolactin levels in contraception: oral contraceptives and intrauterine devices. Contraception 17: 7, 1978.

Tamaya T, et al.: The mechanism of action of the copper intrauterine device. Fertil Steril 27: 767, 1976.

Tatum HJ, Zipper JA: The T-intrauterine contraceptive device and recent advances in hormonal anticonceptional therapy. Proc Northeast Obst Gyn Cong Bahia Brazil 6: 7885, 1968.

Thompson JE: The IUD and prostaglandins: a review of the evidence. J Obstet Gynecol 42: 4, 1973.

Timonen H: Intrauterine contraception with copper-T, Academic dissertation, Helsinki, 1976.

Timonen H: Copper release from copper-T intrauterine devices, Contraception 14: 1, 1976.

Timonen H, et al.: Use effectiveness of the copper T-300 during the first year. Am J Obstet Gynecol 120: 466, 1974.

Tredway DR, et al.: Effects of intrauterine devices on sperm transport in the human being: preliminary report. Am J Obstet Gynecol 123: 734, 1975.

Wynn RM: Intrauterine devices: effects on the ultrastructure of human endometrium. Science 156: 1508, 1967.

Zielske F, et al.: Studies on copper release from copper-T devices (T-Cu 200) and its influence on sperm migration in vitro. Contraception 10: 561, 1974.

Zipper JA, et al: Toxic action of copper and zinc on implantation rates in rabbits. World Cong Fertil Steril 6: 154, 1968.

Zipper JA, et al.: Suppression of fertility by intrauterine copper and zinc in rabbits. Am J Obstet Gynecol 105: 529, 1969.

Zipper JA, et al.: Human fertility control through the use of endo-uterine metal antagonisms of elements. Nobel Symp 15: 199-218, 1970.

Zipper JA, et al.: Contraception through the use of intrauterine metals I: copper as an adjunct to the T-device: the endouterine copper-T. Am J Obstet Gynecol 109: 771, 1971.

11. COPPER IUDs IN NULLIPAROUS WOMEN

R. Percival Smith

> The use of copper intrauterine devices in nulliparous women remains a controversial topic.
>
> Editorial, *British Medical Journal*, 22 July 1978.

Prior to the introduction of the Cu-7-200 and the Cu-T200 IUDs, the small plastic devices, Lippes Loop, Saf-T-Coil and Dalkon Shield, were not accepted as well by nulliparous women as by parous women, there being higher rates of pregnancy, and of expulsion and removal due to bleeding and pain. Results obtained in nulliparous women with the Cu-7s and Cu-Ts were only marginally different from those achieved in parous women with respect to expulsion and removals for bleeding and pain. The pregnancy rate with copper IUDs does not differ between nulliparous and parous women. The controversy lies in the possible effect that the copper IUDs may have on the future fertility of the young nullipara who chooses the IUD as her method of contraception. Nobody will dispute the fact that pelvic inflammatory disease (PID) is more frequent in nulliparous IUD wearers compared to women using other methods of contraception (Westrom et al. 1976). Furthermore, the copper IUD may be one of the factors contributing to an increased prevalence of ectopic pregnancies (Tatum and Schmidt 1977), although this has been disputed in a recent review of the subject (Sivin 1979). Both these events would be expected to have an effect on the future fertility of young nulliparous women. In spite of careful counselling about this possible effect, approximately 10 percent of women attending the Student Health Service at the University of British Columbia are using IUDs as their chosen method of contraception. It should be noted that after careful counselling with regard to IUD use approximately 40 percent of the women decide to use another method, of whom only a small number are excluded for medical reasons.

The copper IUD does offer young women some distinct advantages. Many women start contraception with oral contraceptives; the majority of prospective IUD users are changing from these. Both methods have the appeal of being noncoital. At the Student Health Service the IUD is the most continued method of contraception of all, with a five-year continuation rate of 55 percent.

The reason for writing a chapter specifically on nulliparous women is not only to discuss use and effectiveness, but also to discuss some of the special problems encountered with the copper IUD in nulliparous women, and to make a special plea for improved counselling and education for these young women prior to the insertion of their copper IUD.

1. PREGNANCY RATES

Figure 1 shows a cumulative net pregnancy rate of 3.2 at one year and 6.4 at two years, much higher

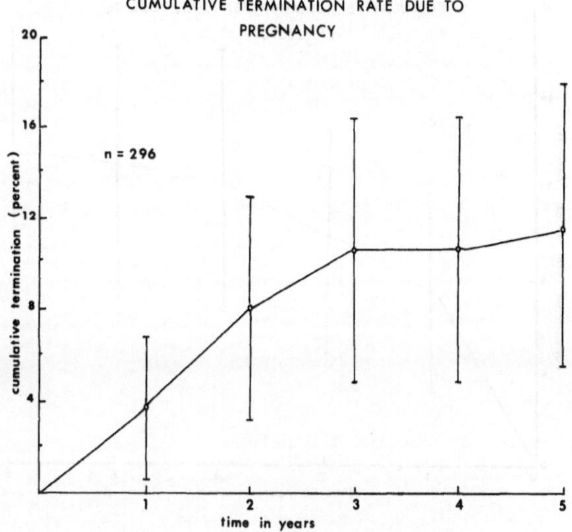

Figure 1. Gross cumulative pregnancy rates with copper IUDs in the Student Health Service over five years, with 99% confidence limits.

than the early studies suggested (Newton et al. 1972; Mishell et al. 1973), but in keeping with more recent reports (Jain 1975a, 1975b; Tatum 1978; Liedholm et al. 1974) on copper IUDs in nulliparous women. A number of variables are now known to affect pregnancy rates. The younger the woman the higher the rate (Jain 1975a, 1975b; Weiner et al. 1978); the shorter the uterine length the higher the rate (Gibor et al. 1973); a retroverted uterus has a lower rate than the anteverted uterus (Cheng Chi et al. 1978); and the timing of insertion after an abortion affects the rate (Jain 1975a, 1975b), in that immediate insertion and waiting ninety days both carry lower rates than insertion between ten and ninety days post-abortum. Most studies are now in agreement that nulliparous and parous women's rates do not differ.

II. EXPULSION RATES

The expulsion rate of 8.9 percent at 24 months (Figure 2) are similar to other studies; comparative studies show no difference between nulliparous and parous women. Randomized double-blind studies done in the same clinic have shown the Cu-7 significantly more likely to be expelled than the Cu-T (Mishell 1978; Shaila et al. 1974). However, it should be pointed out that the expulsion rate after a second insertion is very low, so that the problem is more likely a problem of the inserter. In the Student Health Service clinic 29 women (10%) had expulsion after first insertion and of these 20 had a second insertion of whom only one expelled the second device.

III. REMOVALS

III.A. Bleeding or pain

Bleeding and pain are major reasons for discontinuing use of the IUD (Figure 3). There are two factors which affect the removal rate: nulliparity and age. A young nulliparous woman is more likely to require removal of her IUD because of bleeding and pain. The suggestion of Newton et al. (1972), that nulliparous women are less likely to develop menorrhagia, has not been followed up in other studies. In the Student Health Service no IUDs were removed because of menorrhagia in nulliparous women. The gross rates for removal of IUDs for bleeding and pain shown in Figure 3 are similar to those found in other studies on nulliparous women (Newton et al. 1972; Mishell et al. 1973; Jain 1975a, 1975b; Liedholm et al. 1974; Weiner et al. 1978; Shaila et al. 1974).

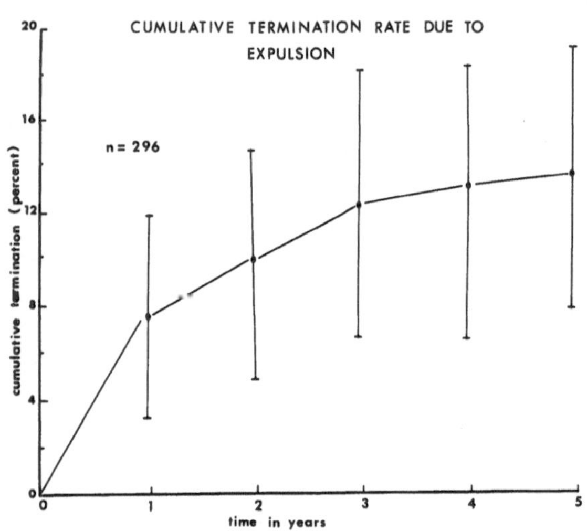

Figure 2. Gross cumulative expulsion rates with copper IUDs in the Student Health Service over five years, with 99% confidence limits.

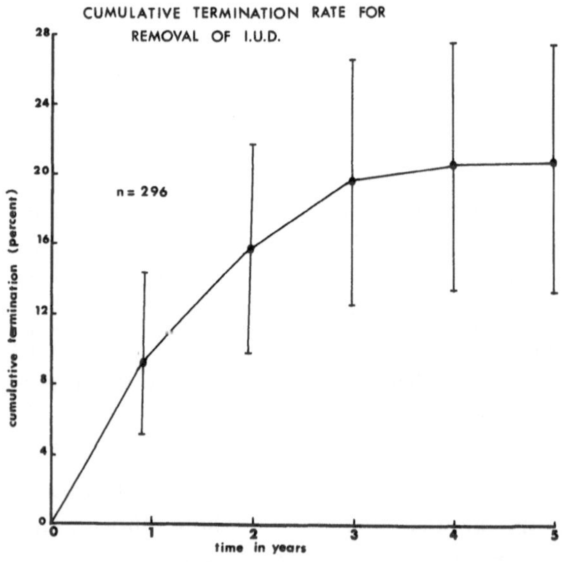

Figure 3. Gross cumulative rates for removal of the Cu IUD for bleeding or pain in the Student Health Service over five years, with 99% confidence limits.

III.B. Other medical reasons

III.B.1. Pelvic inflammatory disease (PID)

Clearly PID is associated with women using an IUD. Retrospective and prospective (Westrom et al. 1976; Eschenbach 1976) studies have shown that PID occurs more frequently in IUD users than in women using other methods of contraception. Furthermore Westrom et al. (1976) showed that nulliparous women were at greater risk than parous women using IUDs. In the Student Health Service problems with PID have not been common; the presented symptoms and other data are shown in Table 1. It is notable that five out of six occurred within thirty days of insertion of the IUD. Liedholm et al. (1974) also reported a high incidence within one month of insertion. It is interesting to note that one woman who had a tender adnexal mass was treated with the IUD in place. Subsequently she had the IUD removed and had a normal intrauterine pregnancy. None of these women were admitted to hospital for laparoscopic confirmation of the diagnosis, so the diagnosis of PID can only be considered presumptive. In one woman out of the six the PID developed secondarily to gonorrhea; the IUD was removed and routine treatment was given for gonorrhea.

Cupric salts have been shown to inhibit the growth of *Neisseria gonorrhea* in vitro (Fiscina et al. 1973), but when this hypothesis was tested clinically there was no evidence of this effect in vivo (Spellacy et al., 1974). There was one case of PID caused by gonorrhea (patient 3 in Table 1) and one case of endocervical gonorrhea treated in the Student Health Service group. Copper IUDs have no adverse effect on endocervical flora and do not interfere with the bacterial sensitivity to antimicrobial agents (Salmi et al. 1976).

III.B.2. Other diseases

Rarely, copper is capable of causing eczematous allergic contact dermatitis; at the Student Health Service two women required removal of their IUDs for this reason. Two reports of a generalized systemic pruritic dermatitis from internal exposure to a copper IUD have appeared in the literature (Barranco 1972; Byrnes 1978).

A report that copper IUDs produced changes of acute cervicitis in 25 percent of women with a healthy cervix at the time of insertion raised the question of possible increased cervical dysplasia and carcinoma in situ. At the Student Health Service there has not been a difference in incidence of class-II cells (dyskaryotic squamous cells) in copper IUD users compared with women using other methods of contraception. The oncogenic potential of copper IUDs is being studied (Misra et al. 1977) but at present there is no evidence of increased incidence of carcinoma in situ in this group of women. The incidence of cervical dysplasia in women wearing copper IUDs in a study by Luthra et al. (1978) has not increased over the expected incidence, although the follow-up time of three years is too short to be conclusive.

Table 1. The clinical symptoms and signs present in those women considered to be suffering from acute pelvic inflammatory disease.

Patient	*To > 38°*	*A*	*B*	*C*	*Raised erythrocyte sedimentation rate*	*Raised white blond cell court*	*IUD removed*	*Within one month of insertion*	*Subsequent pregnancy*
1	yes	yes	yes	no	yes	yes	yes	yes	yes
2	yes	yes	yes	no	yes	yes	yes	yes	no
3	yes	yes	yes	no	not known	yes	yes	no	no
4	yes	yes	yes	yes	not known	not known	no	yes	yes
5	no	yes	yes	no	yes	yes	yes	yes	no
6	yes	yes	yes	yes	not known	yes	no	yes	no

A: Lower abdominal tenderness with guarding.
B: Tenderness on moving the cervix during examination.
C: Palpable tender adnexial mass.

III.C. Planning pregnancy

> Can IUD use affect future fertility? This is an important question which needs to be answered, particularly in relationship to nulliparous women.
>
> Editorial, *British Medical Journal*, 22 July 1978.

As would be expected removal of the IUD for a planned pregnancy occurred with increasing frequency over five years. All women in this small group of ten achieved a live birth. There have been few studies of fecundity following IUD use, and no study has been done on the fecundity of nulliparous IUD wearers. An important paper (Jain and Moots 1977) on the Taiwan study population has shown a decreased fecundity in women over thirty years in correlation with duration of use. The fecundity of women under thirty years did not show this trend, but their numbers were smaller.

The relevant termination rate over five years at the Student Health Service of 44.8 percent is a low one when compared with other methods of contraception (Figure 4). The copper IUD is not usually a first method of choice and the average age at insertion was 21.6 years (range 17-32); for oral contraceptives it was 19.4 years. Even taking this into account a net continuation rate of 55.2 percent over five years is a comparatively high rate and all ten women who planned pregnancy intended to use the IUD as a spacing contraceptive.

IV. COUNSELLING NULLIPAROUS WOMEN REQUESTING A COPPER DEVICE

> The aim is to arrive at a position where teaching of psychological techniques would parallel teaching of insertion skills.
>
> Reading et al. (1977)

Most young women who come to the Student Health Service requesting an IUD are not well informed about it; most have been influenced by a friend who has been wearing an IUD successfully, rather than by any more objective literature or discussion. At the health service approximately 60 percent of the women counselled will have the IUD inserted; of the 40 percent who reject the IUD only a small number do so for medical reasons. Conversely, a number of young women believe that they cannot use the IUD until they have been pregnant.

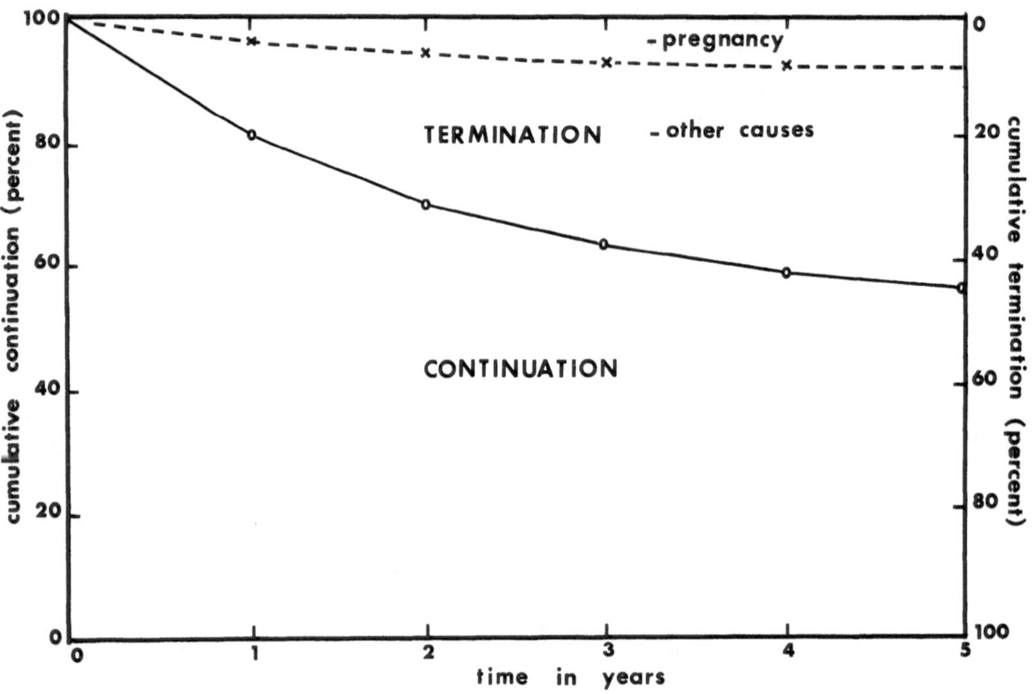

Figure 4. Net cumulative continuation, termination and pregnancy rates in women using Cu IUDs over a five-year period in the Student Health Service.

All women coming for contraceptive advice should have the opportunity to discuss all methods of contraception before making a final choice for themselves. Since controversy exists about the use of IUDs in nulliparous women it is important that the counselling process systematically covers all the controversial issues.

Several authors have commented on various aspects of counselling in relation to use-effectiveness and acceptability of IUDs. Both the technical skill and the counselling skill of the doctor have been shown to be important (Bernard 1969). Different clinics get different results, and even different clinics run by same staff get different results (Snowden et al. 1973), with seemingly the only variable being the time spent in patient contact. Close family members affect the termination rate (Measham et al. 1974), as indeed does the eagerness with which women want to continue the method and accept some discomfort (Willson et al. 1967). The plea for contraceptive providers to pay greater attention to the counselling aspect has been coming for many years and it has now been shown that even the postinsertion pain can be lessened by proper psychological preparation (Reading et al. 1977).

Counselling of nulliparous women about IUD use is an ongoing process through three phases. Counselling is required about:

1. The pros and cons of IUD use;
2. Preinsertion and insertion;
3. Postinsertion.

IV.A. The pros and cons of IUD use

All information should be as accurately and as plainly stated as possible. The counsellor should adjust the discussion to take into account the age and special circumstances (post-abortion, position of uterus, etc.) of each woman counselled in the following areas:

IV.A.1. Pregnancy

1. Rates.

2. What would you do if you became pregnant?

3. The importance of early diagnosis of pregnancy and removal of the device before the strings retract into the uterus.

IV.A.2. Expulsion

1. Rates.

2. Importance of self-examination of the vagina to feel the cervix and IUD strings.

3. If the first device is expelled a second insertion is advised.

IV.A.3. Removal for bleeding and pain

1. Information with regard to expectation of heavy periods, particularly during the subsequent three menstruations.

2. Cramping and spotting are common following the insertion up to first menstruation.

3. If she cannot tolerate the IUD because of pain and bleeding, removing the device is easier than inserting it.

IV.A.4. Risk factors

1. Rarely fundal perforation can occur and would necessitate a surgical operation for removing the device.

2. The importance of early recognition of uterine perforation by self-examination.

3. Cervical perforation can occur with partial expulsion of the device.

4. Ectopic pregnancy may be more common with the IUD in place; a surgical operation would be needed.

5. She should know that PID is more likely to occur in women using an IUD than other methods and that it is more likely to occur in the first month after insertion.

6. She should appreciate that PID after the first month may be related to sexual transmission and that there is evidence that women with multiple sexual partners are at a greater risk. She should know that a prophylactic approach to sexually transmitted disease might be taken in the case of a sexual indiscretion.

IV.A.5. Pros

1. There are some advantages to the IUD, you know! It is noncoital, usually comfortable, has a smaller range of complications than oral contraceptives; the mortality-benefit ratio is excellent (Jain 1975a, 1975b).

2. The IUD is the most continued method in nullipara; when they are good they are very, very good.

3. The pregnancy rate is low when compared with no contraception.

4. Each person having an IUD is treated as an individual trial; statistics mean very little when dealing with the individual.

IV.B. Preinsertion and insertion

Prior to the insertion procedure young nulliparous women should be examined by the prospective inserter. This allows a sense of confidence to develop between them, and it is an important opportunity for education (Percival-Smith 1978). At the examination the uterus and adnexa may be assessed, and a discussion of the insertion procedure can be completed. She can then be asked to return by appointment during her next menstrual cycle for the insertion of her IUD. If an infection is detected on the culture, this should be treated before insertion. Class-II cervical cytology (dyskaryotic squamous cells) does not preclude the insertion of an IUD.

Since it is now clear that the risk of infection at the time of insertion is as great as at any other time, it is not acceptable to insert an IUD into a nulliparous woman without a proper aseptic technique. Use of surgical gloves, sterile instruments, proper nursing assistance and careful antisepsis of the vagina are essential to the insertion procedure. A fast-acting (dental) anesthetic like prolocaine should be used on the anterior lip of the cervix before it is grasped with the tenaculum. An intracervical local anesthetic can be performed at three, six and nine o'clock around the cervix. This will allow for a pain-free sounding of the internal cervical os; and if the sound will not itself dilate the internal os, then dilatation may be performed up to the equivalent of a No. 4 Hagar dilator, thus allowing a Cu-T200 to pass through the internal os. If the No. 3 Hagar dilator or equivalent does not pass easily into the uterine cavity, the woman is best advised against continuing with the procedure. When the sound touches the fundus of the uterus the woman will experience a menstrual-like cramp; on removal of the sound this will settle down. She should be warned of this discomfort prior to the touching of the fundus. If the cramping is very severe and does not settle quickly she should be advised against continuing with the procedure. The IUD may then be removed from its package by the nurse and inserted into the uterus using the manufacturer's suggested procedure. In the case of the Cu-T200 a high fundal placement can be assured if, after releasing the arms of the device, the inserter tube is again advanced into the uterus so that the arms are pushed up against the fundus. The strings are then trimmed to about 2 cm. The records concerning the IUD insertion should include the uterine length, the type of IUD inserted, any problems encountered at insertion, and the length of the IUD strings.

IV.C. Postinsertion

1. The importance of feeling for the strings should be stressed and she should be encouraged to feel the strings before she leaves the clinic.

2. There is some concern that using a tampon after insertion may inadvertently pull the IUD out. Sanitary napkins are advisable for the first 24 h postinsertion.

3. Mild analgesic medication may be needed during the first few days postinsertion.

4. The minimum follow-up for IUDs of once within three months and yearly thereafter is suggested.

5. It is helpful to have the counselling information summarized into a 'take-home' information pamphlet to reinforce the postinsertion advice and to summarize some of the important features of the preinsertion counsellings (i.e. expected bleeding patterns and so on).

IV.D. Some special considerations

During the first five years of using copper IUDs in the Student Health Service, inability to insert the device occurred in 28 women, which represents 8.6 percent of first insertions. In twenty women cervical stenosis of the internal os precluded insertion of the device. Of these twenty, six decided not to continue with the device and fourteen were referred to a gynecologist who inserted the IUD using a local anesthetic and dilating the cervix before insertion. In the other eight women pain prior to insertion caused discontinuation of the procedure. Four women developed severe pain on grasping the cervix with the tenaculum; four women developed pain with vasovagal syncope. Partly as a result of this experience and partly to make the insertion procedure more acceptable it was decided to use an intracervical local anesthetic routinely in nulliparous women.

Insertion problems were encountered in 31 women (9.6%). In five women technical difficulty was encountered. Three women had a very small cervix with a small external os which could not be sounded without risk of trauma; two women had acutely anteflexed uteri. A short uterus (less than 5 cm) is a contraindication to using an IUD since the results are poor (Gibor et al. 1973).

Ten women developed pain, pallor, sweating and bradycardia. They were treated with atropine sulphate 0.2 mg i.v. and 0.2 mg s.c. They made a prompt recovery with their pulses rising and colour improving within two minutes.

Three women developed syncope with their pain and were treated with atropine and Demerol 100 mg i.m. to control the bradycardia and pain. In two of the women the IUD had to be removed.

One woman developed pain, syncope and then developed a *grand mal* seizure from the severe bradycardia. She required treatment with oxygen, atropine, resuscitation and removal of the IUD. She was kept in hospital for observation for 24 h.

Since using routine local anesthetics, women have not needed referral from the clinic for insertion. Whilst the numbers are too small for statistical analysis, the trend appears to be toward fewer vasovagal attacks, less pain at and after insertion, and a lower removal rate for pain and bleeding in the first year.

Whilst the mode of action of the IUD is of interest to many women it was not considered an essential part of the counselling. The results of a study showing that human chorionic gonadotropin was detectable in 15 percent of the luteal phases of women wearing IUDs (Beling et al. 1976) were reported in the local news media. This raised an important ethical issue for a number of women wearing IUDs. Since that time a similar study (Klein et al. 1977) has failed to confirm these findings. That some women would distinguish between preventing implantation and causing an early abortion came as an unexpected surprise. It is important that women be given the opportunity to discuss ethical issues and IUD contraception.

The copper IUD may be used as a postcoital method of contraception with good results (Lippes et al. 1976) and certainly offers an alternative to the chemical methods available.

V. CONTRAINDICATIONS IN NULLIPAROUS WOMEN

V.A. Absolute

1. A uterus less than 5.5 cm in length.
2. Acute anteflexion or retroflexion of the uterus.
3. A small cervix and external os; cervical diameter of less than 1 cm.
4. Congenital anomalies of the uterus.
5. Possible pregnancy.
6. Suspected vaginal or cervical infection at the time of insertion.
7. Undiagnosed pelvic mass at the time of insertion.
8. Undiagnosed medical illness at the time of insertion: anemia, blood dyscrasia, and so on.

V.B. Relative

1. Previous history of PID.
2. Cervical dysplasia (class-II cervical cytology).
3. Severe emotional disorder.
4. History of severe dysmenorrhea.
5. Under 19 years of age.

REFERENCES

American Journal of Obstetrics and Gynecology: Study of the Copper-T200 and Copper-7 intrauterine devices with modified insertion techniques. Am 5 Obstet Gynecol 120: 110, 1974.

Barranco VP: Eczematous dermatitis caused by internal exposure to copper. Arch Dermatol 106: 386, 1972.

Beling CG et al: Demonstration of chorionic gonadotropin during the second half of the cycle of women using IUD contraception. Am J Obstet Gynecol 125: 855, 1976.

Bernard RP: Factors governing IUD performance. Am J Public Health 61: 559-567, 1969.

British Medical Journal: Editorial: the nulliparous patient, the IUD and subsequent fertility. Br Med J 2(6132): 233, 1978.

Burnhill MS: Prescriptive approaches to IUD usage. In: Intrauterine devices, Wheeler RG et al (eds.), New York, Academic Press, 1974.

Byrnes AJ: Allergy to copper in intra-uterine devices. Med J Aust 2(11): 532-533, 1978.

c01Cheng Chi I et al: An epidemiologic study of intrauterine contraceptive devices: a preliminary report. In: Risks, benefits, and controversies in fertility control, Sciarra JJ et al (eds.), New York, Harper and Row, 1978.

Eschenbach DA: Acute pelvic inflammatory disease etiology, risk factors, and pathogenesis. Clin Obstet Gynecol 19: 147, 1976.

Fiscina B, et al: Gonococcicidal action of copper in vitro. Am J Obstet Gynecol 116: 86, 1973.

Gibor Y, et al: Uterine .length: a prognostic indicator for successful use of the Copper-7 IUD. J Reprod Med 11(5): 205-208, 1973.

Jain AK: Safety and effectiveness of intrauterine devices. Contraception 1(3): 243, 1975a.

Jain AK: Comparative performance of three types of IUD in the United States. In: Analysis of intrauterine contraception, Hefnawi F, Segal SD (eds), Amsterdam, North-Holland Biomedical Press, 1975b.

Jain AK, Moots B: Fecundability following the discontinuation of IUD use among Taiwanese women. J Biosoc Sci 9 (2): 137-152, 1977.

Klein TA, et al: Absence of circulatory chorionic gonadotropin in wearers of IUDs. Am J Obstet Gynecol 129 (6): 626-628, 1977.

Liedhom P, et al: Two years experience with Copper-T200 in a Swedish population: a comparison between nulliparous and parous women. Contraception 10 (1): 55-61, 1974.

Lippes J, et al: The post-coital Copper-T. Adv Plann Parent 11(1): 24-29, 1976.

Luthra VK et al.: Role of Cu IUD in cervical carcinogenesis: a followup of 36 months. Indian J Med Res 68: 78-83, 1978.

Measham AR, et al: The role of the family in post-partum family planning acceptance. Int J Gynaecol Obstet 12: 66-71, 1974.

Mishell DR Jr: In: Risks, benefits and controversies in fertility control, Sciarra JJ, et al (eds), New York, Harper and Row, 1978.

Mishell DR Jr, et al.: Pregnancy related complications and bleeding problems with IUDs. A study of the Copper-T intrauterine device (T-Cu-200) in nulliparous women. Am J Obstet Gunecol 116: 1092, 1973.

Misra JS, et al: Cytological studies in women using copper intrauterine devices. Acta Cytol Scand 21(4): 514-8, 1977.

Newton JR, et al: Intrauterine contraception using the copper-7 device. Lancet 2: 951, 1972.

Newton JR, et al: In: Analysis of intrauterine contraception, Hefnawi F, Segal SJ (eds), Amsterdam, North-Holland Biomedical Press, 1975.

Osser S, et al: Is development of PID in women using IUDs equal regardless of parity: one-year follow-up. Contraception 17(6): 563, 1978.

Percival-Smith R: An educative approach to pelvic examination in young women. Can Family Physician 24: 357-361, 1978.

Reading AE, et al: The effects of psychological preparation on pain at intrauterine device insertion. Contraception 16(5): 523-532, 1977.

Reading AE, et al: Psychological factors in IUD use: a review J Biosoc Sci 9: 317-323, 1977.

Rubinstein E: The Cu-7 device in chronic and IUD-induced acute cervicitis treated with oral estriol. Contraception 10(6): 673-683, 1974.

Salmi T, et al: Cervical Bacterial flora in women fitted with a copper-releasing intrauterine contraceptive device (IUD). Acta Obstet Gynecol Scand 55: 317, 1976.

Shaila NG et al: A comparative randomized double blind study of copper T 200 and copper 7 intrauterine contraceptive devices with modified insertion techniques. Am J Obstet Gynecol. 120 (1): 110, Sept 1974.

Sivin I: Copper-T IUD use and ectopic pregnancy rates in the United States. Contraception 19(2): 151-174, 1979.

Snowden R, et al: Social and medical factors in the use and effectiveness of IUDs. J Biosoc Sci 5: 31-49, 1973.

Spellacy WW, et al: The effect of copper intrauterine devices on endocervical gonococcicidal cultures. Fertil Steril 25: 772, 1974.

Tatum H: Clinical aspects of intrauterine contraception: circumspection 1976. Obstet Gynecol Annu, 1978.

Tatum H, Schmidt F: Contraceptive and sterilization practices and extrauterine pregnancy: a realistic perspective. Fertil Steril 24(4): 407-421, 1977.

Weiner E, et al: Copper intrauterine contraception devices in adolescent nullipara. Br J Obstet Gynaecol 85: 204-206, 1978.

Westrom L, et al: The risk of pelvic inflammatory disease in women using intrauterine contraceptive devices as compared with non-users. Lancet 2: 221, 1976.

Willson JR, et al: IUD: a comparison between their use in indigent and private patients. Obstet Gynecol 29: 59-66, 1967.

12. IMMEDIATE POSTPLACENTAL INSERTION OF AN IUD

M. Thiery

The desirability of initiating contraception soon after delivery is self-evident (Echeverry 1973; Zatuchni 1970: virtually no puerpera desires a new pregnancy right away and, except in women who are breast-feeding or taking a long-acting steroid preparation to inhibit lactation (van Bogaert et al. 1977), resumption of ovulation may take place early (Zarate et al. 1974).

Regrettably, puerperal application of some of the currently available contraceptive methods involves disadvantages. Before the involution of the genital tract is completed the risk inherent in tubal sterilization is increased (Ministry of Health 1969) and the effectiveness of the operation less than optimal (Prystowsky and Eastman 1955). The diaphragm fit must be checked after resumption of pelvic integrity. Many women still find pill-taking unattractive during a period when they do not have sexual intercourse. Laymen share with too many professionals the belief not only that the pill interferes with lactation but also that steroidal contraception may have adverse effects on the baby because the steroid compounds pass the blood-milk barrier (Nilsson and Nygren 1979). Injected medroxyprogesterone acetate, besides only requiring periodic motivation, reportedly has a beneficial effect on lactation (Zanartu et al. 1976). However, the reversibility of the antifertility effect of the method is entirely unpredictable (Karim et al. 1971), and the medication, when administered at the time of discharge after confinement, will sometimes produce unacceptably prolonged and distressing metrorrhagia (Staelens et al. 1979). Finally, the Federal Drug Administration ban on this compound for contraceptive purposes has probably affected the acceptance of this method in many countries.

According to classical views, IUD insertion is only safe and effective after uterine involution is complete (Snowdon et al. 1977; Pollock 1979), and most doctors hold to this principle because of the fear of specific complications (for example uterine perforation and pelvic inflammatory disease) and the risk of expulsion. Undoubtedly, hazards of earlier IUD insertion have been overrated (Banharnsupawat and Rosenfield 1971), the high incidence of uterine perforations reported for example from Singapore (Tow et al. 1967) being in fact restricted almost entirely to IUD insertions performed six or more weeks after delivery. Nonetheless, the main obstacle to early postpartum IUD insertion remains the inverse relationship between the delivery-to-insertion interval and the expulsion rate (Zatuchni 1970; Pollock 1979). However this phenomenon has been documented for first-generation IUDs and must be checked for the newer IUD models.

An entirely new approach is to insert the IUD on the delivery table immediately after expulsion of the placenta and membranes. The advantages and disadvantages of this approach, called immediate postplacental insertion (IPPI), are discussed in this chapter.

I. DEFINITIONS

An IUD can be inserted at various times (Table 1). Apart from the introduction of a device through the uterine incision at abdominal delivery, three categories of postpartum (puerperal) insertion can be distinguished; (1) immediate postplacental insertion, that is placement of an IUD immediately after delivery of the afterbirth while the woman is still lying on the delivery table; (2) early postpartum or predischarge insertion, that is, from the first postpartum day on but before the women leaves the

Table 1. Timing of IUD insertion.

In cycling women (interim or interval insertion)
1. during menstruation
2. second half of menstrual cycle

In noncycling women
1. duting pathologic amenorrhea
2. during physiologic amenorrhea
   - 2.1 postabortion insertion
     - 2.1.1. after first-trimester abortion (< 12 weeks gestation): immediate, early or delayed insertion
     - 2.1.2. after second-trimester abortion (12-18 weeks gestation): immediate, early or delayed insertion
   - 2.2 postpartum or puerperal insertion (> 28 weeks gestation)
     - 2.2.1 at cesarean section
     - 2.2.2 immediate postplacental insertion
     - 2.2.3 early (predischarge) postpartum insertion
     - 2.2.4. delayed (postdischarge) postpartum insertion

maternity clinic, usually between days 4 and 6 ; and (3) delayed puerperal or postdischarge insertion, that is after discharge but before the first menstrual period, including the period of lactation and amenorrhea.

II. BENEFITS

Theoretically, IPPI offers several advantages over predischarge and delayed puerperal insertion :(1) because even in developing countries a high proportion of gravidas deliver in hospital settings, albeit on an outpatient basis, so the method reaches a large number of women, is applied at a moment when the woman's contraceptive motivation is very high, and confers protection before the resumption of sexual activity and ovulation, two events which in practice show tremendous individual variability; (2) the IUD is easily inserted under sterile conditions through a patent cervical canal; (3) signs of the puerperium and afterbirth pains mask the postinsertion symptoms; and (4) in contrast with oral contraception, IPPI asks for almost no repeat motivation and the financial burden is small.

III. EXPERIENCE

III.A. Reported experience

In the literature details concerning the timing of postpartum IUD insertion are often vague and terminology is sometimes misleading. For example, the term 'immediate [contraception] acceptor' (Zatuchni 1970) corresponds in most instances to our category of 'early' IUD application. Reported experience with IPPI is scanty and usually combined with that of other categories of puerperal insertion. In fact, it is limited to the results of two international programmes and to a few smaller reports, mainly on pilot or feasibility studies.

Between 1966 and 1968, the Population Council sponsored the International Postpartum Family Planning Program (Zatuchni 1970; Castadot et al. 1975). Only the Lippes D Loop was used, and very few of the insertions belonged to the genuine IPPI category. When the IUD was placed within 24 h of delivery, expulsion rates amounted on average to 27 percent and in some centers initially even to 50 percent. The poor results were ascribed to lack of experience with the method (device inserted in the lower uterine segment) and the use of too short an inserter. Bangkok participated in this study (Banharnsupawat and Rosenfield 1971): the loop was inserted on the first postpartum day in only 0.7 of the subjects (N=48) and in this subgroup, which includes IPPI, the rate of first expulsions amounted to 19 per hundred users at one year. Largely because of the good follow-up, the rate of pregnancy was low (1.3 percent at one year). More recently, the WHO launched a multicentre trial (Trial No. 74,059) to evaluate randomly the Cu-T200, the Cu 7-200, and the Lippes Loop D inserted immediately after the delivery of the placenta. For this study, which terminated in August 1977, only preliminary and unpublished results are available (P. Rowe, personal communication, 1979). They indicate that for all of the devices studied the expulsion rate was high (20-30% of insertions) in all but two centres (which had a 10-15% expulsion rate); it also cannot be excluded here that partially expelled devices were reinserted. Of the 280 expulsions, 247 (88%) occurred within three months of insertion.

Zerzavy (1967) published the results of a pilot study on IPPI. In fifteen women a large Birnberg

Bow was inserted manually immediately after completion of the third stage of labour; a few devices (number not stated) were placed at Cesarean section. This series is very small and the data concerning genuine IPPI were not given separately. For the entire postpartum group, with IPPI including insertion at Cesarean section plus early and delayed insertions, a total of 63 subjects and 813 woman months of experience, the expulsion rate was low (1.6%) but the pregnancy rate high (8.0%). The single case of expulsion was discovered three weeks postpartum. Neither infection, interference with uterine involution, unusual increase in lochial flow nor cramps immediately after insertion were observed, there was no effect on the menstrual cycle. From Beth Israel Hospital, New York, Rashbaum and Wallach (1971) reported splendid results with the Petal or Lem device, a radioopaque inert polyethylene IUD provided with a monofilament polyethylene thread tied to the stem (Figure 1). The authors performed IPPI in 125 subjects. Up to 21 months of observation (life table analysis was not used) five expulsions (4%) and one pregnancy (0.8%) were recorded; in 5.6 percent of the subjects the device had to be removed because of pain or bleeding. There were no serious complications. In contrast, a larger IPPI trial (1,359 insertions and 8,613 woman-months of use) in which the same device was inserted according to the same technique, has yielded less favourable results (Apelo et al. 1976): at 12 months, the net cumulative pregnancy and expulsion rates amounted to 5 and 20 percent respectively. However the one-year removal rate for bleeding or pain was quite low (2.2%).

Within twenty minutes of delivery of the placenta, Newton et al. (1977) applied one of the following IUD models: the Lem device (N= 100); the Cu-7-200 (N = 123); and the Progestasert system (N = 51) using a somewhat longer (25 cm) inserter. In the first six weeks after the insertion there were 7 percent expulsions of the Lem, 7.3 percent of the Cu-7-200, and 2 percent of the Progestasert. Uterine perforations were not diagnosed and there was no difference in puerperal morbidity between the propositae and their matched controls.

A variety of IUD models, some of them specially designed and others only adapted for immediate postplacental insertion, are being or have been tested, but no hard data are available. In addition, a new principle, the so-called suture devices, aiming at better IUD retention within the involuting uterine cavity is under study. It consists in the addition of short sutures of chromic catgut to the upper cross-arm of the Lippes Loop or to the horizontal bar of a T-shaped device (Figure 1). The projections embed in the endometrium of the fundus uteri, biodegrade, and vanish in approximately the same

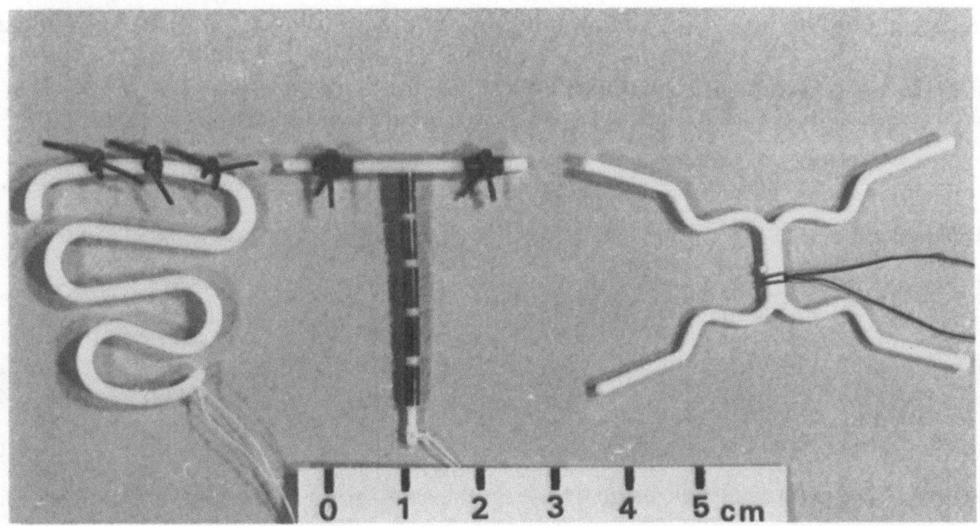

Figure 1. Left: two types of suture device: the suture Lippes Loop D and the suture Cu-T220C. Right: the Petal of Lem IUD.

time interval needed for the uterus to regain its original size (Potts 1978). Preliminary results are encouraging. The six-month net life table expulsion rate amounts to 5.3 percent for the sutured Lippes Loop, (N = 341), and to 8.6 percent for the sutured Cu-T220c N = 324 (Laufe et al. 1979; B. Taylor, personal communication, 1979).

III.B. Personal experience

The low expulsion rate observed during interim application of the ML Cu 250, a new copper-wired IUD (Thiery et al. 1978a, prompted us to assess this device for IPPI as well. Since the preliminary results were encouraging (van Os et al. 1976; Thiery et al. 1978b), the straight trial was expanded and eventually extended to provide a randomized comparative study.

III.B.1. Straight evaluation of the ML Cu 250

Six hundred devices were inserted with the usual 20-cm inserter immediately after delivery of the placenta in women who had given birth at or about term (Thiery et al. 1979a). Thirty months after the insertion, the data, covering 9,843 woman-months of experience, were computerized and analyzed according to the life table method (Table 2, Figure 2). The gross cumulative pregnancy and expulsion rates amount to 1.3 and 6.0, respectively. More than half of the expulsions occurred within the first six months after insertion, and the expulsion rate did not increase after the first year. Six unwanted pregnancies occurred, all of them within the first year, but there were no ectopics. The removal rates for bleeding and pain suggest an inverse relationship with the age of the acceptor. Parity had no marked effect on the pertinent event rates. No IUDs had to be removed for medical reasons other than bleeding or pain. We were aware of translocation in utero in eight instances. Seven of these were properly diagnosed (three by radiography and

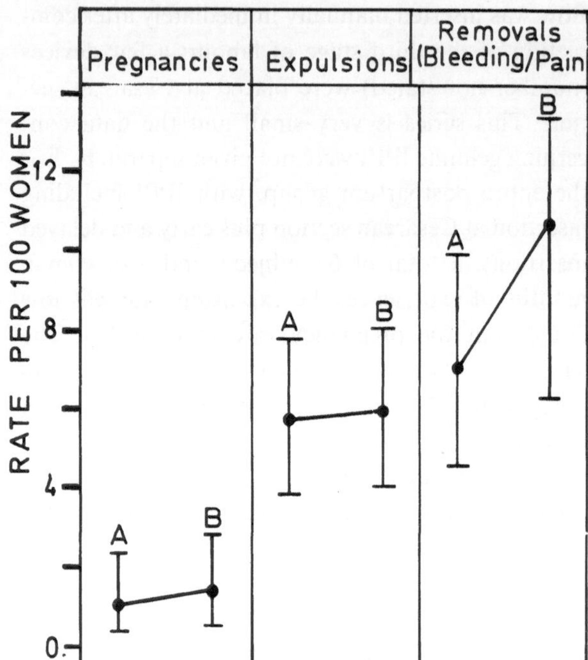

Figure 2. Immediate postplacental insertion of the ML Cu 250: gross cumulative event rates (and 95% confidence limits) per 100 users, at one (A) and two (B) years (Thiery et al. 1979a).

Table 2. Immediate postplacental insertion of ML Cu 250 (N = 600): gross cumulative event rates per 100 users at six-month intervals, with upper and lower confidence limits at the 95-percent level in parentheses. (Thiery et al. 1979a.)

	6 months	*12 months*	*18 months*	*24 months*	*30 months*
Woman-months of use	3,315	5,895	7,770	9,138	9,843
Events					
Accidental pregnancy	0.6(0.1-1.7)	1.0(0.3-2.3)	1.3(0.5 2.8)	1.3(0.5 2.8)	1.3(0.5 2.8)
Expulsions	3.7(2.1-5.2)	5.8(3.8-7.8)	6.0(4.0-8.1)	6.0(4.0-8.1)	6.0(4.0-8.1)
Removals					
– bleeding/pain	4.3(2.4-5.5)	7.1(4.5-9.8)	9.1(5.7-11.9)	10.7(6.3-13.2)	11.8(7.2-14.8)
– planned pregnancy	0.6(0.1-1.6)	7.3(4.8-9.8)	12.8(9.5-16.1)	15.9(12.2-19.7)	18.0(14.0-22.1)
– other personal reasons	3.6(2.0-5.1)	5.1(3.2-7.0)	6.0(3.9-8.)	6.4(4.2-8.7)	7.1(4.7-10.0)
– investigator's choice	1.6(0.7-3.0)	1.6(0.7-3.0)	1.9(0.9-3.5)	1.9(0.9-3.5)	1.9(0.9-3.5)
Continuation rate	87.2	72.7	64.0	59.7	55.8
Lost to follow-up	1.5(0.6-2.9)	4.5(2.6-6.3)	5.9(3.7-8.0)	11.4(8.0-14.8)	15.0(11.0-19.1)
Released from study	0.4(0.0-1.3)	0.6(0.1-1.8)	0.9(0.2-2.3)	1.3(0.4-3.0)	1.3(0.4-3.0)

four by hysteroscopy) and removed. One inversion within the uterine cavity was diagnosed at removal of the IUD for unwanted pregnancy. The method had no significant effect on uterine involution, puerperal pyrexia, or bleeding, and did not influence the return to normal menstruation. Therefore, we consider the ML Cu 250 a fair candidate for IPPI, the only theoretical risk associated with the method being intrauterine translocation of the device, which could lead to erosion and ultimately to perforation of the uterine fundus by the stem of the device. Consequently, it is our, unsupported, opinion that translocation should be actively detected and managed by removal of the IUD.

Recently, Ruiz-Velasco et al. (1978) have reported comparable preliminary results with IPPI in 200 women using the ML Cu 250.

III.B.2. Comparative assessment of the ML Cu 250 and the Cu-T200

This randomized comparative IPPI trial (Thiery et al. 1979b) is being performed in 562 women, 293 of whom were fitted with an ML Cu 250 (Table 3). At two years, 8.036 woman-months of experience had accumulated. At that time, the gross cumulative pregnancy rate for the CU-T200 and the ML Cu 250 amounted to 1.2 and 2.4 respectively. At two years, the gross cumulative expulsion rates for the Cu-T200 and the ML Cu 250 were 11.2 and 9.9 respectively. The removal rates for bleeding and pain did not differ significantly between the two devices tested.

Figure 3 shows the cumulative pregnancy and expulsion rates at two years for both devices inserted into a nonpregnant uterine cavity (interim insertion) as well as immediately after the delivery of the placenta. It is evident that only the expulsion rate is significantly affected by the time of insertion.

Figure 4 shows the cumulative expulsion rates

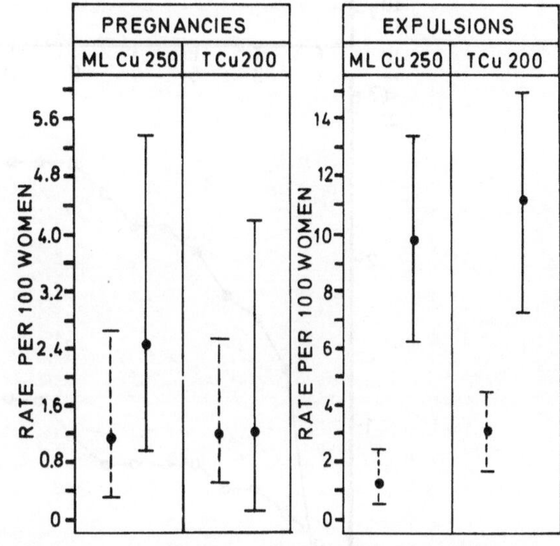

Figure 3. Immediate postplacental (solid line) and interim (broken line) insertion of the ML Cu 250 and the Cu-T200 gross cumulative pregnancy and expulsion rates (and 95% confidence limits) per 100 users, at two years (Thiery et al. 1979b.).

Table 3. Immediate postplacental insertion: randomized study of Cu-T200 (N = 269), against ML Cu 250, (N = 293), with upper and lower confidence limits at the 95-percent level in parentheses (Thiery et al. 1979b).

	12 months Cu-T200	ML Cu-250	*24 months* Cu-T200	ML Cu-250
Woman-months of use	2,632	2,902	3,796	4,240
Events				
Accidental pregnancy	0.5(0.0-2.6)	2.4(0.9-5.3)	1.2(0.1-4.2)	2.4(0.9-5.3)
Expulsions	11.2(7.3-15.1)	9.9(6.3-13.5)	11.2(7.3-15.1)	9.9(6.3-13.5)
Removals				
– bleeding/pain	1.8(0.5-4.5)	3.6(1.6-7.1)	5.2(2.1-10.7)	5.9(2.4-9.3)
– other medical reasons	0.4(0.0-2.3)	0.9(0.1-3.1)	0.4(0.0-2.3)	0.9(0.1-3.1)
– planned pregnancy	8.6(4.7-12.5)	5.6(2.5-8.7)	16.0(10.4-21.6)	12.9(7.6-18.1)
– other personal reasons	1.2(0.2-3.6)	3.2(1.4-6.3)	1.2(0.2-3.6)	6.7(3.0-10.4)
– investigator's choice	0.4(0.0-2.2)	1.1(0.2-3.2)	0.4(0.0-2.2)	1.1(0.2-3.2)
Continuation rate	77.2	77.3	67.2	66.5
Lost to follow-up	2.0(0.5-5.1)	1.6(0.4-4.1)	2.0(0.5-5.1)	3.1(1.0-7.2)
Released from study	0.8(0.1-3.0)	0.8(0.1-3.1)	4.2(1.3-9.8)	2.1(0.4-6.2)

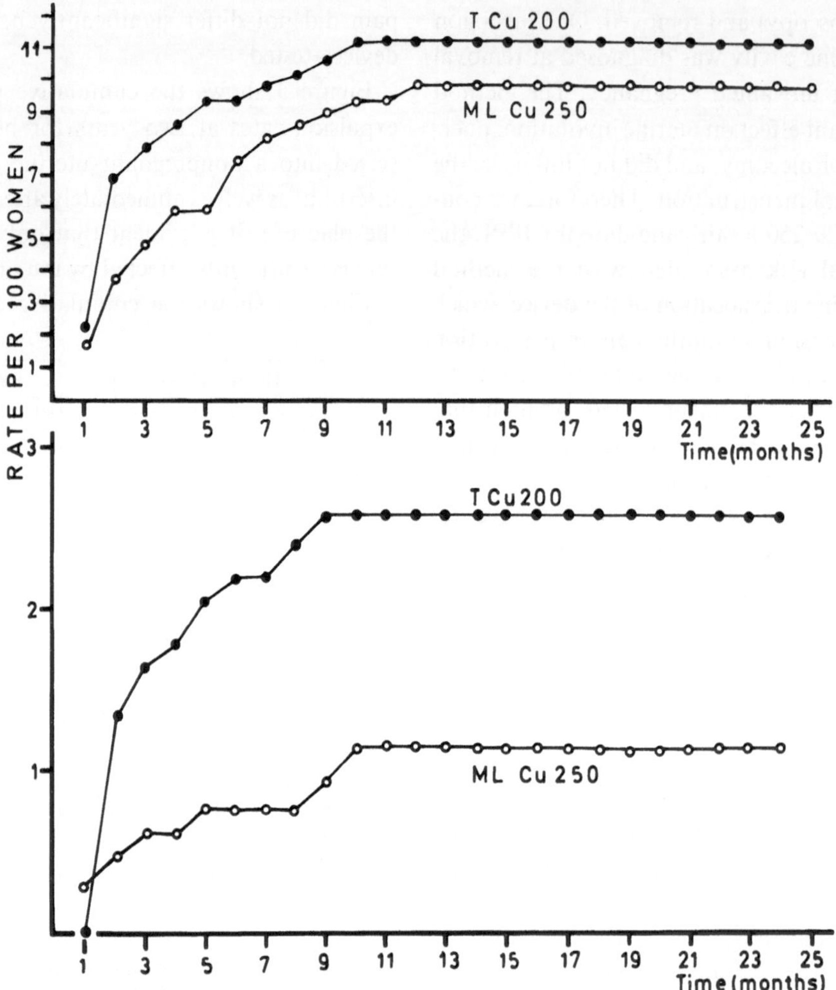

Figure 4. Gross cumulative expulsion rates (per months) of the ML Cu 250 (circles) and the Cu-T200 (spots) after, top: immediate postplacental insertion; and bottom interim placement (Thiery et al. 1979b).

per month after IPPI: the ML Cu 250 was retained slightly more often than the Cu-T200 but the trend of the expulsion is comparable for the two devices. After interim placement, the expulsion rates characterizing the two IUDs differ significantly, but under these conditions too the trend toward early expulsion observed after IPPI is clearly present.

IV. INSERTION TECHNIQUE

Immediate postplacental insertion of an IUD (ML Cu 250 or Tmodel) is a very simple procedure. Our standard technique is as follows. After delivery of the placenta and the membranes, we routinely insert the blade of a bayonet speculum into the anterior vaginal vault, grasp both the anterior and the posterior lips of the cervix with one or two ring forceps and draw the cervix down for close inspection. If no tears are found and before episiotomy repair is undertaken, we insert the IUD. For this purpose the loaded inserter tube is slipped along the palmar aspect of two fingers inserted into the uterine cavity until it is felt that the IUD has reached the fundus. In case of doubt, we check with the flat right hand on the abdominal wall covering the fundal region. The inserter is then withdrawn very gently, taking care not to pull on the strings, which are left uncut. Steadying of the uterus with ring forceps is also advocated by other investigators (Rashbaum and Wallach 1971; Apelo et al. 1976) but the WHO programmers have questioned the necessity for this procedure (P. Rowe, personal communication, 1979). Newton et al. (1977) use a comparable insertion technique, albeit with slight variations:

> The patient or the assistant places the flat of the hand over the fundus of the uterus and exerts gentle downward pressure thus bringing the open cervix to a lower level. The IUD in the inserter tube is taken into the right hand: two fingers of the left hand are then inserted into the vagina and against the inner surface of the posterior wall of the open cervix. The IUD is then inserted into the uterus with the left hand as a guide. The resistance of the firmly contracted uterus is easily felt so that the IUD can be correctly placed in the fundus. When the IUD is at the fundus the tread is released (the authors use a tube provided with a slit) and the inserter tube withdrawn. The mobile uterus is controlled during this procedure by the hand of the patient or assistant.

We use the standard inserter for both the ML Cu 250 and the CU-T200 for the latter with the plunger removed. The tube acts merely as a pusher (push in technique). Laufe et al. (1979) prefer manual insertion, at least for the Lippes Loop. Because it is impossible to place a device in the fundus without the hand first coming into contact with the vaginal flora, H.J. Tatum (personal communication, 1979) is firmly opposed to manual placement on the grounds of the increased chance of introducing bacteria. In our experience, a standard inserter of about 20 cm permits fundal placement of both an ML Cu 250 and a T device. However, the high expulsion rates observed with Lippes Loop D (Zatuchni 1970; Castadot et al. 1975) prompted several hospitals to introduce king-size inserters. Subsequently, expulsion rates fell in centres using this device but it could not be determined whether this drop was the result of the inserter or the increased experience with early postpartum insertion. More recent experience has not shown any relationship between the use of long inserters and lower expulsion rates (Castadot et al. 1975), but Newton et al. (1977) believe that the introduction of a 25-cm inserter tube improved their expulsion rate.

As mentioned, we do not cut the strings short after the insertion, and we urge the woman not to use tampons before the first follow-up visit. However, missing strings may be a problem (Millen et al. 1978; Lancet 1979) and may indicate expulsion, perforation,translocation in utero, or simply that the thread has become wound around the device. Recently, several devices such as a Karman catheter (Goh 1978) or a flexible flat helix of plastic (Husemeyer and Gordon 1979) have been proposed for retrieval of IUD threads from within the uterine cavity. Our management of this situation is as follows. If the threads cannot be seen at the first postpartum visit, a cautious attempt is made to extend the tailpiece with a platinum loop or a blunt-ended suction catheter. If these manoeuvres fail, the patient is reexamined after her first menstrual period and if the tailpiece is still invisible at that time, a radiographic control (flat plate) is performed with Allis forceps as a marker clamped to the anterior lip (Figure 5). One coauthor has recently resorted to hysteroscopy to assess patients with unextruded tailpieces. The problem of retracted threads might be solved by affixing longer strings to devices used for IPPI or by using the following trick. To prevent loss of the threads, Rashbaum and Wallach (1977) and Apelo et al. (1976) attach an absorbable catgut suture to the permanent thread of the Lem device, cutting it beyond the external os immediately after insertion; after 6-14 days, the suture is expelled, leaving the nonabsorbable thread extending through the cervix.

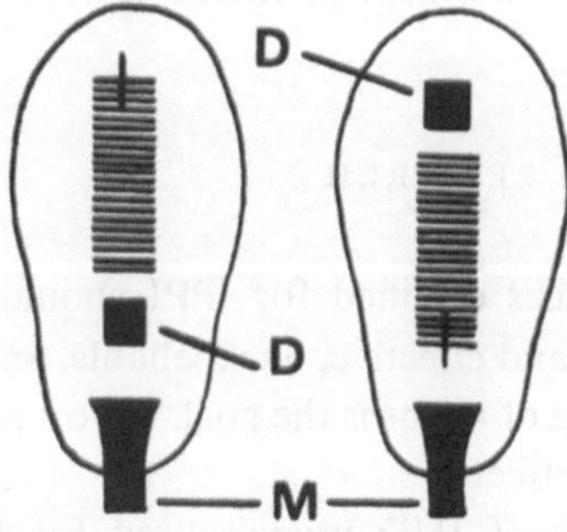

Figure 5. The ML Cu 250 in correct position (left) or inverted within the involuted uterine cavity (right). The position of the device is correct when the dot of solid metallic copper (D) is found pointing toward the marker (M).

V. FOLLOW-UP

Originally we checked all our *patients* radiographically at the time of hospital discharge. Because all of the devices (N =about 200) could be visualized, the procedure was discarded, and at present we check for expulsion simply by digital examination at the time of discharge. In addition, women are asked to refrain from using tampons, and were instructed to inspect pads for an expelled IUD before discarding them.

At the first postpartum visit (5-6 weeks), the nylon thread is usually found protruding from the uterine os and is shortened. If the tailpiece cannot be seen the situation is handled as described above. Only when the IUD is found inverted in utero is it removed, using forceps or a hook; a new device is immediately inserted.

As stated, inversion is probably the only risky condition after IPPI, because of the possibility of fundal perforation. Inversion of the ML Cu 250 is easily diagnosed by radiography. When an ML Cu 250 has been inserted the use of a marker is important because the plastic skeleton of these devices is not radio-opaque but the two ends of the copper thread clearly have a different appearance (Figure 5). Ultrasound is not helpful for this purpose, but one of our coinvestigators recently found that hysteroscopy offers a simple method to clarify the cause of missing strings and especially to diagnose an inverted IUD. Other investigators have reported comparable experience with this technique (Valle et al. 1977). Management of intrauterine translocation consists of withdrawal followed by immediate replacement of the device.

VI. FUTURE RESEARCH

Ideally, devices destined for IPPI should be 100-percent safe and effective, unexpellable, and, except when spacing of births is the goal, have a prolonged antifertility effect.

The safety of IUD models used for IPPI has generally been found to be adequate. However, at least theoretically the innocuity of intrauterine translocation of a stemmed device may be questioned, and therefore both the prevention and the early diagnosis of this phenomenon must be improved. No way to prevent asymmetrical IUD models from inverting within the involuting uterus has been proposed yet. Insertion of the device at Cesarean section through the uterine incision and holding it in place with an absorbable catgut suture placed in the myometrium of the fundus, as proposed by Zerzavy (1967) for the Birnberg Bow, is easy enough but when attempted immediately after vaginal delivery the procedure was found to be extremely difficult and even dangerous. However, it seems possible that providing the horizontal bar of a T-shaped IUD with chromic catgut sutures (Potts 1978; Laufe et al. 1979) will not only decrease the risk of expulsion but also prevent the device from somersaulting.

The IUD models assessed for IPPI have been well tolerated by the uterus, as indicated by the acceptable rates of removal on account of bleeding, pain or both. Bleeding remains an obnoxious side effect in some women, but is not related to the time of insertion and the management of menorrhagia and metrorrhagia in IUD wearers is currently being tackled on a worldwide scale.

Effectiveness of intrauterine contraception and the threat of expulsion of the device, although both influenced by correct fundal placement, are not strictly related. After both interval placement and IPPI the majority of the expulsions occur soon after insertion (Figure 4). This implies that after IPPI the time of expulsion will largely coincide with a period in which the woman is still refraining from sexual activity or is still protected by breast-feeding or the effect of a steroidal lactation inhibitor. In any case, the crux of effectiveness remains early diagnosis of spontaneous expulsions, whether complete or partial. Measures that enhance early diagnosis include inspection of pads by the patient, digital self-examination and, above all, an early first follow-up visit. Moreover, patients should be cautioned against the use of vaginal tampons prior to the first postpartum visit and against pulling on threads protruding outside the vagina. As already mentioned, retention of postplacentally placed IUDs is improved by introduction high into the fundal area of the uterus, but the preferability of manual placement or the use of longer inserters is still questionable. Even when correctly placed, current IUD models are far from being unexpellable. The benefit to be derived from designing specific IUD models for the purpose of IPPI is a moot question, as indicated by the data of the various studies conducted with, for example, the Lem device. Nor has modification of existing IUDs produced the answer, one tentative exception being the sutured devices which, according to preliminary data, are significantly less expellable from the involuting uterus (Laufe et al. 1979).

Finally, there is the question of the intrauterine lifespan of the device. In this respect inert IUDs are no doubt supreme, and if the suture loop (Potts 1978; Laufe et al. 1979) fulfils its promise, a great advance will have been made. The lifespan of copper-wired devices, although still unknown, is 'expanding', as indicated in a paper by Zipper et al. (1977), who found a continuation rate of at least six years for the CU-T200. Nonetheless multisleeved copper devices, such as the CU-T220C, with an antifertility effect lasting at least twenty years may prove a valuable acquisition. (Tatum 1973).

VII. CONCLUSIONS

Intrauterine contraception initiated immediately after the delivery of the placenta is gaining attention from both the medical profession and from those responsible for family planning programmes. The procedure is technically simple, well-accepted, and safe. Although compared with interval placement, immediate postplacental insertion of second-generation IUDs yields significantly higher expulsion rates, the method effective provided the expulsions, most of which occur very early, are diagnosed soon and managed properly. Intrauterine translocation of stemmed devices remains a potential though unproved hazard. Future research should be directed at (1) providing us with devices which are less expellable and more stable within the involuting uterine cavity, and (2) expanding the effective intrauterine lifespan of biodegradable IUDs in order to meet the demands of women wishing to refrain from further procreation and do away with the burden of follow-up and periodic IUD replacement.

ACKNOWLEDGEMENT

This work was supported by the Population and Family Study Centre (CBGS) of the Belgian Ministry of Public Health and the Family.

REFERENCES

Apelo R, Ramos R, Thomas M: The LEM device in an immediate postpartum contraceptive program. Fertil Steril 27: 517, 1976.

Banharnsupawat L, Rosenfield AG: Immediate postpartum IUD insertion. Obstet Gynecol 38: 276, 1971.

Bogaert LJ van, de Ridder V, van der Pas H: First postpartum ovulation in women treated with a combination of ablactating steroids. Contraception 15: 319, 1977.

Castadot RG, Sivin I, Reyes P, Alers JO, Chapple M, Russell J: The International Postpartum Family Planning Program: eight years of experience, Reports on population and family planning 18, New York, Population Council, 1975.

Echeverry G: Family planning in the immediate postpartum period. Stud Fam Plan 4: (2) : 33, 1973.

Goh TH: The use of a Karman cannula and suction to manage a retained IUD with retracted thread. Int J Gynaecol Obstet 16: 80, 1978.

Husemeyer RP, Gordon H: Retrieval of contraceptive device threads from within the uterine cavity. Lancet 1: 807, 1979.

Karim M, Ammar R, El Mahgaub S, El Granzoury B, Fikri F, Abdon I: Injected progestogen and lactation. Br Med J 1: 200, 1971.

Lancet: Review: missing threads. Lancet 1: 811, 1979.

Laufe LE, Wheelers RG, Friel PG: Modification of IUDs for postpartum use. Am J Obstet Gynecol, 1979.

Millen A, Austin F, Bernstein GS: Analysis of 100 cases of missing IUD strings. Contraception 18: 485, 1978.

Ministry of Health: Confidential enquiries into maternal deaths in England and Wales, 1964-1966, Ministry of Health reports on public health and medical subjects 119, London, HMSO, 1969.

Newton J, Harper M, Chan KK: Immediate post-placental insertion of intrauterine contraceptive devices. Lancet 2: 272, 1977.

Nilsson S, Nygren KG: Transfer of contraceptive steroids to human milk. Res Reprod 11 (1): 1, 1979.

Os W van, Thiery M, van der Pas H, Rhemrev P, Kosasih F, van Kets H, Amy J-J: Experience with a combined Multiload Cu250 intrauterine contraceptive device. Proc Int Cong Asian Fed Obstet Gynaec 1:217, 1976.

Pollock M: The time of insertion of IUDs: a discussion. Br J Fam Plan 5(1): 11, 1979.

Potts M: Postpartum IUD: the suture loop. IPPF Med Bull 12 (6): 4, 1978.

Prystowsky K, Eastman NJ: Puerperal tubal sterilization: report of 1830 cases. JAMA 158: 463, 1955.

Rashbaum WK, Wallach RC: Immediate postpartum insertion of a new intrauterine contraceptive device. Am J Obstet Gynecol 109: 1003, 1971.

Ruiz-Velasco V, Vargas MM, Goldsmith A: Aplicacion del MLCu250 postalumbriamiento: reporte preliminar. Presented at the Mexican conference of obstetrics and gynecology, 1978.

Snowdon R, Williams M, Hawkins D: The IUD: a practical guide. London, Croom Helm, 1977.

Staelens R, Thiery m, Cliquet R: Psychologic-sexual assessment of sterilization [in Dutch]. T Geneesk, 1979.

Tatum HJ: Metallic copper as an intrauterine contraceptive agent. Am J Obstet Gynecol 117: 602, 1973.

Thiery M, van der Pas H, van Os WAA, Tauber PF, Dombrowic N, MacDonald JS, Haspels AA, Drogendijk AC, van Kets H, Boogers W: Three years experience with the MLCu250, a new copper-wired intrauterine contraceptive device. Adv Planned Parenthood 13: 35, 1978a.

Thiery M, van der Pas H, van Os WAA, van Kets H: Clinical experience with two never copper-loaded IUDs (TCu220C) and MLCu250): simultaneous use of an IUD and a spermicide; postplacental insertion of the MLCu250. In: Human Fertilization, Ludwig H, Taube PF (eds), Stuttgart, Thieme, 1978b, p 253ff.

Thiery M, van der Pas H, Delbeke L, van Kets H: Immediate post-placental insertion of the MLCu250. Br J Obstet Gynaecol, 1979a.

Thiery M, van der Pas H, Delbeke L, van Kets H: Randomized comparative trial of immediate postplacental insertion of MLCu250 and TCu200. Int J Obstet Gynaecol, 1979b (submitted).

Tow SH, Goon SM, Lean TH: Translocation of an intrauterine device: an analysis of 125 cases. Presented at the Second International Postpartum Family Planning Program Meeting, New York, 1967.

Valle RF, Sciarra JJ, Freeman DW: Hysteroscopic removal of intrauterine devices with missing filaments. Obstet Gynecol 49: 55, 1977.

Zanartu J, Aguilera E, Munoz G, Peliowsky H: Effect of a long-acting contraceptive progestogen on lactation. Obstet Gynecol 47: 174, 1976.

Zarate A, Canales ES, Soria J, Leon CN, Garrido J, Fonseca E: Refractory post-partum ovarian response to gonadal stimulation in non-lactating women. Obstet Gynecol 44: 819, 1974.

Zatuchni GI: Postpartum Family Planning: a report of the international program, New York, McGraw-Hill, 1970.

Zerzavy FM: Use of intrauterine contraceptive devices in the postpartum period. Am J Public Health 57: 28, 1967.

Zipper J, Medel M, Goldsmith A, Edelman DA: Six-year continuation rates for Cu-T200 users. J Reprod Med 18: 95, 1977.

13. POST-ABORTUM IUD INSERTION

L. Andolšek

In recent years many countries have liberalized the laws on medical termination of pregnancy and, consequently, a significant increase in legally induced abortions was observed throughout the world. The large abortion studies (Tietze and Lewit 1972; Andolšek 1974; Andolšek et al. 1977; Cheng et al. 1977) confirmed the safety of first-trimester abortion performed in the hospital. On the other hand, there are more reports on serious complications of hormonal as well as intrauterine contraception, which are considered to be the most popular fertility regulation methods. All these findings strengthen the old dilemma: abortion or contraception. In evaluating this dilemma, not only should medical effects be compared with various methods, but the acceptability of these methods should also be considered.

In some countries abortion, even if legalized, is still considered as a necessary evil, yet women use it simply as a fertility-regulating method. In these countries a new category of women called *repeat aborters*, was created. According to Tietze (1978) the appearance of this category of women is expected approximately two years after the liberalization of abortion law. The incidence of repeaters varies significantly from country to country and even within the same country. It is related to different factors, among which the definition of repeat abortion plays an important role.

The importance of immediate and effective use of contraception following abortion must be stressed particularly in the high-risk patient groups. Among the reasons for immediate post-abortal use of contraception, two of them seem to be the most important: the fact that ovulation after MTP may occur as early as ten days after abortion (Boyd and Homstrom 1972; Greenhalf 1973; Last 1973) and the possibility of increased risk of medical complications following repeat abortions (Subcommittee on the Study of Induced Abortion 1966; Czeizel 1970; Wright 1972).

The hypothesis about the higher risk of these complications was confirmed only recently. Significantly lower birthweights and a higher rate of premature birth were observed among repeat aborters (World Health Organization 1979) than in the women who had had one abortion only. These findings are important for all women who have not reached the desired family size, and particularly for the increasing number of aborters among adolescent girls. Bracken et al. (1972) analyzed some characteristics as race, residency, religion, and so on among first and repeat aborters. They found that the rate of repeat aborters was slightly higher among black women; repeat aborters were more than three times more likely to be from urban areas; and women with no religion preference were more than twice as likely to have repeat abortions. No statistically significant difference in contraceptive history between the two groups of women was found. The women having a repeat abortion were more likely to seek the abortion in the first trimester than women having the first abortion.

Characteristics of the repeaters differ in various parts of the world, although they are found most often in the low socioeconomic groups (Newton et al. 1973; Rao et al. 1974). Knowledge of contraceptive practice is no guarantee that contraception will be used; motivation and the ease with which supplies can be obtained is equally important.

I. CONTRACEPTION FOLLOWING ABORTION

The initiation of high use-effective contraceptive methods immediately following abortion has advantages for women as well as for the health service. Usually the women are more highly motivated to accept contraceptives immediately after abortion than in other situations. Other reasons for post-abortum contraception are: convenience of the patient being already on the operating table, and the ensurance that the contraceptive method will be started before the patient leaves the hospital. Besides the medical advantages, the cost of providing such contraceptive advice is minimal.

A woman's decision to accept contraceptives at the time of an abortion may be influenced by a number of factors including the advice of her physician, her anxiety to avoid future unwanted pregnancy, and the availability of contraceptive services (Goldsmith et al. 1974). The decision is related also to counselling. The counselling provides an excellent opportunity for communication about motivation toward the use of more effective contraception. If the counselling is adequate, persistent usage of the different contraceptive methods is more common.

I.A. The choice of contraceptive method

Although some physicians prescribe oral hormonal contraceptives immediately after abortion, the main methods recommended (Goldsmith et al. 1974) during this period still remain IUD insertion and sterilization. Post-abortum IUD insertion is optimally timed, particularly for repeat aborters. In one study of IUD acceptance among women with one or more previous induced abortions, about two thirds who accepted intrauterine contraception as their method preferred immediate post-abortion insertion in comparison with less than fifty percent of such insertions in women with only one induced abortion (Randić et al. 1974).

Rao et al. (1974) concluded that sterilization or the IUD appeared to be advisable for abortion patients who had not effectively used any pre-abortion contraception.

Information regarding the desire for additional children should be considered in connection with the patient's socioeconomic status and educational level in recommending IUD or sterilization.

The IUD was generally the method of choice for women who expressed a desire for additional children; sterilization is recommended only for those who have already obtained their desired family size. There is still some disagreement whether or not surgical sterilization should be performed together with an induced abortion, but this is not the topic of this paper.

Many physicians prefer not to insert IUDs after an evacuation of the uterus. This hesitation can be explained by the concern about increased rates of complications and a higher expulsion rate, expressed especially in now already 'classic' IUD literature (Ishihama 1959; Lippes 1962).

I.B. IUD post-abortum

After renewed interest in intrauterine contraception appeared in 1959, the post-abortion IUD insertions were not recommended because of Ishihama's negative experience (Ishihama 1959, 1962). These articles reported slightly increased risk of complications (bleeding, pregnancy with IUD in situ, endometritis) when metallic rings were inserted immediately after abortion. On the basis of his results he recommended to avoid insertion of an IUD immediately after induced abortion in general, while Lippes (1962) recommended insertion no earlier than 60 days after it.

In spite of the fear of increased complication rates associated with post-abortal IUD insertion, especially the higher expulsion and perforation rates, some investigators (Gostin 1966; Cabrera 1969; Koukal and Nemec 1970; Szereday and Szontàgh 1970; Viel and Lucero 1970: Andolšek 1971) started to experiment with this new timing of insertion.

Some years later appeared in the literature the first preliminary reports of IUD insertion immediately after induced as well as after incomplete and febrile abortion (Gostin 1966; Andolšek 1967; Choudhuri 1967; Koukal and Nemec 1970). In these articles authors reported on immediate post-abortion insertion of the IUD, that is, right after evacuation of the uterus, as well as on early post-abortal insertion – during the first, second or even the third post-evacuation day. Although the conclusions about the best time for insertion after abortion were different, the first results showed no increased rates of complication. These results were later confirmed in much larger studies using inert as well as bioactive IUDs.

The most important advantage of immediate post-abortion contraception is the prevention of repeat abortion. Beside this there are some other advantages too: at the time of abortion the cervix is already dilated, and side effects like bleeding and pain are frequent also after abortion alone.

Immediate post abortion IUD insertion must be evaluated in two ways:

- by comparison with complications after abortion alone;
- by comparison with the complications after postmenstrual insertion.

In the following a review of the published literature on immediate post-abortion IUD insertion will be presented.

II. IMMEDIATE POST-ABORTION IUD INSERTION VERSUS ABORTION ALONE

II.A. Immediate insertion of an IUD after illegally induced abortion

The first studies of immediate insertions of IUD after illegally induced abortion date back to 1965, when in Chile a group of doctors started to study this timing of insertion. Viel (1970) was one of the first authors to report about this timing for insertions done during 1966 and 1967 in Santiago Hospital. They inserted the IUD either immediately after the curettage or 2-3 days later.

In these series slightly higher expulsion and removal rates for immediate post-curettage insertion in comparison with insertion performed during next 24 h were found, although the difference in continuation rate 35 days after insertion did not differ essentially (92,8% versus 95.8%).

They recommended, however, immediate insertion after the curettage 'because a great number of those who have not been inserted immediately, reject the later insertion, promising to go to an outpatient clinic in due time, a promise rarely kept'.

At the same time a large study by the Population Council was performed in seven hospitals in different countries. In the overview of the programme, Zatuchni (1970) reported on 2672 post-abortion Lippes Loop insertions. Of these 27 percent were done immediately after evacuation, 43 percent in the first 24 h, 17 percent on the second day and 3.2 percent on days three, four and five. They did not observe in these series higher incidences of inflammation, perforation and expulsion than in patients having devices inserted postmenstrually.

Analyzing these data further Phatak and Chandorkar (1970) found a continuation rate of 72 percent after three years. The retention rate is then similar to that in postmenstrual insertions.

Ben Cheikh (1971) compared 1000 insertions of the Sterilet IUD performed after abortion with 1000 insertions of the same type done after menstruation. She observed in the post-abortion group a slight increase in leukorrhea (13.5% versus 11.8%) and expulsion (9.2% versus 8.6%) while other events did not differ significantly.

Goldsmith et al. (1972) compared in a double-blind study women having Lippes Loop D inserted immediately after incomplete (spontaneous or illegal) abortion and women with abortion only. They did not find serious complications for either group during the first months after abortion. Differences were significant only for the interval between curettage and first menses, and for the quantity of flow in relation to previous menstruation. The event rates shown in this study were perfectly acceptable, although higher than the event rates for intermenstrual insertions done in the same hospital (see Table 1). Tatum (1972) reports on 2388 patients. In 1209 of them an IUD was inserted directly after curettage; 1179 were inserted at the follow-up visit

Table 1. Net cumulative event rates per 100 Lippes Loop D users by time of insertion for selected periods of use: San Juan de Dios and Felix Bulnes hospitals, Santiago, Chile.

	Months since insertion			
Events	*After incomplete abortion*		*Postmenses*	
	3-5	*6-11*	*3-5*	*6-11*
Pregnancy	0.5	0.9	0.6	1.7
Expulsion	8.9	10.7	5.7	7.9
Removal				
medical	1.4	6.3	1.6	1.5
personal	2.6	8.1	2.6	3.6
Continuation	86.6	72.0	90.6	84.2
Number of first insertions	1470		14577	

Source: Goldsmith et al. (1974).

after four weeks. There were no significant differences between the groups regarding temperature ranges or length of the hospitalization. These and other data suggest that insertion of an IUD after the evacuation of the uterus can in most instances be done very safely.

Hue et al. (1974) studied the post-abortal insertion of Lippes Loop D in a self-selected group of women having an MTP (medical termination of pregnancy) covered with parenteral antibiotics and medication for more rapid shrinking of the uterus. They did not observe significant difference in the gross incidence of complications in the two groups, although acceptors experienced significantly increased leukorrhea and back pain.

Of the IUD acceptors 56 percent in comparison with only 33 percent of nonacceptors returned for at least one visit. From this the conclusion was drawn that patients with an IUD inserted at abortion were more likely to return for a checkup; this is in disagreement with previous findings (Newton et al. 1973).

Quan et al. (1975) reported on study of over 500 first insertions of a standard-size Dalkon Shield in patients treated for an incomplete abortion mostly (91.9%) in the first trimester. The usual pertinent event rates – pregnancy, expulsion and bleeding – were at acceptable levels although compared with studies of the Dalkon Shield in intermenstrual insertions and insertions after induced abortion statistically significant higher rates of pregnancy and expulsion were found. The authors explained this difference with possible differences in age-parity distribution, gestational age and physicians' experience.

II.B. Immediate insertion of an IUD after legally induced abortion

While the studies of immediate insertions of IUDs after illegally induced abortions were mostly carried out in Chile, almost at the same time in some of the Eastern European countries, such as Yugoslavia, Czechoslovakia and Poland, some authors were studying the immediate insertion of IUDs after a legally induced abortion. Later authors from Scandinavia and other countries performed similar studies with new devices. These studies mostly compared IUD event rates with complications after abortion only. In a few studies the events of immediate IUD insertion after abortion were compared with the events of postmenstrual insertions.

Andolšek (1967, 1971) did not find any increase in the frequency of early complications from this timing of insertion. The net cumulative expulsion rate for a group of 661 women having Lippes Loop D inserted immediately after induced abortion was significantly lower, and the rates of pregnancy and for removals for bleeding or pain were insignificantly lower, when compared with a corresponding group of women who had had Lippes Loop D inserted in the postmenstrual period (see Table 2).

Malec et al. (1969) inserted in 238 women the

Table 2. Net cumulative event rates per 100 Lippes Loop D users by time of insertion for selected periods of use: Family Planning Institute, Ljubljana, Yugoslavia.

	Months since insertion					
Events	*After artificial abortion*			*post Menses*		
	6	*12*	*24*	*6*	*12*	*24*
Pregnancy	1.1	2.0	4.5	2.5	3.8	5.6
First expulsion	1.8	2.8	3.9	12.1	16.1	19.6
Removals						
Bleeding/pain	2.1	2.9	5.2	2.3	4.0	5.3
Other medical	1.2	1.4	2.2	0.2	0.6	1.3
Other personal	0.2	0.5	1.5	0.4	0.6	1.3
Continuation rate	94.4	91.4	83.0	89.5	83.9	76.0
Number of first insertions		661			unknown	

Source: Goldsmith et al. (1974).

Dana 2, Super Dana 2 or Dana 1 device immediately after induced abortion. Their conclusion was that the complication rate is not greater than in the women who have abortion only, and the events ascribed to IUDs are not more frequent than those known for insertion of the IUD in the postmenstrual period.

Koukal and Nemec (1970) also found a lower expulsion index in 66 post-abortal insertions with Dana S-3 device if compared with 1545 intermenstrual insertions with the same device. All other complications were of similar frequency.

In a comparison of 331 post-abortion Lippes C insertions with 344 cases of same IUD inserted postmenstrually, Randić (1975) has found that one-year net cumulative rates for pregnancy and bleeding/pain removal were similar in both groups (2.0% versus 2.2% for pregnancy and 3.0% versus 2.6% for bleeding/pain removal), while the expulsion rate was considerably lower in women with immediate post-abortion IUD insertion (6.9% versus 14.9%).

When the second generation of IUDs became available, different authors started to insert new devices immediately after abortions. Nygren and Johansson (1973) reported similar rates of complications for patients having first-trimester MTP combined with Cu-T200 IUD insertions and those having first-trimester abortion alone. They observed slight lowering of complications rates when compared with published results for the Lippes Loop D. The general conclusion was that the insertion of the IUD immediately following MTP does not represent an additional hazard for women.

Newton et al. (1974) inserted in 121 women after MTP either the Dalkon Shield or the Cu-7; after twelve months of observation no differences in complication rates were found between the two devices studied.

Timonen and Luukkainen (1974) found out that the immediate post-abortal insertion of the Cu-T200 did not increase the frequency or type of early somatic complications if compared with the group of women who had abortion only. After eighteen months of FU (follow up) they found lower expulsion and higher continuation rates than in the similar study where the IUD was inserted postmenstrually. Data from the various studies are summarized in Table 3 and Table 4.

In one other study conducted in Ljubljana and Maribor, Andolšek (1975) compared the Dalkon Shield with the Lippes Loop D either postmenses (Ljubljana) or post-abortion (Maribor). Nine months after insertion it was shown that for both devices the protection was greater for postmenses

Table 3. Selected post-abortion IUD insertion studies.

Investigators	*Type of abortion (MTP, incomplete)*	*No. post-abortion insertions*	*Type of device*	*Control group (PMI: postmenses insertion; AO: Abortion only)*
Andolšek (1967, 1971)	MTP	815	Lippes C, D	? PMI
Malec et al. (1969)	MTP	238	Dana 2, 1, Super 2	–
Viel and Lucero (1970)	incomplete	1561	Lippes D	–
Zatuchni (1970)	incomplete	2672	Lippes	–
Koukal and Nemec (1970)	MTP	66	Dana	1545 PMI
Ben Cheikh (1971)	incomplete	1000	Sterilet	1000 PMI
Goldsmith et al. (1972)	incomplete	242	Lippes D	248 AO
Tatum (1972)	incomplete	1209	Lippes D	1179 PMI
Nygren and Johansson (1973)	MTP	196	Cu-T200	436 AO
Newton et al. (1974)	MTP	121	Dalkon Shield/Cu-7	144 AO
Timonen and Luukkainen (1974)	MTP	154	Cu-7-200	144 AO
Hue et al. (1974)	incomplete	1104	Lippes D	1124 AO
Andolšek (1975)	MTP	415	Lippes D/Dalkon Shield	641 PMI
Quan et al. (1975)	incomplete	259	Dalkon Shield	? AO
Larsson and Hamberger (1975)	MTP	594	Cu-7	? AO
Lauersen et al. (1975)	MTP	548	Antigon-F, Y, Cu-T200	2733 PMI
Randić (1975)	MTP	331	Lippes C	344 PMI
Solheim and Rydnert (1976)	MTP	143	Cu-7	163 AO

Table 4. Data from some immediate post-abortion IUD insertion studies, compared with data from the same centres on intermenstrual IUD insertions.

Investigators	*IUD*	*No. of cases*	*Time period (months)*	*Post-abortum insertion*			*Intermenstrual insertion*		
				C	*P*	*E*	*C*	*P*	*E*
Viel (1970);	Lippes D	1,470	11	72.0	2.9	10.7	–	–	–
Viel and Lucera (1970)	Lippes D	14,577	11	–	–	–	84.2	1.7	7.9
Andolšek	Lippes D	664	24	83.0	4.5	3.9	–	–	–
(1976, 1971, 1974, 1975)	Lippes D	?	24	–	–	–	76.0	5.6	19.6
	Lippes D	664	36	77.0	5.8	4.4	–	–	–
	Lippes C	187	36	70.4	5.7	10.4	–	–	–
Phatak and Chandorkar	Lippes	200	36	71.9					
(1970)	Lippes	842	36	–	–	–	73.0	–	–
Randić (1975):	Lippes C	331	12	88.1	2.0	6.9	–	–	–
Randić et al. (1974)	Lippes C	344	12	–	–	–	80.3	2.2	14.9

Key: C: Continuation rate, *P:* pregnancy rate; *E:* expulsion rate.
Source: Modified from Edström (1972).

than for post-abortion insertions (the pregnancy rate for Lippes Loop D inserted postmenses was 1.0% versus 2.3% post-abortion; for the Dalkon Shield the figures were 2.8% against 3.2%). The expulsion rates were similar for Lippes Loop D inserted either post-abortionally or postmenstrually (4.1% versus 4.8%); a virtual absence of expulsion for the Dalkon Shield (0.4% versus 1.6%) in both groups was noted. (see Table 5). The distribution of pertinent events in the Dalkon Shield group was much lower than in the Lippes Loop series; only IUD removal through investigator's choice was more frequent.

Larsson and Hamberger (1975) inserted Cu-7 in 601 women after first-trimester MTP with or without cervical dilatation. They did not observe any increase in complications and the incidence of infection was lower than in the control group having abortion only. This low risk of complication is ascribed to good analgesia and to exact knowledge of the shape of the uterine cavity before insertion.

Lauersen et al. (1975) compared in their study the pertinent event rates of three different devices, the Antigon-F, the Ypsilon and the Cu-T200, in postmenstrual and post-abortal insertions. As can be seen from Table 6 they found slightly higher event rates in the post-abortion group for all three IUDs studied, except for the pregnancy rate for Antigon-F. It should be noted however that this was not double-blind trial; comparison was made at the end of the follow-up period with multiparous and nulliparous women and tabulated as Pearl's index. The Tietze-Potter-Viel life table method would probably have given slightly higher event rates.

Van Os et al. (1975) found in 1975 that ML Cu-250, inserted immediately after second-trimester abortions, showed a lower expulsion rate and a better continuation rate than Lippes Loop D, the standard Dalkon Shield, the Cu-T200 and the Gravigard.

Table 5. Nine months gross cumulative rates of pertinent events per 100 women for two blind trials comparing the Dalkon Shield with the Lippes Loop D in Ljubljana and Maribor, Yugoslavia, 1972-1974.

Event	*Ljubljana DS*	*Ljubljana LL*	*Maribor DS*	*Maribor LL*
Pregnancy	2.8	1.0	3.2	2.3
Expulsion	0.4	4.1	1.6	4.8
Bleeding/pain	2.8	1.4	2.4	4.9
Other medical reasons	0.8	1.0	0.4	0.5
planning pregnancy	0.8	0.0	0.4	1.4
Other personal reasons	0.0	0.0	0.4	0.0
At investigator's choice	0.0	0.0	0.4	0.0
Released from follow-up	0.0	0.5	0.0	0.0
Lost to follow-up	1.5	1.3	0.8	0.9
Total terminations	8.8	8.9	9.3	14.0

Table 6. Comparison of pertinent event rates of postmenstrual and post-abortion insertion of three different IUDs: Observation period 1 March 1972 to 28 February 1974.

Type of IUD	*No. of insertions (PM: postmenses; PA: post-abortion)*	*Rates per 100 women years, tabulated as Pearl's index*		
		Pregnancy	*Expulsion*	*Continuation*
Antigon-F	PM: 884	0.88	5.1	79.8
	PA: 214	1.3	4.5	84.5
Ypsilon	PM: 910	1.8	1.9	88.9
	PA: 194	1.3	2.2	90.3
CU-T200	PM: 939	0.85	1.8	88.4
	PA: 140	0.0	1.1	90.8

Source: Adapted from Lauersen et al. (1975).

Solheim and Rydnert (1976) reported on immediate insertion of IUD performed on 143 women having first-trimester abortions. The control group was composed of 163 women who chose alternative contraceptive methods after abortion. Insertion of Cu-7 IUDs did not change the incidence of somatic complications during an observation of four weeks. They measured the blood loss during the first hours as well as the first week after MTP and found that this was not dependent on the presence of absence of the Cu-7 IUD. The latest data on this topic came from the WHO special programme on human reproduction with multicenter trials using Lippes Loop D and Copper-T220 C for either postmenstrual or post-abortion insertion (1979). Data on a 5 025 subjects, providing 81 414 woman months of experience, have been analyzed so far. They found after two years of use significantly higher discontinuation rates with Lippes Loop D, regardless of the time of insertion. The Lippes Loop D has a significantly higher removal rate for pain and/or bleeding than the Copper-T220, except after IUD insertion immediately after MTP. The IUP rate in Lippes Loop D users is at least twice that of Copper-T220 C users and the expulsion rate is at least one half time that for the Copper-T220 during the same period. The Lippes Loop is also associated with a greater increase in menstrual blood loss following insertion than Cu-T220. The data from these multicenter trials show not only the device related effects, but also the inter-centre differences in IUD performance. Because of the superior effectiveness of the Copper-T220 C use and the smaller increase in menstrual blood loss, the WHO Steering Committee recommended consideration of the Cu-T220 C as a suitable alternative for national family planning programmes.

III. CONCLUSIONS

From these studies one can draw the following conclusions:

1. Abortion in general seems to increase motivation for accepting contraceptive methods, especially those available at the time of pregnancy termination, and thus prevent the repeat abortions.

2. Immediate IUD insertion after induced abortion is generally safe: there is no increase in inflammatory processes among women with an immediate post-abortion IUD insertion when compared with

Table 7. WHO HR CCCR multicenters Comparative study: Lippes D vs Cu-T220 C, MTP vs Interval/Multip, 14 Centers, 5.025 ♀, 81.414 months of use.

Timing of insertion	*MTP*	*Interval*
Nb of Insertion		
Lippes D	777	894
Cu-T220 C	791	889
% LFUP		
Lippes D	9,3%	10,1%*
Cu-T220 C	8,3%	6,4%

NS – non significant
* – p < 0.01

Source: Modified from World Health Organization, Special Programme of Research, Development and Research Training in Human Reproduction. An assessment of the Lippes Loop D and the Copper-T220 C, HRP/79.1 Rev 1, April 1979.

Table 8. Lippes D vs Cu-T220 C. Net cumulative life table discontinuation rates per 100 women.

Reasons	*MTP* *Two years*		*Interval Multip* *Two years*	
	Lippes D	*Cu-T220 C*	*Lippes D*	*Cu-T220 C*
All Reasons	36.6 ± 2.0**	28.4 ± 1.8^{NS}	33.4 ± 1.8	29.8 ± 1.7
IUP	4.7 ± 1.0*	2.0 ± 0.6	3.3 ± 0.7*	1.2 ± 0.4
EXP	9.3 ± 1.2	3.9 ± 0.8	10.0 ± 1.1	6.6 ± 1.0
Re B/P	14.9 ± 1.6^{NS}	11.2 ± 1.4	12.9 ± 1.5*	8.8 ± 1.2
Number of M Observation	11.276	12.683	14.822	16.576

NS = not significant * $p < 0.05$ ** $p < 0.01$ *** $p < 0.001$

Source: Modified from World Health Organization, Special Programme of Research, Development and Research Training in Human Reproduction. An assessment of the Lippes Loop D and the Copper T220 C, HRP/79.1 Rev 1, April 1979.

women who have abortion only. As shown from the studies reviewed, the results of post-abortion IUD insertions are slightly different in different countries.

3. Studies from Chile found higher expulsion rates, while in the studies in Czechoslovakia and Yugoslavia the reverse result was obtained. This difference can be ascribed to the type of abortion – whether illegally or legally induced. The lower expulsion rate in induced abortion groups was later confirmed by different authors. In most of the studies reviewed the rates of two other pertinent events, i.e. pregnancy and bleeding/pain removals, were not significantly different between women with post-abortionally and postmenstrually inserted IUDs of the same type and size.

4. When comparing the effectiveness of post-abortion versus postmenstrual IUD insertion we should take into account also the differences in age and parity distribution of women, because these factors may considerably influence IUD performance in general, regardless of timing of insertion, as well as the type of IUD and the experience of the person who performed the insertion.

5. It is unknown how many of almost 65 million IUD users in the world were inserted with IUD immediately after abortion. If the number of post-abortion IUD insertions is only that published in the literature, and even if it is somewhat higher, than there can be no question that post-abortion IUD insertion should be used more frequently.

REFERENCES

Andolšek L: Insertion of IUDs after abortion: preliminary report. Proc Int Conf Planned Parenthood Fed 8: 285, 1967.

Andolšek L: Experience with immediate post-abortion insertions of the IUD. In: Abortion techniques and services: proceedings of a symposium. New York, June 1971.Amsterdam, Excerpta Medica, p 65ff.

Andolšek L: The Ljubljana abortion study 1971-1973, Ljubljana, National Institute of Health Centre for Population Research, 1974.

Andolšek L: The Ljubljana IUD experience: ten years. In: Analysis of intrauterine contraception, Hefnawi F, and Segal SJ (eds), Amsterdam, North-Holland Publishing, 1975, p 205ff.

Andolšek L, Cheng M, Hren M, Ogrinc-Oven, M, Ng A, Ratnam S, Belsey M, Edström K, Heiner P, Kinnear K, Tietze C: The safety of local anesthesia and outpatient treatment: a controlled study of induced abortion by vacuum aspiration. Stud Fam Plann 8: 118, 1977.

Ben Cheikh B: Étude comparative de 1000 cas d'insertion de Sterilet dans le post-abortum immédiat et de 1000 cas d'insertion de Sterilet dans les conditions normales. Paper presented at the Journées medicales, Tunisia, 1971.

Boyd EF, Homstrom EG: Ovulation following therapeutic abortion. Am J Obstet Gynecol 113: 469, 1972.

Bracken MB, Hachamovitch M, Grossman G: Correlates of repeat induced abortions. Obstet Gynecol 40: 3, 1972.

Cabrera R: Aplicación postaborto del D.I.U. Saf-T-Coil 33 S. Rev Chile Obstet Ginecol 33: 215-220, 1969.

Cheng M, Andolšek L, Ng A, Ratnam S, Hren M, Ogrinc-Oven M, Belsey M, Edström K, Heiner P, Kinnear K, Tietze C: Complications following induced abortion by vacuum aspiration: patient characteristics and procedures. Stud Fam Plann 8: 125, 1977.

Choudhuri PK: Loop in postpartum and postabortal period. J Indian Med Assoc 49: 32, 1967.

Czeizel A: Changes in mean birth weight and proportion of low-weight births in Hungary. Br J Prev Soc Med 24: 146, 1970.

Edström K: Post-abortum contraception: a review of current experience: working paper for consultation on abortion care, Turku, 1972.

Goldsmith A, Goldberg R, Eyzaguire H, Lizana L: Immediate postabortion intrauterine contraceptive device insertion: a double-blind study. Am J Obstet Gynecol 112: 957, 1972.

Goldsmith A, Edelman DA, Brenner WE: Contraception immediately post-abortion. Paper presented at the Twelfth annual meeting of the association of planned parenthood physicians. Memphis. 1974.

Gostin L: Nueva modalidad de anticonceptión mediante dispositivo intrauterino. Inserción precoz post-aborto. Rev Chile Obstet Ginecol 31: 256-265. 1966.

Greenhalf JO: When to begin contraception after pregnancy. Lancet 1: 1243, 1973.

Hue K, Kwon HY, Michael PH, Watson W: A comparative study of the safety and efficacy of postabortal intrauterine contraceptive device insertion. Am J Obstet Gynecol 118: 975, 1974.

Ishihama A: Clinical studies on intrauterine rings, especially the present state of contraception in Japan and the experiences in the use of intrauterine rings. Yokohama Med Bull 10: 89, 1959.

Ishihama A: My viewpoints on intra-uterine contraceptive devices. In: Intra-uterine contraceptive devices, Segal SJ, Southam AL, Shafer KD (eds), Amsterdam, Excerpta Medica, 1962, p 21ff.

Koukal J, Nemec M: Insertion of IUD after artificial interruption of pregnancy. Cesk Gynekol 35: 456, 1970.

Larsson B, Hamberger L: Insertion of Copper-7 IUDs in connection with induced abortions during the first trimester. Contraception 12: 69, 1975.

Last P: Contraception after pregnancy. Lancet 1: 1385, 1973.

Lauersen NH, Cederqvist LL, Donovan S, Fuchs F: Comparison of three intrauterine contraceptive devices: the Antigon-F, the Ypsilon-Y, and the Copper-T200. Fertil Steril 26: 638, 1975.

Lippes J: Instructions for the insertion of an intra-uterine loop. In: Intra-uterine contraceptive devices, Amsterdam, Excerpta Medica, 1962, p 145ff.

Malec I, Žak K, Weber I, Hontela S, Pospišil J: Experiences with early insertion of IUD after artificial interruption of pregnancy. Cesk Gynekol 34: 418, 1969.

Newton J, Brotman M, McEvan J, Owens C: Hospital family planning: termination of pregnancy and contraceptive use. Br Med J 4: 280, 1973.

Newton J, Elias J, Johnson A: Immediate post-termination insertion of Copper-7 and Dalkon Shield intrauterine contraceptive devices. J Obst Gyn Brit Cwlth 81: 389, 1974.

Nygren KG, Johansson EDB: Insertion of the endouterine Copper-T (T Cu-200) immediately after first-trimester legal abortion. Contraception 7: 299, 1973.

Phatak L, Chandorkar K: Experience with immediate postpartum and post-abortal IUD insertions. Disappearance of IUD threads. In: Postpartum family planning. Zatuchni GI (ed), New York, McGraw-Hill, 1970, p 299ff.

Os WAA van, Rhemrev PER, Loendersloot EW: Ervaringen met post abortum geplaatste IUDs. Jaarverslag afd Gynaecologie en Verloskunde Elisabeth Gasthuis, 1975.

Quan A, Edelman DA, Goldsmith A, Thomas M, Zappala-Badia D: Immediate post-abortion insertion of the Dalkon Shield. Contraception 12: 23, 1975.

Randić L: Primjena intrauterine kontracepcije i sadržaj bakra u cervikalnoj sluzi. Dissertation, Rijeka 1975.

Randić L, Kogoj-Bakić V, Stanković T: Intrauterina Kontracepcija i višekratni zahtjevi za prekid trudnoće. Jugosl Ginekol Opstet 14: 415, 1974.

Rao SR, Kanitkar SD, Brinton LA: Post-abortal fertility control acceptance: India fertility research programme conference. Paper presented at the Sixth Asian congress on obstetrics and gynecology, Kuala Lumpur, Malaysia, 20-27 July, 1974.

Solheim F, Rydnert J: Vacuum aspiration at therapeutic abortion: effect of Cu IUD insertion at operation on postoperative blood loss. Contraception 13: 707, 1976.

Subcommittee on the Study of Induced Abortion: Harmful effects of induced abortion, Tokyo, Family Planning Federation of Japan, 1966.

Szereday Z, Oroján I, Szontágh F: Terhességmegszakitással egyidôben felhelyezett IUD- val (fogamzásgátló hurok) Szerzett tapasztalataink. Orv Hetil 111: 2299-2300, 1970.

Taum H: Intrauterine contraception. Am J Obstet Gynecol 112: 1000, 1972.

Tietze C: Repeat abortions: Why more? Fam Plann Respect 10: 286, 1978.

Tietze C, Lewit S: Joint program for the study of abortion (JPSA): early medical complications of legal abortion. Stud Fam Plann 3: 97, 1972.

Timonen H, Luukkainen T: Immediate post-abortion insertion of the Copper-T (T Cu-200) with eighteen months follow-up. Contraception 9: 153, 1974.

Viel B: The hospital and its function in a family-planning program. In: Postpartum family planning, Zatuchni GI (ed), New York, McGraw-Hill, 1970, p 193ff.

Viel B, Lucero S: An analysis of 3 years' experience with intrauterine devices among women in the western area of the city of Santiago, July 1, 1964 to June 30, 1967. Am J Obstet Gynecol 106: 765, 1970.

World Health Organization: Ab task force on the sequelae of induced abortion. Unpublished studies, Geneva 1979.

World Health Organization: Special programme of research, development and research training in human reproduction: an assessment of the Lippes Loop D and the Copper-T 220 C. HRP/79.1. Rev 1 April, 1979.

Wright CS: Second-trimester abortion after vaginal termination of pregnancy. Lancet 1: 1278, 1972.

Zatuchni GI: Overview of program: two years experience. In: Postpartum family planning, Zatuchni GI (ed), New York, McGraw-Hill 1970, p 30ff.

14. INTRAUTERINE CONTRACEPTION WITH THE PROGESTASERT ® SYSTEM

Y. GIBOR

The idea of continuous intrauterine administration of progesterone for contraception, as originally presented by Dr. Antonio Scommegna, is based on four observations:

- The estrogenic component of oral contraceptives is not essential for contraception.
- Progestin-only mini-pills achieve satisfactory levels of contraception without inhibiting ovulation.
- The mini-pill interferes with nidation and may change the cervical mucus, thus interfering with sperm penetration.
- Most contraceptive failures associated with the mini-pill can be traced to poor patient compliance.

These observations suggest low-level, continuous intrauterine administration of progesterone, a naturally occurring hormone with strong antiestrogenic effect, would be an effective contraceptive. Furthermore, this method would not depend on patient compliance, nor would it cause systemic side effects.

The Progestasert intrauterine progesterone contraceptive system (Figure 1) delivers progesterone to the uterus at a rate of 65 μg/day for one year. The delivery rate was selected after studies with prototype system releasing 5-110 μg/day of progesterone. A 65 μg/day release rate significantly reduced the incidence of proliferative endometria as well as maximizing suppression of the endometrium. Dr. Howard Tatum originally designed the system's T shape.

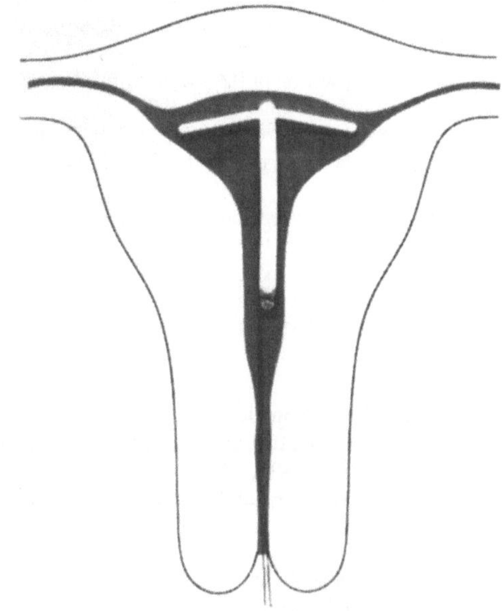

Figure 1. Representation of the Progestasert intrauterine progesterone contraceptive system in the uterus. (Copyright 1976 ALZA Corp.)

I. DATA BASE

Studies with the Progestasert system cover 127,580 woman-months of use in 12,008 women, of whom 3,310 were nulliparous. The studies were conducted in more than forty centers worldwide, and included patients from both public health clinics and private practices.

II. RESULTS

II.A. Systemic effects

The endometrium readily metabolized progesterone. Systems were inserted in women scheduled to undergo hysterectomy (Sievers and Dallenbach-Hellweg 1976); a local progesterone effect was found only in the endometrium. Progesterone and its metabolites were measured in the uterine and peripheral veins of baboons. Essentially no difference was found between progesterone levels, and mainly progesterone metabolites were found in the uterine vein. Plasma follicle-stimulating and luteinizing hormone levels during the menstrual cycle have been examined to determine the effects of progesterone on the hypothalamic-pituitary-ovarian axis (Tillson et al. 1975). This axis, which is very sensitive to changes in systemic progesterone levels, was essentially unaffected.

In a preliminary report, Spellacy et al. (1978) indicated that changes in prolactin levels occur in patients wearing the Progestasert system; however, further research by the authors did not support these findings (Spellacy and Buhi 1979). Another report from this group indicates a difference from preinsertion levels in second-hour blood glucose following the oral glucose tolerance test in women who had used the stystem for one year (Spellacy et al. 1977).

II.B. Bleeding and pain

During our Phase III trials, it became clear that the system – like oral contraceptives, but unlike other IUDs – reduced menstrual blood loss and pain. Patients who reported having heavy blood loss upon admission to the study later reported a significant reduction in this. Patients with severe menstrual cramps upon admission also reported a lessening of their symptoms (Figure 2). Quantitative studies of blood loss, reported by ourselves and others, indicate that while all other IUDs increase the amount of blood loss by from 50 percent (copper IUDs) to 100 percent (inert IUDs), progesterone-releasing IUDs decrease bleeding by an average of 50 percent (Figure 3).

Three factors observed during use of the system may be responsible for decreases in menstrual bleeding and cramps:

- suppression of the endometrium significantly reduces the endometrial hyperemia that is typical of the secretory phase;
- fibrinolytic activity in the endometrium – an effect known to increase menorrhagia during use of other IUDs – decreases;
- $PGF_{2\alpha}$ concentrations in menstrual blood, which affect blood loss and uterine contractility, also fall to significantly below preinsertion levels (Trobough et al. 1978; Zahradnik et al. 1978).

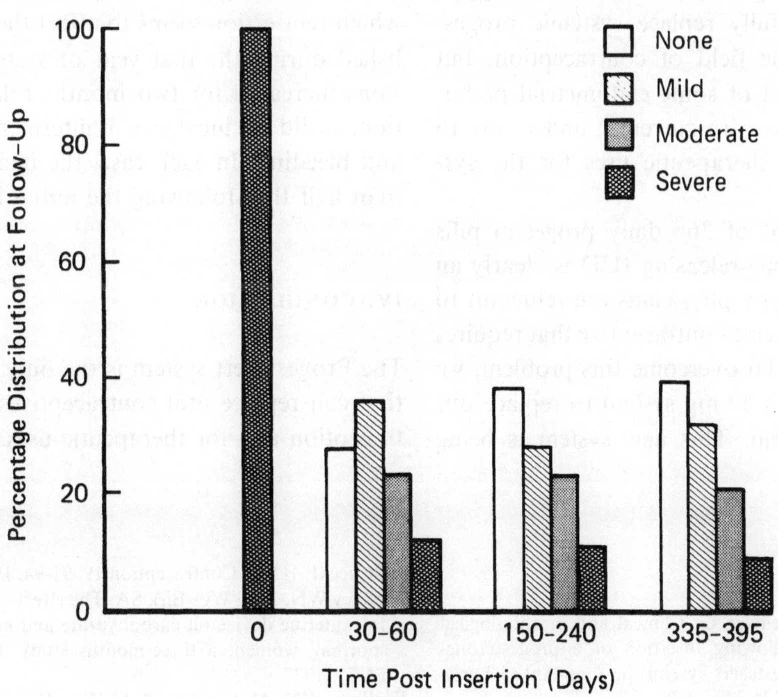

Figure 2. Menstrual cramps in 253 women with severe cramps at insertion of the Progestasert system. (Copyright 1976 ALZA Corp.)

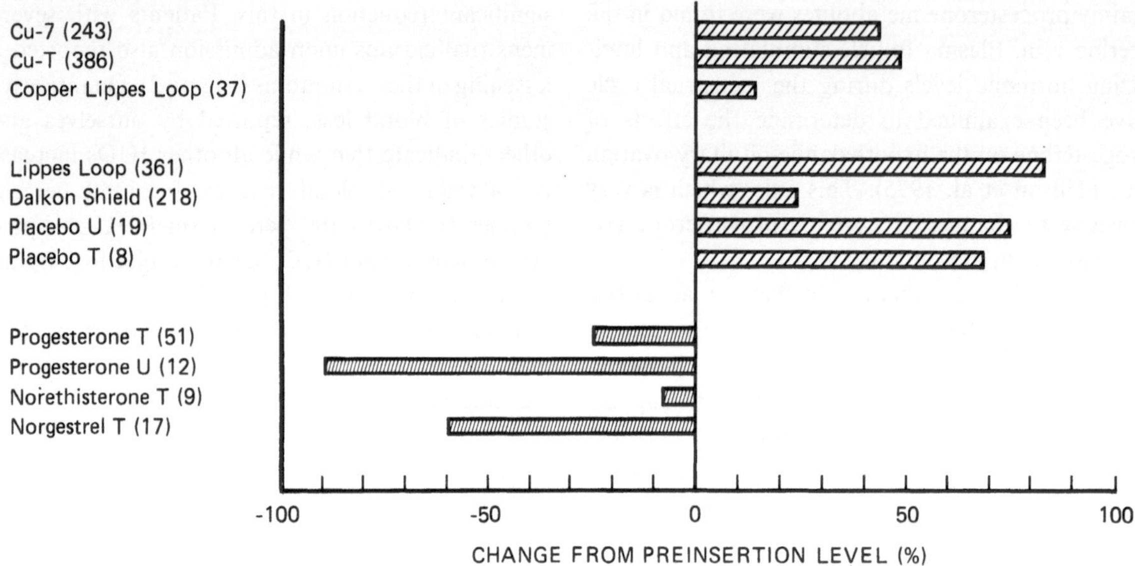

Figure 3. Change in menstrual blood loss for various medicated and nonmedicated intrauterine devices. (Copyright 1979 ALZA Corp.)

III. DISCUSSION

The significant antiestrogenic effect of the Progestasert system on the endometrium, as well as its reduction of bleeding and pain, strongly suggest that it can successfully replace systemic progestins not only in the field of contraception, but also in the treatment of some endometrial pathologies. Several studies are currently under way to examine additional therapeutic uses for the system.

While replacement of 365 daily progestin pills with one progesterone-releasing IUD is clearly an accomplishment, many physicians are reluctant to prescribe an intrauterine contraceptive that requires annual reinsertion. To overcome this problem, we are now producing a 52-mg system to replace our current 38-mg system. This new system is being tested for a contraceptive efficacy of three years; its actual effectiveness may be longer.

We have also analyzed our data to quantify the incidence of complications associated with reinsertion. This analysis has revealed only two areas in which reinsertion seems to affect the pattern established during the first year of system use. Expulsions increased for two months following reinsertion, as did the incidence of intermenstrual spotting and bleeding. In each case, the incidence was less than half that following the initial insertion.

IV. CONCLUSION

The Progestasert system is the only IUD available that can replace oral contraceptives both for contraception and for therapeutic uses.

REFERENCES

Sievers S, Dallenbach-Hellweg G: Clinical and morphological studies in patients following insertion of a progesterone-containing IUD (Progestasert system) [in German] Geburtshilfe Frauenheilkd 36: 334-340, 1976.

Spellacy WN, Buhi WC: A prospective study of plasma prolactin levels in women using the progesterone-releasing intrauterine device (P-IUD). Contraception 19: 91-94, 1979.

Spellacy WN, Buhi WC, Birk SA: The effect of a progesterone-T intrauterine device on carbohydrate and lipid metabolism in 'normal' women: a three-months study. Contraception 15: 65-73. 1977.

Spellacy WN, Mahan CS, Buhi WC, Dumbaugh VS: Plasma prolactin levels and contraception: oral contraceptives and intrauterine devices. Contraception 17: 71-77,1978.

Tillson SA, Marian M, Hudson R, Wong P, Pharriss B, Aznar R. Martinez-Manautou J: The effect of intrauterine progesterone on the hypothalamic-hypophyseal-ovarian axis in humans. Contraception 11: 179-192, 1975.

Trobough G, Guderian AM, Erickson RR, Tillson SA, Leong P, Swisher DA, Pharriss BB: The effect of exogenous intrauterine progesterone on the amount and prostaglandin-$F_{2\alpha}$ content of menstrual blood in dysmenorrheic women. J. Reprod Med 21: 153-158, 1978.

Zahradnik HP, Stengele E, Kraut E, Breckwoldt M: New aspects of pathogenesis and treatment of dysmenorrhea: prostaglandin-$F_{2\alpha}$ level in the menstrual blood [in German] Dtsch Med Wochenschr 103: 1280-1273, 1978.

15. INDICATIONS FOR PROGESTERONE-RELEASING IUDs

N.A.M. BERGSTEIN and R.H.M. VAN DER GIESSEN

The progesterone-releasing IUD has a beneficial effect on the amount of menstrual flow, on dysmenorrheal pain and on premenstrual cramp. We were interested in studying the effects of a progesterone-releasing IUD in a particular group of women. These women were complaining of the following side effects at least three months after the insertion of a copper IUD:

- increased menstrual flow,
- irregular bleeding patterns,
- dysmenorrhea,
- headache.

The following criteria were used for the selection of these patients:

1. The women must have had their complaints for more than three months, and must have mentioned them in two follow-up visits.

2. All the women with dysmenorrhea had to be free from any significant pelvic lesion, including tubal pregnancy, pelvic infection, adnexal involvement, gastroenteritis and appendicitis. The dysmenorrhea must have been due to factors intrinsic to the uterus itself. Any patient whose dysmenorrhea was thought to be due solely to psychogenic factors was excluded from the trial.

3. With regard to menstrual flow, the patient must have come to require more pads or tampons than were needed before the insertion of the copper IUD, or the duration of menstruation must have increased.

4. The headache must not have existed before the insertion of the copper IUD and could not be related to a low hemoglobin or iron value.

A total of 120 women who had used a contraceptive pill before changing to a copper IUD were recruited from two family planning clinics. These 120 women were selected on the basis of the criteria mentioned above; 58 had a Cu-T200 and 62 had a Multiload IUD. Table 1 shows the practically identical distribution of age and parity in both groups of women. Some of these 120 women suffered from more than one of the symptoms listed above during the time in which they used a copper IUD (Table 2). The duration use of the copper IUD is shown in Table 3.

Table 1. Distribution of age and parity of patients.

		Cu-T200	*Multiload*
Age	range	21-38	20-38
	average	26	27
Parity	range	1-3	1-3
	average	2.1	2.0

Table 2. Complaints of women before the study.

Complaints	*Cu-T200*	*Multiload*
Dysmenorrhea	24	26
Irregular bleeding	12	14
Heavy menstrual flow	31	33
Irregular bleedings and heavy menstrual flow	6	9
Headache	6	9

Table 3. Duration of in utero presence of copper IUD when women were included in the study.

Type of IUD	*3-6 cycles*	*6-12 cycles*	*> 12 cycles*
Cu-T200	9	42	7
Multiload	10	46	6

A change to the Progestasert was not made in the case of women coming to the family planning clinic and complaining of the symptoms mentioned in our criteria on her first visit after the insertion of a Cu-T200 or Multiload. Attempts were made to persuade these women to continue with the copper IUD for at least three months. If the complaints were still present at the second follow-up visit, the copper IUD was changed to the progesterone-releasing IUD.

I. DYSMENORRHEA

The 50 women who suffered from dysmenorrhea when using a copper IUD had not suffered from this complaint when using a contraceptive pill. The following question was put routinely to these women: 'Do you habitually feel pelvic pain or genital pain during menstruation, or during the three days before menstruation only, or on the days between two menstrual periods?' The results obtained in these 50 women after changing from a copper IUD to progestasert are shown in Table 4.

Only two women in the Cu-T200 group and three women in the Multiload group did not experience some relief of their dysmenorrhea after conversion to the progesterone-releasing IUD. Three women who did not present dysmenorrhea before the insertion of the Progestasert developed this condition after its insertion (Table 4).

Table 4. Effect on the dymenorrhea after switching to the Progestasert.

Type of IUD	Relief after treatment cycles 3	6	9	12	> 12	no result	total
Cu-T200	6	10	4	12	0	2	34
Multiload	5	13	3	2	0	3	26

II. MENSTRUAL FLOW

Many investigators have reported a decrease in menstrual flow in women with progesterone-releasing IUDs, while others (Pizarro et al. 1977) observed no significant difference between the Gravigard and Progestasert with regard to menstrual flow, although there was a higher percentage of irregular menstruations in the Gravigard group than in the Progestasert group.

From our group of 120 women, 105 who had experienced menstrual abnormalities during the period of copper IUD use were selected; 49 had used a Cu-T200 and 56 a Multiload. Among the 49 in the Cu-T200 group, twelve complained of irregular menstrual patterns, 31 of heavy menses and six of both irregular menstruation and heavy menses. Of the 56 women in the Multiload group, fourteen complained of irregular menstruation, 33 of heavy menses and nine of both irregular and heavy menstruation. The results in this group of 105 women changed from a copper IUD to a Progestasert system are shown in Table 5 and Table 6. Twelve of the 105 women reported no change in their menstrual abnormalities after conversion from a copper IUD to Progestasert: seven had used a Cu-T200 and five a Multiload. Eight women who had experienced no menstrual flow complaints when using a copper IUD developed irregular menstruation or spotting during their treatment with the Progestasert. In five of these eight cases this was sufficient reason to terminate this method of contraception.

Table 5. Effect on the menstrual blood loss during treatment with a Progestasert in a group of women who previously used a Cu-T200.

Complaints	Relief after (cycles) 3	6	9	12	no result	total
Irregular bleeding	4	5	1	0	2	12
Heavy menses	12	12	1	1	5	31
Irregular bleeding and heavy menses	2	3	1	0	0	6

Table 6. Effect on menstrual blood loss during treatment with a Progestasert in a group of women who previously used a Multiload.

Complaints	Relief after (cycles) 3	6	9	12	no result	total
Irregular bleeding	5	4	9	1	1	14
Heavy menses	11	12	5	1	4	33
Iregular bleeding and heavy menses	6	1	1	1	0	9

III. HEADACHE

Headache is a difficult complaint to assess. All the women who changed from a copper IUD to a progesterone-releasing IUD had used an oral contraceptive prior to their use of an IUD, and at that time had not suffered from headaches. In our group of 120 women there were fifteen who suffered from headache during their period of treatment with a copper IUD; of these, six had used a Cu-T200 and nine a Multiload. The results obtained after changing to the Progestasert are shown in Table 7.

Table 7. Effect on headache during treatment with the Progestasert.

Type of IUD	*Relief after (cycle)* 3	6	9	12	*no result*	*total*
Cu-T200	4	1	1	0	0	6
Multiload	5	1	1	0	1	9

This group is too small for any conclusion.

IV. DISCUSSION

Pizarro et al. (1977) studied the effect of various types of IUD on menstrual blood flow and dysmenorrhea. The mean number of days of menstrual and intermenstrual bleeding patterns were the same in the group of women with a Gravigard as in those with the Progestasert in their study. Irregular bleeding was higher in their Gravigard group (13.4%) than in the Progestasert group (7.5%). However they mentioned that the results can hardly be considered significant since the bleeding was always slight and did not require IUD removal or special treatment. In their study the total menstrual blood loss was lower among women using the progesterone-releasing IUD than among those using the Gravigard.

The menstrual blood loss is enhanced in women using an IUD which contains copper (Rybo 1976; Rybo and Bergqvist 1980). The percentages vary from 35 to 100 percent. The menstrual blood loss in the group of women with a Progestasert is 15 to 40 percent lower than in women without IUDs. The finding of a suppression of the $PGF_{2\alpha}$ values could explain the good results that we found in our group of women who switched from a copper IUD to a progesterone-releasing IUD. However, our results in the Progestasert group cannot explain the good results obtained by Pizarro et al. (1977) in their group of Gravigard users. There is partial suppression of the endometrium in the Progestasert group so that less tissue is available for prostaglandin synthesis. This could explain the decrease in total blood loss in the Progestasert group.

The increase in menstrual blood loss in the users of copper IUDs has been explained by the observation that there is an increase in fibrinolytic activity, especially at the site where the copper IUD is in contact with the endometrium. Liedholm et al. (1978) demonstrated that there is no increase in fibrinolytic activity in the endometrium after the insertion of a progesterone-releasing IUD. In his group of seventeen women he found on several occasions a decrease or suppression of the endometrium after the insertion of the Progestasert ($p < 0.05$).

The precise cause of dysmenorrhea is unknown. It has been hypothesized that prostaglandins of the $F_{2\alpha}$ group may play an important role in its etiology. Zahradnik et al. (1977) found lower $PGF_{2\alpha}$ values in a group of women with a progesterone-releasing IUD than were found in the menstrual blood of women with a copper IUD. The $PGF_{2\alpha}$ content of the menstrual blood fell from 0.975 ± 0.311 μg/ml to 0.196 ± 0.046 μg/ml. These findings of Zahradnik et al. (1977) have been confirmed by other investigators (Trobough et al. 1979; Trobough 1978).

The beneficial effect of the progesterone-releasing IUD can be explained by the fact that the $PGF_{2\alpha}$ values in the menstrual blood flow are lower in Progestasert users than in women using a copper IUD. The headache which also did not exist when these women were using a contraceptive pill is a prostaglandin-induced headache.

There are many reports which have demonstrated that, according to current laboratory methods, the progesterone of a Progestasert has only a localized effect (Scommegna et al. 1975; Tillson et al. 1975; Wan et al. 1977).

The final assumption that there is no systemic effect could explain the fact that we found galactorrhea in five women during treatment with the progesterone-releasing IUD. The prolactin values were normal in these women (two determinations in each case).

V. CONCLUSION

If a women complains of dysmenorrhea, heavy menstrual blood flow or headache during treatment with a copper IUD, there is sufficient justification to switch from the copper IUD to the Progestasert.

REFERENCES

Liedholm P, Sjöberg N-O, Srivastava K, Ästed B: No increase of the fibrinolytic activity of the human endometrium by progesterone-releasing IUD (Progestasert). Contraception 17 (6): 531-536, 1978.

Pizarro E, Gomez-Rogers C, Rowe PJ, Lucero S: Comparative study of the Progesterone T (65 μg daily) and copper-7 IUD. Contraception 17: 313-323, 1977.

Rybo G: Menstrual blood loss associated with intrauterine contraception with copper and progesterone. Proc world cong gynecol obstet 8: 499, Amsterdam, Excerpta medica international congress series 396, 1976.

Rybo G, Bergqvist A: Comparison of menstrual blood loss with the Progestasert system and the Cu-T200. To be published, 1980.

Scommegna A, Avila T, Luna M, Rao R, Dmowski WP: Fertility control by intrauterine release of progesterone. Obstet Gynecol 43: 769–779, 1979.

Tillson SA, Marian M, Hudson R, Wong P, Pharriss B, Aznar R, Martinez-Manautou J: The effect of intrauterine progesterone on the hypothalamic hypophyseal-ovarian axis in man. Contraception 11: 179-192, 1975.

Trobough G: Pelvic pain and the IUD. J Reprod Med 20 (3): 167-174, 1978.

Trobough G, Gederian AM, Erickson RR, Tillson SA, Leong P, Swisher DA, Pharris BB: The effect of exogenous intrauterine progesterone on the amount and prostaglandin-$F_{2\alpha}$ content of menstrual blood in dysmenorrheic women J Reprod Med 21 (3): 153-158, 1978.

Wan L, Hsu Y, Ganguly M, Bigelow BR: Effects of the Progestasert on the menstrual pattern, ovarian steroids and endometrium. Contraception 16 (4): 417-434, 1977.

Zador G, Nilsson B-A, Nolsson B., Sjöberg N-O, Weström L, Woese J: Clinical experience with the uterine progesterone system (Progestasert). Contraception 13 (5): 559-569, 1976.

Zahradnik HP, Kraut E, Flecken U, Breckwoldt M: Intrauterine progesterone treatment for dysmenorrhoea: measurement of the prostaglandin-$F_{2\alpha}$ level in menstrual blood. Presented at the First European symposium on the intrauterine progesterone-releasing contraceptive, Cologne, 1977.

16. ULTRASONOGRAPHY FOR LOCATING IUDs IN THE UTERINE CAVITY

F.K. BELLER and E.H. SCHMIDT

The contraceptive effectiveness of any intrauterine device depends largely on its correct position in the uterine cavity. Any method capable of monitoring the position is therefore expected to improve the effectiveness of IUDs. Previous methods used for locating IUDs such as identification of the attached thread and probing of the uterus are largely insufficient. Also the use of the beolocator (Fuchs et al. 1965), hysteroscopy, hysterosalpingography and pelvic X-ray are of limited value because they are inadequate, too time-consuming, invasive or inapplicable in the presence of pregnancy.

The method of ultrasonography seemed to have the potential for locating intrauterine contraceptive devices in the architecture of the uterine cavity. We have the method systematically developed (Schmidt et al. 1975; Quakernack et al. 1975) and the results with a consequent follow-up by ultrasonography are reported in regard to pregnancy failure (Schmidt et al. 1979).

Ultrasonography for this purpose was first employed by Winters 1966 using the A-scan mode transvaginally. However this technique did not allow for an exact location of the IUD in the uterine cavity. Nemes and Kerenyi (1971), Ianniruberto and Mastroberadino (1972), Tsai et al. (1973) and Janssens et al. (1973) used the compound B-scan for identifying IUDs with good results when the thread was lost. In contrast Defoort and Thiery (1974) questioned the usefulness of ultrasonography for differentiating of various IUDs in the uterine cavity.

I. MODEL EXPERIMENTS

In early 1973 our study was begun to identify and localize IUDs, preferably Cu-T200s, in the uterine cavity and to diagnose descended location in the cervical canal. The instrument used was a real-time scanner (Vidoson 635S, Siemens, Erlangen). The technique used is schematically presented in Figure 1, where a Lippes Loop is present in the uterine cavity. The ultrasound applicator was applied on the abdominal wall and moved from right to left, resulting in an ultrasound picture of which the cross section is labelled as a in Figure 1. If the applicator is moved up or down in a parallel manner, another cross section is obtained (b Figure 1).

This was the basic application technique used. Early results were, however, disappointing. There were difficulties in relating the IUD properly to the

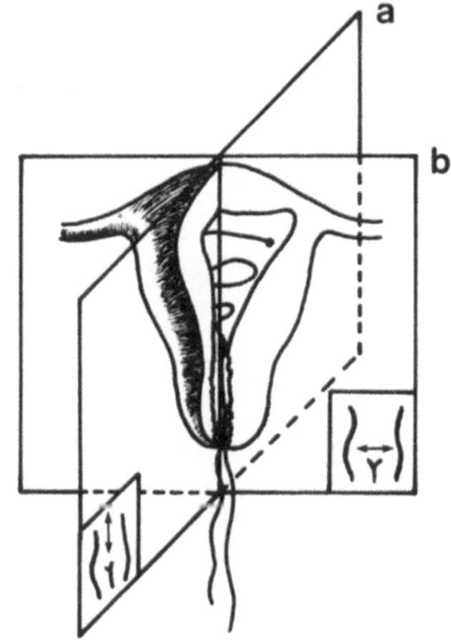

Figure 1. Schematic representation of sections through an anteflexed uterus with inserted Lippes Loop by ultrasonography: (a) longitudinal position of the ultrasonic applicator; (b) transversal position of the ultrasonic applicator. At the lower corners the ultrasonic applicator is shown in relation to the patient. Reproduced from Quakernack et al. (1975), with permission of the publisher.

architecture of the cavity. It became obvious that differentiation of the various parts of the IUD was especially difficult when the uterus was retroflexed.

We then began to study this problem by a model experiment (Schmidt et al. 1975). Various IUDs, such as the Cu-T200, the Lippes Loop and the Dalkon Shield, were selected for study. The IUD was inserted in a uterus before scheduled hysterectomy. Sonographic echoes were obtained and photographed. Following hysterectomy the uterus was fixed in a water tank on a wire frame in front of the ultrasound applicator. The uterus was then systematically placed into the various – anteflexed, retroflexed and intermediate – positions; echograms were obtained again and documented by photography. At the end of the experimentation the uterus was opened to establish the actual location of the IUD. Out of a large number of data a few exemplary figures may explain the various problems. The uterus was clearly distinguished from the surrounding water because of large impedance differences but poorly delineated against the metal support.

In Figure 2 a Cu-T200 is demonstrated in a uterus in middle position. The ultrasound applicator was moved from the fundus to the cervix uteri crosswise to the longitudinal axis of the uterus. A transverse line in the fundus represents the crossbar of the CU-T200. In Figure 2 (d) a pointlike echo corresponds to the transversely struck upright of the device. It is notable that the thread is seen in the transverse section and cannot here be distinguished from the upright of the T (Figure 2,f). Ultrasonography reveals an IUD in the uterine cavity, but the IUD cannot be properly located when the applicator is moved transversely on an extended uterus. The position of the IUD in the uterus is ascertained only when the uterus, with the IUD, is displayed in the longitudinal axis. This is done by placing the applicator longitudinally when the uterus is extended (Figure 3,c). In Figure 3 a Dalkon Shield is seen. If the uterus is retroflexed or anteflexed the crosswise-applied applicator is required to move transversely (Figure 3,a,b). In Figure 3 one may recognize the close relation between the fundus of the uterus and the IUD. This corresponds with a

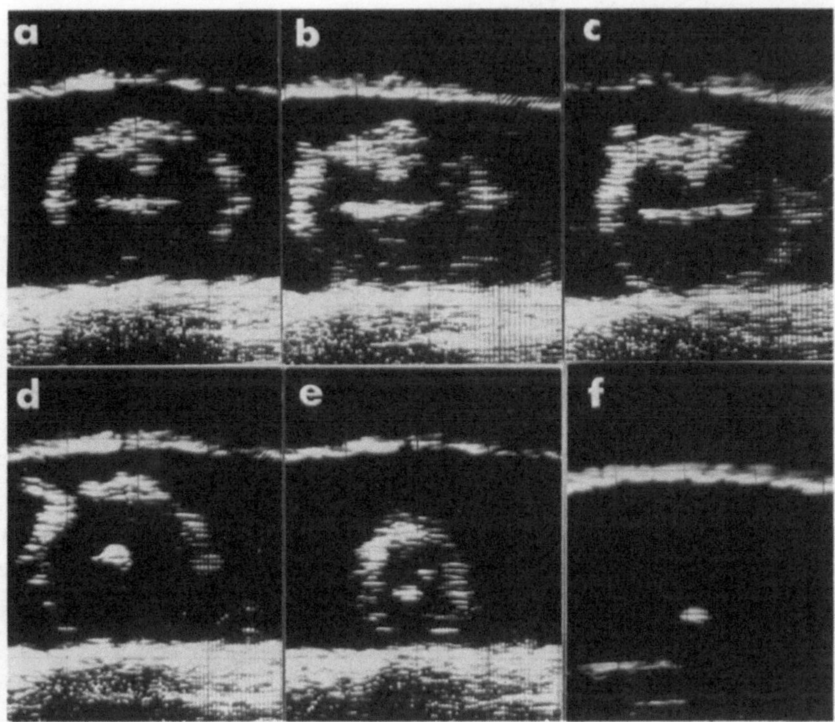

Figure 2. Echograms obtained from an extirpated uterus in a water tank; (a,b,c) the echos correspond to the crossbar of a Cu-T200; (d,e) a pointlike echo, corresponding to the transversely sectioned struck upright of the Cu-T; (f) transverse section of the Cu-T thread. Reproduced from Schmidt et al. (1975), with permission of the publisher.

correct intrauterine placement of the device.

From these model studies three principles emerge: (1) display of the uterus is required in at least two planes for accurate localization of the IUD in the uterine cavity; (2) differentiation of the uterus from neighbouring organs requires a well-filled urinary bladder; (3) the easiest demonstration of the IUD by ultrasound is achieved in the anteflexed or extended uterus. Retroflexed uteri are difficult to delineate because of the large distance from the ultrasound applicator, difficulty in differentiation from intestinal loops and limited topographic relation to the bladder.

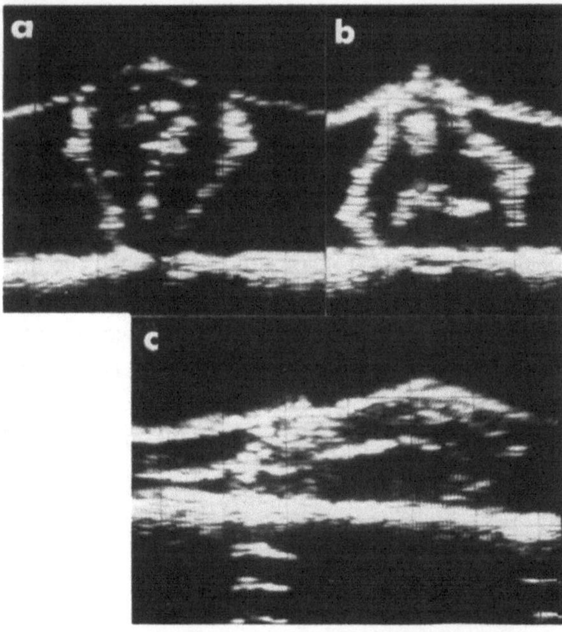

Figure 3. Dalkon Shield: (a,b) uterus in 'ante/retroflexed' position, ultrasonic applicator placed transversely; (c) uterus in 'intermediate' position, applicator placed longitudinally. Reproduced from Schmidt et al. (1975), with permission of the publisher.

II. CLINICAL APPLICATION

By applying these principles to the employment of ultrasonography for determining positions of IUDs in the cavity, the results were so much improved that the technique could be considered as useful (Quakernack et al. 1975). The application of the three principles is demonstrated in Figures 4-8 in women wearing a Cu-T200. In Figure 4 upright of the T is seen in a transverse echogram. The relative position of the IUD in the uterine cavity is not clear in this instance. The extension of the arms of the IUD is difficult to differentiate. It can also not be determined whether the stem of the IUD reaches into the fundus. The correct IUD placement in this instance can be determined only by examining in the longitudinal axis.

The clinical application confirmed the results of the model study. It is easier by ultrasound application in patients to demonstrate an IUD in an anteflexed uterus. The transverse application reveals the T in the uterine cavity, which is confirmed by longitudinal examination (Figure 5, Figure 6). Figure 7 shows an empty fundus. In this instance the IUD has descended into the cervical canal. If this results in a contraceptive failure the Cu-T200 is seen in the cervical canal next to a pregnancy (Figure 8).

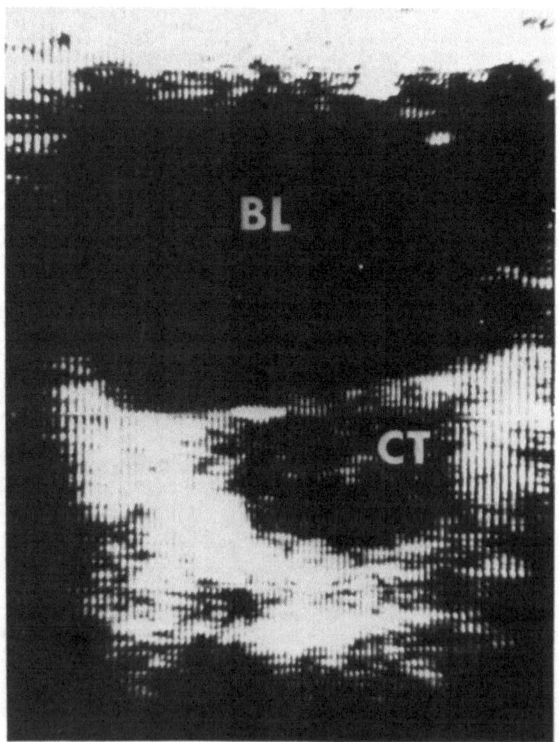

Figure 4. Cu-T200 in an intermediately positioned uterus. BL: urinary bladder; CT: transversely sectioned uterus with struck upright of the Cu-T.

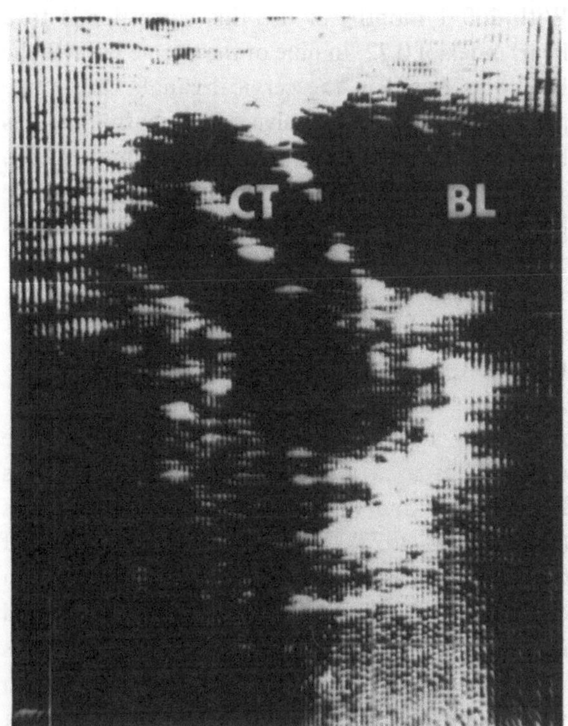

Figure 5. Cu-T200 in an anteflexed uterus, ultrasonic applicator placed longitudinally. BL: urinary bladder; CT: struck upright of the Cu-T.

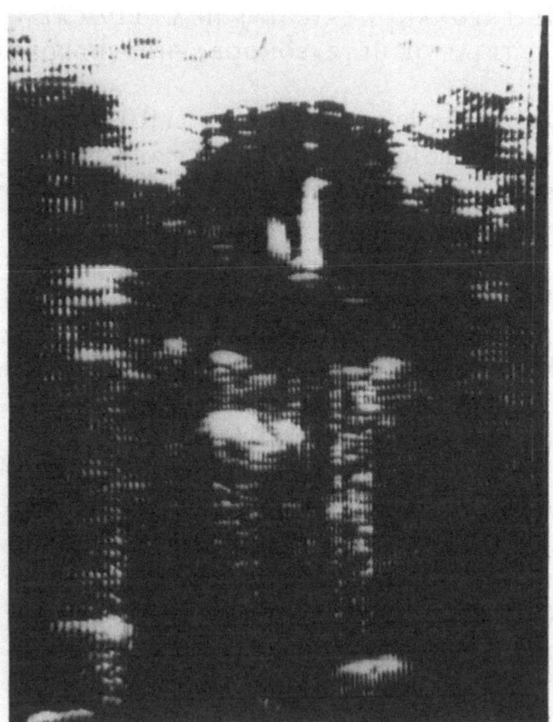

Figure 6. Cu-T200 in an anteflexed uterus, ultrasonic applicator placed transversally.

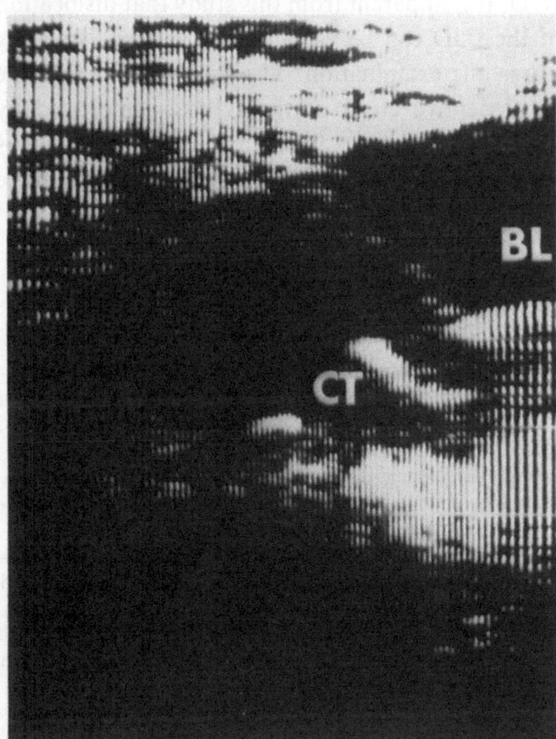

Figure 7. Cu-T200 in an anteflexed uterus. The uterine fundus is empty; the IUD has descended into the cervical canal. BL; urinary bladder; CT; struck upright of the CU-T in the cervical canal.

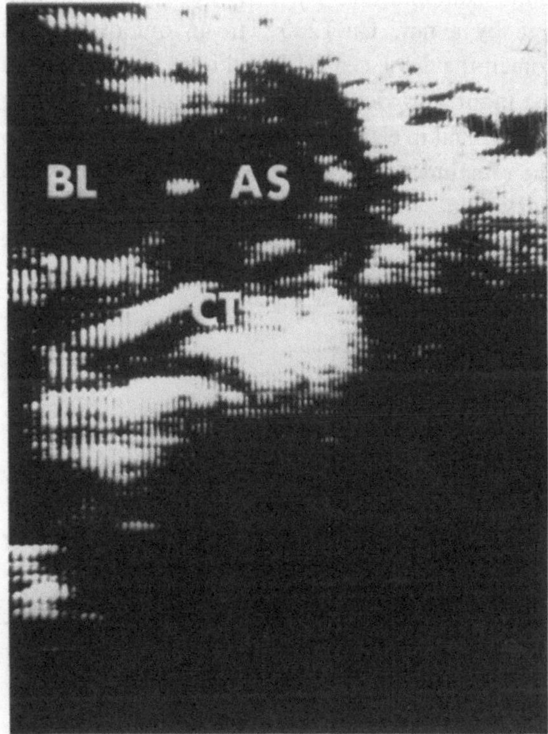

Figure 8. Pregnancy in a case of intracervical dislocation of a Cu-T200. BL: urinary bladder; AS: amniotic sac; CT: Cu-T.

III. PREGNANCY FAILURES IN A CLINICAL TRIAL OF ULTRASONOGRAPHIC FOLLOW-UP

Our working hypothesis was that an IUD correctly placed in the fundus of the uterine cavity should be associated with a lowering pregnancy rate; a descended device in the cervical canal should therefore be associated with a higher frequency of pregnancy failure. Since the descended device can be diagnosed by ultrasonography, ultrasonographical follow-up should be able to improve the contraceptive effectiveness of IUDs. Our clinical follow-up study confirms our assumption (Schmidt et al. 1979).

From 1 September 1973 to 31 August 1977, 1372 women were fitted with a Cu-T200 and controlled by ultrasonography. The average time of IUD use was 14.6 months, corresponding with a total of 20031 menstrual cycles. Ultrasonography was performed one week after insertion, after three and six months and then every six months. The number of ultrasonic examinations performed was 2565. A total of 139 IUD dislocations into the cervical canal were found, including 21 cases being questionable, which could not be confirmed by repeated ultrasound examinations. The IUD was replaced at that time by a new Cu-T200 . In 46 out of the 118 women the displaced IUD had been fitted less than one month previously; in 25 women less than two months and in eleven less than three months before. The remainder were scattered over a period of two years.

Pregnancies were observed in twelve instances. With 20031 months of use this corresponds to a Pearl index of 0.72. In nine of the twelve failures the IUD was found in the cervical canal. Only three patients out of those twelve contraceptive failures followed the advice of regular ultrasonic control. The last preceding examination of each of the twelve women was performed more than six months previously.

IV. CONCLUSION

According to the literature, the pregnancy rate using IUDs as a contraceptive method averages between one and three per 1200 menstrual cycles (Zielske et al. 1977). Therefore a pregnancy rate of 0.72 expressed as a Pearl index can be considered an excellent result, especially since this is a compiled study derived from an outpatient service. The IUDs were inserted by a number of physicians with varying experience. It seems therefore that proper localization of the Cu-T200 is of greater significance than other factors related to pregnancy failures, as for example size, form or surface of the IUD. It is apparent from this study that dislocation of the IUD can be visualized at an early stage by ultrasonic examination. The data suggest that the contraceptive effect of the IUDs is improved by ultrasonic follow-up. The sequence for follow-up is the first week after insertion, after one month, three months and then every six months.

REFERENCES

Defoort P, Thiery M: IUD-typing by ultrasound: an in-vitro study. Contraception 9: 609, 1974.

Fuchs FF, Buchman MJ, Nakamoto M: A new instrument for localization of intrauterine contraceptive devices: the be-olocator. Am J Obstet Gynecol 93: 128, 1965.

Ianniruberto A, Mastroberadino A: Ultrasonic localization of the Lippes Loop. Am J Obstet Gynecol 114: 78, 1972.

Janssens D, Vrijens M, Thiery M, van Kets H: Ultrasonic detection, localization and identification of intrauterine contraception devices. Contraception 8: 485, 1973.

Nemes G, Kerenyi T: Ultrasonic localization of the IUCD. Am J Obstet Gynecol 109: 1219, 1971.

Quakernack K, Schmidt EH, Lieder B, Beller FK: The identification of IUDs by ultrasound in the uterine cavity. J Obstet Gynec Reprod Biol 4: 203, 1975.

Schmidt EH, Quakernack K, Lieder B, Beller FK: Ultraschalluntersuchungen zur Lagediagnostik von Intrauterin-Pessaren im Modellversuch und an Patientinnen. Arch Gynaekol 218: 173, 1975.

Schmidt EH, Wagner H, Quakernack K, Beller FK: Ergebnisse der Lageüberwachung von Intrauterin-Pessaren durch Ultraschall. Geburtshilfe Frauenheilkd 39: 138, 1979.

Tsai WS, Chen HY, Chen YP, Wei PY, Sonographic visualization of coexisting gestation sac and IUD in the uterus and a consideration of a causative factor of accidental pregnancy. Int J Fertil 18: 85, 1973.

Winters HS: Ultrasound detection of intrauterine contraception devices. Am J Obstet Gynecol 95: 880, 1966.

Zielske F, Becker K, Knauf P: Schwangerschaften bei Intrauterin-Pessaren in situ. Geburtshilfe Frauenheilkd 37: 473, 1977.

17. FERTILITY AFTER IUD REMOVAL

I. Batár

Most temporary contraceptive methods are reversible, with fertility returning after discontinuation of use. However, relatively little is known about the length of time that must elapse before complete restoration of fertility or about the possibly negative effects of a specific technique on the reproductive system or on the outcome of a pregnancy commencing after discontinuation. For example, is there any connection between the duration of IUD use and the date of the first conception after removing the device? Does the duration of IUD use or the period of time that elapses between its removal and conception influence the outcome of pregnancy or the type of delivery? Have these parameters any effects on the number and severity of malformations of the offspring? Is there any difference in the sex ratio or birthweight between the newborns of the previous users and nonusers of IUDs?

During the last two decades, the failure rates and side effects directly connected with IUD use have mostly been studied. To survey this literature seems almost impossible. Only a few articles dealt with the events that occurred *after* removing the device, the conception rate and the outcome of first pregnancies conceived after discontinuation.

At the beginning only conception rates after IUD removal were published (World Health Organization 1968; Tietze and Lewit 1970). Later the outcome of first pregnancies (Vessey et al. 1974), characteristics of the offspring born of these pregnancies (Vessey et al. 1976) and average fecundability after removing the device (Jain and Moots 1977) were also studied. The modern methods of prenatal and subnatal diagnostics were also used to compare the newborns of mothers whose pregnancies had started after discontinuing oral or intrauterine contraception (Martynshin et al. 1978). In a recent work, the return of fertility after discontinuation of different kinds of contraceptive methods was measured by means only of delivery rates not conception rates (Vessey et al. 1978).

The data set of almost 14000 IUDs inserted at the family planning centre at Debrecen in Hungary made it possible to study the above questions in detail. Out of these cases of different types of devices, the Szontágh-IUD, having the greatest number of insertions, proved to be the most suitable one for evaluating the connections. The results were not primarily compared to those known from the literature, but rather to the local population standards wherever it was possible.

I. MATERIALS AND METHODS

Because the Szontágh IUD (Szontágh et al. 1967) is used only in Hungary, and as it is not known abroad, it is worthwhile describing it. The device is made of a simple fishing line (Figure 1). The 169-mm thread of 1-mm diameter is joined together at the two ends into a looplike shape, which gives the device a suitable flexibility in two dimensions. In this way it can be accommodated to the given intrauterine space. At the end of the device a tail of 0.1-mm diameter is attached.

During the years between 1972 and 1976, 8536 Szontágh IUDs were inserted at the family planning centre. Of these 1091 were removed for planned pregnancy. After excluding those who used any other kind of contraceptives after the removal, even for a very short period, 1008 women remained in the study. Of these, we were not able to obtain any information about 359 patients. In the end, 649 persons proved to be eligible for evaluation.

The data for this retrospective study were mostly

collected at clinic visits and partly by telephone contacts or mail. The evaluation was carried out by computerization through a medium of specially designed forms. The cumulative conception rate after removal was calculated by using the *life table* technique. Further, linear regression, the χ^2 test and analysis of variance as well as covariance were employed for statistical evaluation. The differences cited in this chapter are significant at the 0.05 level.

II. RESULTS

II.A. Conception rate after IUD removal

Of the 649 women evaluated after IUD removal, 587 reported conception. By the end of the first year following discontinuation, 563 pregnancies were recorded. The number of patients at risk in the twelfth month was 54, so the life table technique could be used to calculate the conception rate for the first year. After this period the number of cases was too small to make statistical evaluations suitable for valid conclusions. The number of terminated cases at the end of the twelfth month was 599 and the cumulative number of woman-months of 'nonuse' was 2177.

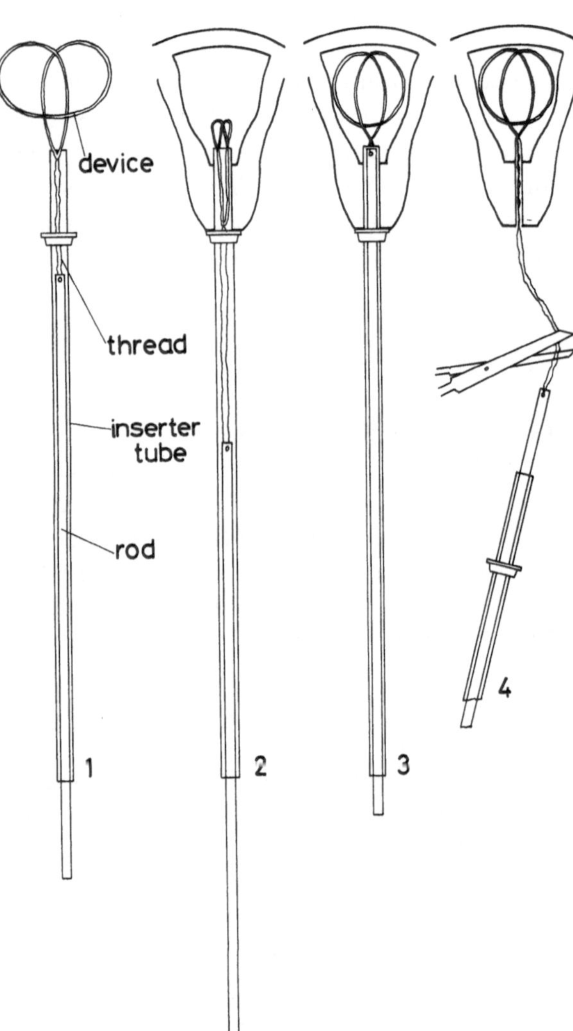

Figure 1. The Szontágh IUD and its insertion.

The distribution of age registered at conception or at termination, or at the cutoff date for patients who did not conceive is shown in Table 1. Within the subgroups, except for those of 21-30 years, the number of cases was not enough to calculate an age-specific life table conception rate in order to compare it with that of the normal population standard. We were able though to compute a cumulative conception rate for all cases for one year (Figure 2).

In the first month after IUD removal almost a third (29.1%) of the patients had conceived; by the end of the second month nearly half of them (48.3%) had done so. After this steep climb the graph of the conception rate levels out and, with a slight rise, reaches 90.5 percent by the end of the twelfth month. These results are similar to those previously published in the literature.

By the end of the first year, conception rates of 91.5 percent and 88.2 percent were reported by the World Health Organization (1968) and Tietze and Lewit (1970), on the basis of evaluating 507 and 378 women respectively. A similar value (85.0%) was published by Jain and Moots (1977). In another study, the conception rate was 33.0 percent after three months and 63.8 percent by the end of the sixth month following discontinuation (Martynshin et al. 1977), but because this data set contains both hormonal contraceptive and IUD cases, it is not

Table 1. Age distribution of total subject population.

Age	*Number*	%
≤ 20	30	4.6
21-25	281	43.3
26-30	256	39.4
31-35	63	9.7
36-40	12	1.8
unknown	7	1.1
Total	649	100.0

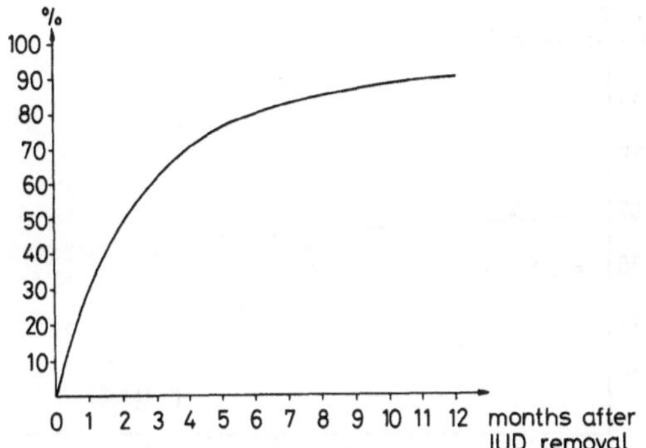

Figure 2. Cumulative conception rate per 100 women after IUD removal.

suitable for comparison. Vessey et al. (1976, 1978) did not regularly record the date of the last menstrual period. In this way only 'outcome rate' could be calculated in their study, and again, this was not suitable to serve as control for our results.

It is worthwhile to analyze the distribution of conceptions registered for the first ordinal month (Table 2). Of the 188 women who conceived only 77 (41.0%) reported menses after IUD removal. The other 111 patients (59.0%) had no more menstruation until conception; calculating its date from the date of the last menstrual period (first day of the last menses + 14 days), it is presumable that 24 of these (12.8) conceived *before* discontinuation. Since these pregnancies were only of 1-8 days at the time of IUD removal, and this period corresponds to the tubal migration of the ova, they were not attributed to the failure of the device.

II.B. Duration of IUD use and date of conception

The data of 585 pregnancies were eligible for studying the connection between the duration of IUD use and the period of time that must elapse after removal until conception. The length of use fell between one and 64 months, but after month 36

Table 2. Distribution of conceptions registered for the first month.

Conception	*Number*	%
Before IUD removal	24	12.8
After IUD removal		
with no menses	87	46.3
with one menses	77	41.0
Total	188	100.0

the number of cases was insufficient to draw valid conclusions.

Among those who employed the IUD for less than one year, 204 women conceived (Group 1). The average number of months until conception was 2.8. After more than one, but less than two years of use (Group 2), 237 women became pregnant with an average of 3.3 months until conception. The latter value was 2.9 months for the 99 women that conceived after more than two, but less than three years of IUD use (Group 3). The other 45 pregnant patients wore the device for 37-64 months (Group 4); the average number of months between discontinuation and conception was 2.2.

Evaluation was made for only 540 women who were in Groups 1-3. The average number of months for conception by the duration of IUD use is shown in Figure 3. A negative correlation of weak medium degree was found between the two characteristics ($r = -0.4$), but it was not statistically significant ($p = 0.217$).

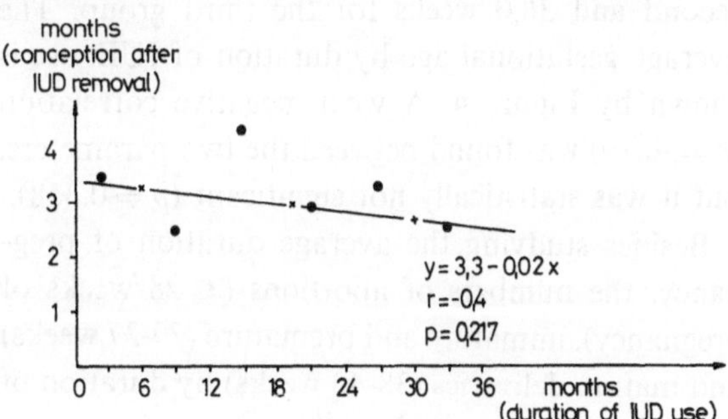

Figure 3. Time of conception by duration of IUD use.

As is seen, most of the conceptions occurred during the first three months and 90.5 percent of the women conceived by the end of the first year. Because of a given sterility rate, not all of the remaining 9.5 percent would become pregnant, and because the period of time that elapsed until the conception showed a wide diversity for the patients who conceived after one year following discontinuation (13-38 months), only those from the three studied groups who conceived within one year of IUD removal were evaluated. In this way data of 516 pregnancies could be analyzed. Studying conception separately within the one, two and three-year users, it was also found that almost a third of the women conceived in the first month and half of them became pregnant by the end of the second ordinal month in each group (Table 3). Statistically there were no significant differences among the three groups ($f = 10.36$, $p = 0.999$), so it is stated that the duration of IUD use, considering no more than three years of use, does not influence the period of time that must elapse until the first conception after discontinuation.

II.C. Duration of IUD use and outcome of first pregnancy conceived after discontinuation

Of the women whose gestational age was known and who wore the device for less than three years, 477 patients are eligible for evaluation. Of these, 176 women used the device for less than one year (Group 1), 214 employed the IUD for more than one but less than two years (Group 2), and 87 wore it for more than two but less than three years (group 3).

At the termination of the first pregnancy conceived after IUD removal, the average gestational age was 36.5 weeks for the first, 37.4 weeks for the second and 36.0 weeks for the third group. The average gestational age by duration of IUD use is shown by Figure 4. A weak negative correlation ($r = -0.19$) was found between the two parameters, but it was statistically not significant ($p = 0.358$).

Besides studying the average duration of pregnancy, the numbers of abortions ($\leqslant$ 28 weeks of pregnancy), immature and premature (29-37 weeks) and mature deliveries (38-43 weeks) by duration of IUD use were also evaluated.

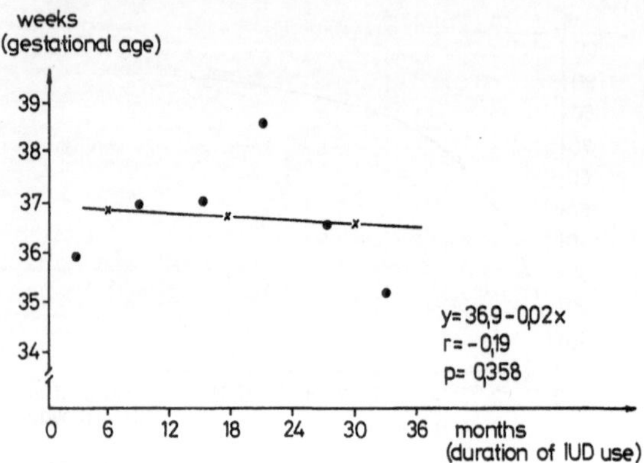

Figure 4. Duration of pregnancy by duration of IUD use.

II.C.1. Abortions

Forty-eight pregnancies (10.1%) were terminated before week 28. Of these nineteen 10.7% were in the first, seventeen (7.9%) in the second and twelve (13.8%) in the third groups. It was found that the frequency of abortions increased as the duration of use advanced (Figure 5). The correlation was positive of a weak medium degree ($r = 0.36$), but it was statistically not significant ($p = 0.242$).

II.C.2. Premature deliveries

The frequency of immature or premature deliveries was in inverse ratio to the duration of IUD use: the longer the wearing period, the lower the rate of prematurity (Figure 6). Of the 56 (11.7%)

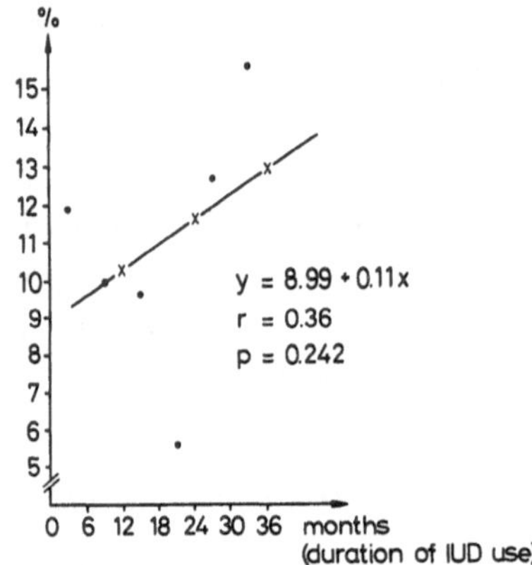

Figure 5. Outcome of pregnancy by duration of IUD use: abortions.

Table 3. Distribution of first conceptions within one year by duration of IUD use.

Duration of IUD use (months)	*Conception (months after IUD removal)* 1 *month(s) after IUD removal*		2		3		4-5		6-7		8-9		10-12		*Total*		*Mean months*
	n	%	*n*	%	*n*	%	*n*	%	*n*	%	*n*	%	*n*	%	*n*	%	
1-12	61	31.6	42	21.8	36	18.7	27	14.0	16	8.3	6	3.1	5	2.6	193	100.0	2.8
13-24	82	35.0	38	16.2	36	15.4	43	18.4	15	6.4	9	3.9	11	4.7	234	100.0	3.3
25-36	27	30.3	25	28.1	12	13.5	14	15.7	6	6.7	3	3.4	2	2.3	89	100.0	2.9
Total	170	32.9	105	20.3	84	16.3	84	16.3	37	7.2	18	3.5	18	3.5	516	100.0	3.0

$f = 10.36$; $p = 0.999$

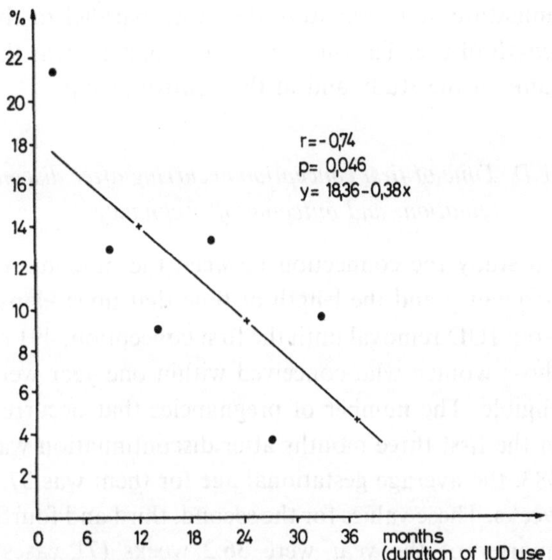

Figure 6. Outcome of pregnancy by duration of IUD use: immature and premature deliveries.

premature deliveries, 28 (15.8%) were in the first, 23 (10.8%) in the second and five (5.8%) in the third group. The correlation was strongly negative ($r = -0.74$) and statistically significant ($p = 0.046$).

II.C.3. Mature deliveries

As the duration of IUD use increased within three years, so did the frequency of mature deliveries (Figure 7). Of the 373 (78.2%) cases, 129 (73.5%) 174 (81.3%) and 70 (80.5%) mature deliveries occurred in Groups 1, 2 and 3, respectively. The correlation was positive of a medium degree ($r = 0.51$), but it was statistically not significant ($p = 0.151$).

Analyzing the gestational age at termination separately for each group (Table 4), we did not find significant differences among them ($f = 0.50$, $p = 0.380$).

The frequency of spontaneous abortions, immature and premature, and mature deliveries for those who used the device for less than three years was compared with the local values of the Department of Obstetrics and Gynecology. As only a small proportion of the first pregnancies conceived after IUD removal (0.7%) was terminated by induced abortion, but at the same time this category had a significantly higher proportion (32.7%) in the control population, abortions of this kind were excluded from both groups. Cases with unknown or uncertain gestational age were also ignored in the study group; furthermore, to avoid duplication, those who had used an IUD before conception and had had the device removed for planned pregnancy were excluded from the control population (Table 5). The number of spontaneous abortions, immature or premature, and mature deliveries was 48 (10.1%), 56 (11.7%) and 373 (78.2%) in the study group and 1819 (10.7%), 1932 (11.4%) and 13263 (78.0%) in the control population, respectively. Analyzing the outcome of pregnancies, it can be stated that there is no significant difference between the two groups ($\chi^2 = 0.24$, $p = 0.887$).

In order to evaluate the frequency of ectopic pregnancies, all conceptions, including those resulting in induced abortions should be considered. Of the 587 pregnancies started after discontinuation of IUD use, 585 (99.7%) were intrauterine and two

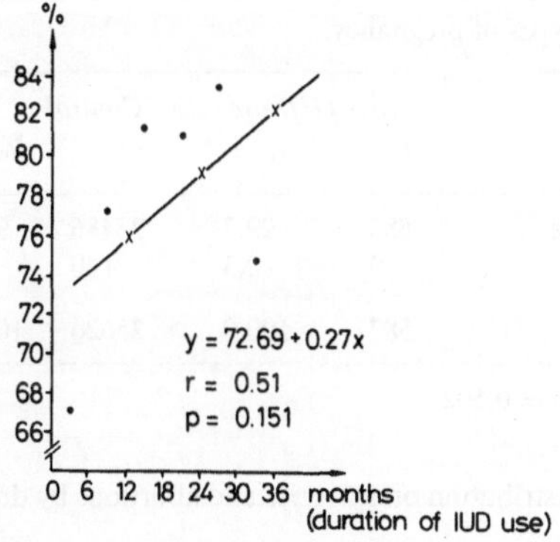

Figure 7. Outcome of pregnancy by duration of IUD use: mature deliveries.

Table 4. Duration of pregnancy by duration of IUD use.

Duration of IUD use (months)	*Gestational age (weeks) at termination (%)* 3-10 (n=16)	11-19 (n=21)	20-28 (n=11)	29-37 (n=56)	38-43 (n=373)	*Average (weeks)*
1-12	4	3	3	16	73	36.5
13-24	3	3	2	11	81	37.4
25-36	2	10	1	6	81	36.0

$f = 0.50$; $p = 0.380$

Table 5. Outcome of pregnancies (percentages).

Gestational age at termination (weeks)	*After IUD use (n=477)*	*Control (N=17014)*
⩽ 28	10	11
29-37	12	11
38-43	78	78

$\chi^2 = 0.24; p = 0.887$

(0.3%) ectopic. Of the 25626 conceptions in the control group, 25486 (99.5%) resulted in intrauterine and 140 (0.5%) in ectopic pregnancies (Table 6). The values were almost the same in both groups and there were no significant differences between them ($\chi^2 = 0.45$, $p = 0.502$).

In order to compare the frequency of all deliveries and abortions in the two groups, the IUD users were divided into six subgroups according to the length of IUD use (Table 7), but statistically significant differences again were not found ($f = 1.62$, $p = 0.714$).

To summarize the results of these evaluations, it can be stated that the duration of IUD use does not influence the outcome of the first pregnancy conceived after discontinuation. The only significant change found was the decrease in numbers of immature and premature deliveries parallel to the length of use. The outcome of pregnancies was the same in the study and in the control group.

Table 6. Types of pregnancy.

Type of pregnancy	*After IUD use* *n*	*%*	*Control* *n*	*%*
Intrauterine	585	99.7	25486	99.5
Ectopic	2	0.3	140	0.5
Total	587	100.0	25626	100.0

$\chi^2 = 0.45; p = 0.502$

Table 7. Distribution of deliveries and abortions by duration of IUD use.

Duration of IUD use (months)	*Deliveries* *n*	*%*	*Abortions* *n*	*%*
1- 6	70	89.7	8	10.3
7-12	110	92.4	9	7.6
13-18	117	91.4	11	8.6
19-24	88	93.6	6	6.4
25-30	50	86.2	8	13.8
31-36	30	88.2	4	11.8
Nonusers (control)	15195	89.3	1819	10.7

$f = 1.62; p = 0.714$

II.D. Time of first conception occurring after discontinuation, and outcome of pregnancy

To study the connection between the outcome of pregnancy and the length of time that must elapse from IUD removal until the first conception, 491 of those women who conceived within one year were eligible. The number of pregnancies that occurred in the first three months after discontinuation was 383; the average gestational age for them was 37.0 weeks. These values for the second, third and fourth quarter of the year were 36.2 weeks (71 cases), 34.4 weeks (20 cases) and 37.2 weeks (17 cases), respectively (Figure 8). A weak negative correlation ($r = -0.14$) was found between the time of first conception and the outcome of pregnancy, but it was not statistically significant ($p = 0.430$).

The frequency of abortions, immature or premature, and mature deliveries was analyzed in this connection too.

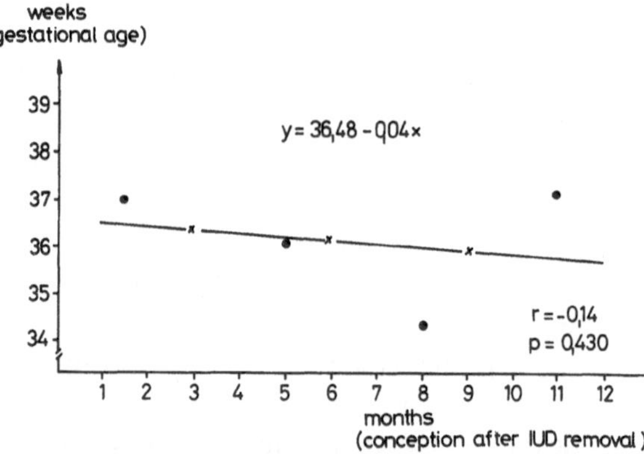

Figure 8. Duration of pregnancy by time of conception after IUD use.

II.D.1. Abortions

A positive correlation of medium degree ($r = 0.65$) was found between the frequency of abortions and the period of time that elapsed until conception (Figure 9). The number of abortions in the first, second, third and fourth quarter was 35 (9.1%), seven (9.9%), three (15.0%) and two (11.8%), respectively. This correlation was not significant ($p = 0.175$).

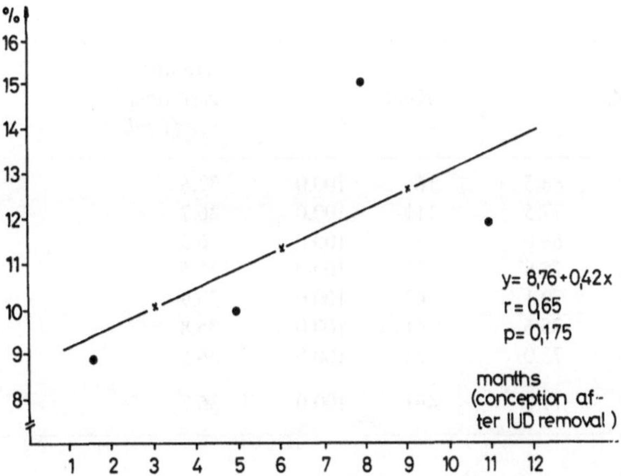

Figure 9. Outcome of pregnancy by time of conception after IUD use: abortions.

II.D.2. Immature or premature deliveries

Of pregnancies resulting in immature or premature delivery 49 (12.8%) were conceived in the first three months, eight (11.3%) in the second, and five (25.0%) in the third quarter. Among those conceived in the fourth quarter, there were no immature or premature deliveries (Figure 10). A weak negative correlation ($r = -0.30$) was found between the two parameters, but it was not statistically significant ($p = 0.351$).

II.D.3. Mature deliveries

The frequency of mature deliveries was lower among those who became pregnant earlier than those who conceived later (Figure 11). The number of these deliveries was 299 (78.1%), 56 (78.9%),

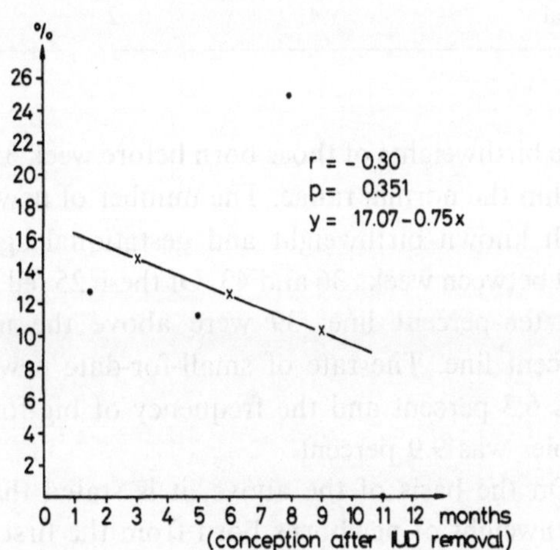

Figure 10. Outcome of pregnancy by time of conception after IUD use: immature and premature deliveries.

twelve (60.0%) and fifteen (88.2%), respectively, in the first, second, third and fourth quarters. The weak positive correlation ($r = 0.11$) found between the two characteristics was not significant ($p = 0.444$).

The distribution of these three obstetrical events by time of conception is shown in Table 8. As to the outcome of pregnancies, there were no statistically significant differences among those who became pregnant during the first year after discontinuation of IUD use ($f = 1.21$, $p = 0.639$).

II.E. Malformations

Of the 502 deliveries, six malformations (1.20%) were registered. Two of those were major and four minor. Between January 1977 and June 1978, the frequency of malformations was 1.22 percent in the local control population. The comparison of the two groups is given in Table 9. The values were almost the same and statistically there was no significant difference between them ($\chi^2 = 0.002$, $p = 0.966$).

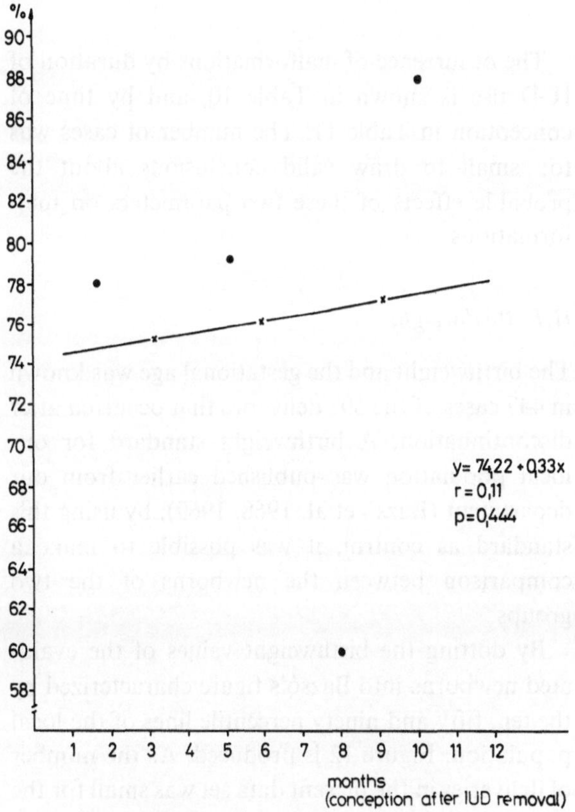

Figure 11. Outcome of pregnancy by time of conception after IUD use: mature deliveries.

Table 8. Outcome of pregnancies by time of conception.

Month of conception	Gestational age at termination (weeks) ⩽ 28 n	%	29-37 n	%	38-43 n	%	Total n	%	Average gestational age (weeks)
1	12	7.3	15	9.1	137	83.5	164	100.0	37.6
2	11	9.9	14	12.6	86	77.5	111	100.0	36.7
3	8	10.7	16	21.3	51	68.0	75	100.0	36.5
4	4	12.1	4	12.1	25	75.8	33	100.0	35.5
5	5	11.6	4	9.3	34	79.1	43	100.0	35.9
6- 8	4	9.8	6	14.6	31	75.6	41	100.0	35.8
9-12	3	12.5	3	12.5	18	75.0	24	100.0	36.5
Total	47	9.6	62	12.6	382	77.8	491	100.0	36.7

$f = 1.21; p = 0.639$

Table 9. Malformations.

Type of malformation	After IUD use n	%	Control n	%
None	496	98.80	5194	98.78
Minor	4	0.80	42	0.80
Major	2	0.40	22	0.42
Total	502	100.00	5258	100.00

$\chi^2 = 0.002; p = 0.966$

Table 10. Malformations by duration of IUD use.

Duration of IUD use (months)	Malformation Minor	Major	Diagnosis
6	1	–	Unspecified slight heart murmur
8	1	–	Acetabular dysplasia
10	–	1	Esophagostenosis
17	–	1	Mucoviscidosis
18	1	–	Talipes, unspecified
19	1	–	Unknown

The occurrence of malformations by duration of IUD use is shown in Table 10, and by time of conception in Table 11. The number of cases was too small to draw valid conclusions about the probable effects of these two parameters on malformations.

Table 11. Malformations by time of conception.

Month of conception	Malformation Minor	Major
1	1	–
2	1	–
3	1	1
6	–	1
14	1	–
Total	4	2

II.F. Birthweight

The birthweight and the gestational age was known in 447 cases of the 502 deliveries that occurred after discontinuation. A birthweight standard for our local population was published earlier from our department (Bazsó et al. 1968, 1969); by using this standard as control, it was possible to make a comparison between the newborns of the two groups.

By dotting the birthweight values of the evaluated newborns into Bazsó's figure characterized by the ten, fifty and ninety percentile lines of the local population, Figure 12 is produced. As the number of deliveries in the present data set was small for the pregnancies terminated before week 38 of gestation, a complete statistical evaluation could not be made. The birthweights of those born before week 35 were within the normal range. The number of newborns with known birthweight and gestational age was 349 between weeks 36 and 43. Of these 25 fell under the ten-percent line; 39 were above the ninety-percent line. The rate of small-for-date newborns was 6.3 percent and the frequency of big-for-date babies was 9.9 percent.

On the basis of the above, it is stated that the birthweight of newborns born from the first pregnancies conceived after discontinuation of IUD use corresponds to that of the local control population.

II.G. Sex of the newborn

The sex of newborns was known in 467 cases; of these 239 (51.2%) were male and 228 (48.8%) female. The male-female ratio was 1.05. In 1977, 3693 newborns were registered at our Department of Obstetrics and Gynecology. The number of males and females was 2059 (55.8%) and 1634 (44.2%), respectively (Table 12) with a male-female ratio of 1.26, but there was statistically no significant difference in the sex ratio between the two groups ($\chi^2 = 3.51$, $p = 0.061$).

Table 12. Sex of newborn.

Sex	*After IUD use* n	%	*Control* n	%
Male	239	51.2	2059	55.8
Female	228	48.8	1634	44.2
Total	467	100.0	3693	100.0

$\chi^2 = 3.51; p = 0.061$

II.H. Management of delivery

The type of management was known in 456 cases of the 502 deliveries. The number of spontaneous vaginal deliveries was 437 (95.8%); three vacuum extractions (0.7%) and sixteen Cesarean sections (3.5%) were made in the study group (Table 13). Between January 1977 and June 1978, 5251 deliveries were registered at our department; these served as control. In this population there were 4750 spontaneous vaginal deliveries (90.5%), 39 vacuum extractions (0.7%) and 462 Cesarean sections (8.8%). The ratio of vacuum extractions was the same in the two groups, but the frequency of Cesarean sections was significantly lower in the study group, and consequently, the proportion of spontaneous deliveries was significantly higher among the former IUD users than in the control population. The difference was strongly significant ($\chi^2 = 15.39$, $p = 0.00046$).

Table 13. Management of delivery.

Type of delivery	*After IUD use* n	%	*Control* n	%
Spontaneous	437	95.8	4750	90.5
Vacuum extraction	3	0.7	39	0.7
Cesarean section	16	3.5	462	8.8
Total	456	100.0	5251	100.0

$\chi^2 = 15.39; p = 0.0005$

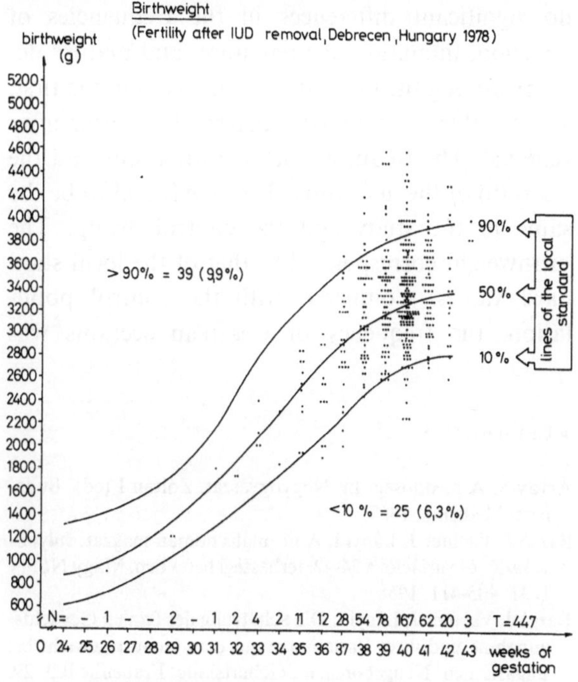

Figure 12. Birthweight after IUD removal and in standard population, by weeks of gestation.

III. SUMMARY

Analyzing the data of 649 women, 587 pregnancies and 502 deliveries after discontinuation of IUD use, the return of fertility was investigated in a retrospective study. The inert, Szontágh-type device was removed for planned pregnancy in every case and after the removal the women did not use any kind of contraception until the first conception. Using the life table technique for calculation, the cumulative conception rate was 90.5 at the end of the first year after discontinuation. It corresponds to the values of literature, and the 9.5-percent rate of infertility is identical with that of the Hungarian woman population (Árvay 1967). The duration of IUD use did not influence the length of time that elapsed until the first conception after removal; and, except for immature and premature deliveries, it had no effect on the outcome of pregnancy: there were no changes in the frequencies of abortion and mature delivery, but a significant decrease was found in the rate of immature and premature deliveries parallel to the duration of IUD use. The outcome of pregnancies was the same in the study and the local control group. The period of time between discontinuation and first conception also did not influence the length of gestation and there were statistically no significant differences in the frequencies of abortion, immature or premature, and mature delivery among the pregnancies conceived in the first, second, third and fourth quarter of the year after removal. The frequency of malformations and the sex ratio of the newborns also were found to be the same in the study and the control group. The birthweight corresponded to that of the local standard values. Compared with the control population, the frequency of Cesarean sections was significantly lower and consequently a significantly higher rate of spontaneous delivery was found in the study group.

Summarizing the results, it is stated that, as for the return of fertility, the Szontágh IUD fulfils the requirement established for all temporary contraceptive methods. After removing the device the fertility was restored and no negative effects on conception, course and outcome of pregnancy were observed. In our opinion, the conclusions drawn from these results may apply to ther inert IUDs, but instead of this, further investigation of the question of studying more cases and different types of IUD should be made.

REFERENCES

Árvay S: A meddöség. In: Nögyógyászat, Zoltán I (ed), Budapest, Medicina, 1967.

Bazsó J, Vachter J, Lányi I: A normális human magzati sulynövekedés és variációi a 24-42. terhességi hetekben. Magy Nőorv L 31: 405-411, 1968.

Bazsó J, Vachter J, Lányi I: Die Schätzung der fetalen Gewichtszunahme und ihrer Variationen aus dem Geburtsgewicht bei ungarischen Neugeborenen. Geburtshilfe Frauenheilkd 29: 845-852, 1969.

Jain AK, Moots B: Fecundability following the discontinuation of IUD use among Taiwanese women. J Biosoc Sci 9: 137-151, 1977.

Martynshin M Ya, Kryzhanovskaya-Kaplun EF, Nikolaeva AM: The course of pregnancy and the state of the intrauterine fetus after the use of various contraceptives [in Russian]. Vopr Okhr Materin Det 22: 60-62, 1977.

Szontágh F, Zelenka L, Szereday Z: Contraception with a simple intrauterine device. In: Preventive medicine and family planning, Hartford, Conn, Austin and Sons, 1967, p 127-130.

Tietze C, Lewit S: Evaluation of intrauterine devices: ninth progress report of the cooperative statistical program. Stud Fam Plann 55, 1970.

Vessey MP, Johnson B, Doll R, Peto R: Outcome of pregnancy in women using an intrauterine device. Lancet 495-498, 23 March 1974.

Vessey M, Doll R, Peto R, Johnson B, Wiggins P: A long-term follow-up study of women using different methods of contraception: an interim report. J Biosoc Sci 8: 373-427, 1976.

Vessey MP, Wright NH, McPherson D, Wiggins P: Fertility after stopping different methods of contraception. Br Med J 1: 265-277, 1978.

World Health Organization: Intra-uterine devices: physiological and clinical aspects, WHO technical report series 397, Geneva, WHO, 1968.

18. PSYCHOLOGICAL FACTORS: COUNSELLING AND MOTIVATION OF CONTRACEPTIVE PATIENTS

B.N. Barwin

Compliance in the use of contraception is directly related to the amount and intensity of counselling and the degree of motivation.

In the study of fertility and sterility, researchers have directed their attention to the physiological factors, as these were most obviously relevant and could be studied rigorously with available techniques. Some factors, previously not unnoticed but of less vital importance, have become of greater significance now that the technical side of fertility control has come closer to being mastered. If basic research has provided man with an adequate means for the accomplishment of family planning and if it promises even better controls in the future, then success of the actual application of these controls depends entirely on the intrapersonal and interpersonal factors that are relevant to the problem. Therefore, while the study of basic physiology and fertility continues to move forward, it is necessary that the sociological and psychological factors involved be subjected to systematic study.

The specific means of contraception, as well as the manner in which the physician advises his patients, are of considerable importance. There is a great deal of literature discussing the social, economic, and cultural situations in various countries and the effect these have on the population's orientation toward birth control. The orientation of various religious groups with regard to birth control has received much attention. While such observations are of great importance, the area of psychological involvement of the individuals applying methods of family planning remains largely neglected. The individual personality traits of husband and wife, their personality interactions, and the wife's relationship with her physician may be especially relevant to the effectiveness of contraception.

A survey of the opinions of general practitioners and obstetrics and gynecology specialists concerning contraceptives showed that oral contraceptives are currently most often prescribed (Wallach and Garcia 1968), but many women abandon them because of distressing side effects (Ryder 1973). This has prompted many physicians almost to give up prescribing them. It is reasonable to assume, however, that women who go to the trouble of starting on a contraceptive programme are highly motivated to prevent pregnancy.

I. PERSONALITY CHARACTERISTICS

Persons who are efficient and effective users of contraceptives have been characterized as mature, responsible, and self-reliant. They establish and appreciate long-range goals and have a capacity to establish good communication and usually good sexual adjustment with their partners. They have a good self-image, assume responsibility with ease and confidence, control their impulsiveness, and have the capacity to tolerate frustration (Sandberg 1975).

The user of the rhythm method is characterized as somewhat rigid regarding her religious and social attitudes. She frequently feels 'overworked, unappreciated and lonely'; she denies her sexual instincts and denies her partner as well. Because of its precarious inefficiency, the rhythm method 'suits her fatalism' and her desire for martyrdom (Tourkow et al. 1973).

The user of the withdrawal method is characterized as having an excessive faith in luck, a denying attitude regarding fertility, and feelings of guilt if she prepared for coitus with a contraceptive. She feels a 'doomed dependence' on men. She must inspire sexual activity that she does not want. Compelled to indulge, she can still mentally and emotionally reject sex and the male as well. Withdrawal deprives each partner of pleasure, but, inasmuch as pleasure and orgasms are not her goals, the method is punitively directed. Furthermore, if withdrawal fails, and she becomes pregnant it is obviously his fault, and her feelings about men are verified. Use of any other method implies an interest and a consent she denies (Sandberg 1975).

Characteristically, women who enforce use of the condom are angry at men and distrustful. They consider men to be weak, disappointing, and unable to equal the strength and qualities of women. The condom is convincing visual evidence of protection from man and sex (Sandberg 1975).

Those women employing intravaginal foams and jellies are described as passive, motherhood/family-directed, and highly satisfied with their femininity. Such women are joyfully dependent on men and see them as strong, supportive, protective and responsible (Sandberg 1975).

The diaphragm users are considered independent, self-reliant, logical, career-oriented and competitive with men. She likes to be in control of herself and her sexuality and the males in the world about her. She may feel 'superior to men and contemptuous of them, but at the same time she retains a need for romance, love, male attention and approval. The diaphragm is under her reassuring observation and direct control. It allows her to dictate the sexual scene, prevents any unbecoming, uncontrolled and unstructured spontaneity and suits her work ethic (Sandberg 1975).

The user of the intrauterine device is not as completely characterized as users of other methods of contraception. Many women feel uncomfortable about having a foreign body in their womb. With women who need to have control over themselves and who become anxious in the passive position of having their fertility controlled by the physician, an IUD is contraindicated. The IUD is the only contraceptive that does not allow a woman to change her mind. It is the somewhat passive, comfortable, trusting woman who adjusts best to an IUD (Tourkow et al. 1973).

Obviously, a person who is required to take medication daily needs to be reasonably well organized, intelligent and regular in habits. Motivation is particularly important with the use of the pill because it is open to conscious and unconscious manipulation by taking risks or forgetting. Oral contraceptives are used most effectively by women who are more responsible than their husbands but who are comfortable with them. There are wide variations in side effects and psychological reactions to the pill; full understanding can be reached only through the study of positive side effects as well as negative ones (Tourkow et al. 1973).

Every contraceptive technique creates some particular psychodynamic stress, requires some anxiety-provoking act, minimizes attention to some other sort of vulnerability and provides some relief. Some people need to feel in control and some need to forget that they contracept while having sex; some, to demonstrate their fertility or secure their adult status, will need to keep on having babies. While it is reasonable to assume that we can significantly increase the percentage of people who successfully control their fertility, some people will fail; some will have unacceptable side effects; some will switch methods; and some will end up trusting in fate, because the psychodynamics of sex and contraception are not entirely rational (Lidz et al. 1976).

II. COUNSELLING

One of the basic limits of contraception is the effectiveness of communication. As there are no laws existing that the world contracept, the issue is an elective one. The problem is one of persuasion and as such make it one of communication and counselling.

From the recognition that there are many nuances, circumstances and forces that can exist one can see an incredible number of situations in which contraception is misused or rejected for psychological reasons. There are probably more reasons not to use contraception than to use it. These all speak to the fact that contraceptive knowledge and immediate availability cannot and do not ensure contraceptive use. As long as conception control is volitional and despite the fact that many persons prefer to deny that contraception pertains to them, each person must come to a personal decision as to where and when contraception fits into his or her psychological structure of life.

The counsel and opinion of physicians are sought with as much or greater frequency than their diagnostic and therapeutic skills. Too frequently, the physician's attitude toward contraceptive use by others is coloured by his own moral, religious and social philosophy. Contraceptive information and counselling should be and can be dispensed to persons of all ages, but honest ignorance is a very uncommon cause of contraceptive nonuse. Physicians can help to provide insight for persons who are avoiding contraception in order to express themselves. Concern over potential side effects, subsequent fertility and use of medication is significant, as is information received from the patient's physician, peers and the news media. Without doubt, the provision of information to all persons regarding all aspects of contraception and the provision of insight into the psychological makeup of themselves and their partners is a prerequisite for optimal decision making.

The physician's role in patient education is based on the patient's 'right to know' the choices available to her, so that she can make intelligent, informed decisions. There is no method of contraception which is universal in its application, individual motivation and selection.

We can postulate a series of logical steps in the process of selection:

1. Establish patient interest in and attitudes toward learning about birth control.
2. Determine the patient's current knowledge of family planning and any previous experience with it. Explore misinformation, misconceptions and myths and deal with them.
3. Provide accurate, detailed information on methods, effectiveness, safety, costs, side effects and resources.
4. Individualize the approach for each patient – adapt to her level of knowledge and understanding.
5. Allow time for the patient to decide.
6. Supplement discussion with appropriate patient literature.
7. Involve male in discussion (if patient desires).
8. Listen – to spoken and unspoken communication and be ready to act on what you see and learn.

Discussion of the woman's feelings and conflicts is recommended in selecting the type of contraception available to her, in alleviating possible sexual problems, including partial frigidity, and in helping the couple to remain aware of the consequences of giving up contraception impulsively.

III. MOTIVATION

The main and unquestionable motivating factor is the avoidance of conception and the fear of pregnancy. It has become evident in recent years that the woman's motivation is the essential ingredient of successful contraception. That all is not well with *that* motivation is shown in the large dropout rates, within weeks in birth control clinics, and complaints of depression, lack of libido, marital strife, and repeated abortion requests from women supposedly on the pill (Hales-Owen and Hawkins 1972).

Unconscious motives for and against contraception can exist side by side in the same individual. Conscious reasons for wanting contraception are that they have all the children they want or could afford, or that husbands are irresponsible, absent or do not want any more children. On the one hand resentment of parental responsibilities may favour the use of birth control, while at the same time realization that contraception is a hostile act directed toward the unborn infant produces guilt and rejection of contraception. Many patients are accustomed to living with the 'monthly insecurity', their ambivalence about pregnancy is helpful in adjusting to unplanned pregnancies.

It appears that the difference between the actual number of children and the number desired has diminished, because (1) parents are more likely to begin practising some form of contraception; (2) they are less likely to take risks by occasionally skipping contraception; and (3) they have a lower rate of unwanted conception while contracepting. If we assume that *desired minus actual* family size is a rough inverse index of the strength of *motivation* to avoid conception we may infer that the stronger the desire to avoid conception the more effective will the contracepting be. However, even with higher user motivation the method and acceptability of a contraceptive will not ensure contraceptive success.

In a study by Lidz et al. (1977) important facts emerged: (1) the complaints of women on the pill were quite similar to those of women with an IUD, indicating that these complaints were not so much due to hormonal changes but rested on psychological grounds; (2) the attitudes and feelings of their mates had tremendous influence on the woman's motivation to continue using or to drop contraception.

Women's psychological complaints may be considered under three headings: (1) guilt and anxiety, (2) frustration and depression, and (3) sexual and marital problems. Vague feelings of guilt and anxiety are common. Some women feel it is unhealthy to fool with nature. Many feel guilty in rejecting motherhood and consider themselves 'selfish' and lazy to do so. A woman may be uneasy feeling that she has become aggressive by controlling her fertility, is denying her husband the 'self-expression' or 'right' to father a child, or has a feeling of guilt over rejecting a child.

Even when both partners are well-motivated, the conflict of not wanting more offspring while wishing for the fulfilment and creativeness of pregnancy can be great. For a woman with little self-esteem, pregnancy is often the only way to prove herself and it can have the meaning of power or potency. Even if women do not want children, interference with their fertility is resented as depriving and degrading. They may have to prove their ability to themselves and society. The effectiveness of the contraception separates the sexual act from pregnancy and having a baby. Many men and women still consider the sexual act for procreation and need to feel fertile to enjoy sex. They feel sex is for 'no purpose' and do not feel like getting 'started'. They feel depressed, avoid marital relations, with resultant marital discord, conflict and estrangement, or the woman abandons contraception. In contrast certain women who are more or less purged manage to remain reasonably comfortable by controlling the frequency of sexual intercourse though using the fear of impregnation: Not this week, I am afraid I might get pregnant'. When this woman loses her control over the frequency of sexual intercourse and over her husband because of effective contraception she can become severely upset or depressed, because she is forced to recognize her sexual problems. The rational and successful utilization of contraceptive pills would seem to require that both spouses seek and gain pleasure from sexual relationships.

The men's complaints can be considered under three headings: (1) fears, (2) fertility needs and (3) sexual problems.

1. Some men become upset when their wives assume responsibility for contraception and feel they have lost control over their wives. When using a condom a man may feel he is being generous, good and self-sacrificing in protecting his wife from impregnation, but should he wish he can impregnate her and make her stay at home and keep her from working or competing with him. With loss of such control, he may become fearful of his wife's independence and her aggressiveness, and the balance of power in the marriage is upset.

2. Many men consider their ability to impregnate as part of their potency and may even confuse the two (Lidz et al. 1976).

3. A man can also lose sexual interest in his wife when she is infertile; consistent lack of consequences from sexual relations when there is no hope of impregnation disturbs him (Lidz et al. 1976).

An often less consciously motivated hostility can be seen in cases of frigidity or impotence which are tied specifically to contraceptive utilization. To have a woman physically and psychologically ready for coitus and then not respond can be an expression of the hostility matched only by the degree of anger felt by the woman on such an occasion.

IV. CONCLUDING REMARKS

Prevention of conception touches on mental complexes which are affectively changed; the use of contraceptive regimens to interfere with fertility induces significant mental reactions in patients.

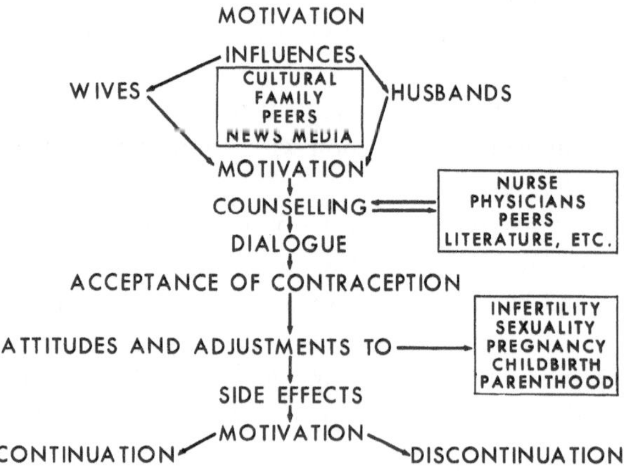

Figure 1. Psychological parameters of contraceptive use.

Attitudes and feelings related to procreation are often conflicting and inevitably contain unconscious and emotional components.

Ryder (1973), in the analysis of the 1970 national fertility study, concluded that 'success in contraceptive use depends in a large part on the degree of motivation of the couple concerned'. Prevention of pregnancy by contraceptive means requires that a well-motivated person actively intervene in a natural process, hopefully with a partner of like intent. Patients have the basic right to be fully counselled and informed. The minimal goal in prescribing a contraceptive regimen should be to make no iatrogenic contribution to contraceptive failure or to reactive symptom development. The contraceptive method should be associated with such confidence in its efficiency and harmlessness as to cause no anxiety attendant on sexual intercourse (Tourkow et al. 1973).

Compliance in the use of contraception is directly related to the amount and intensity of counselling and the degree of motivation. Figure 1 summarizes the psychological parameters involved.

REFERENCES

Hales-Owen J, Hawkins D: Factors affecting the motivation of patients with intrauterine devices. Med Gynecol Sociol 6: 24, 1972.

Lidz RW, Rutledge AL, Tourkow LP: Intrapsychic aspects. In Regulation of human fertility, Moghessi KS, Evans TN (eds), Detroit, Wayne State University Press, 1976, p 132-136.

Ryder N: Contraceptive failure in the United States. Fam Plann Perspect 5: 133, 1973.

Sandberg EC: Psychological aspects of contraception. In: Comprehensive textbook of psychiatry 2: 24, Freedman AM, Kaplan HI, Sadock BJ (eds), Baltimore, Williams and Wilkins, 1975, p 1487-1496.

Tourkow L, Lidz R, Marder L: Psychiatric consideration in fertility inhibition. In: Human reproduction, Hafez ESE, Evans TN, Hagerstown, Harper and Row, 1973, p 615-627.

Wallach EE, Garcia CR: Psychodynamic aspects of oral contraception. JAMA 203 (11): 284, 1968.

19. CONTRACEPTION FOR ADOLESCENTS

H. Amirikia

Contraception for teenagers is beginning to gain some degree of acceptance as an appropriate topic of concern among physicians, parents, educational institutions and the public at large.

The teenage population in the United States (age 15-19) has risen sharply, with an almost fifty-percent increase from 1958 to 1969 (United States Department of Health, Education, and Welfare National Centre for Health Statistics 1974). The average age at onset of puberty shows a secular trend toward earlier occurrence that cuts across geographic and ethnic lines, so the age of initial sexual experience appears to be declining. Moreover, there are firm data that indicate that sexual activity among teenage women is high (Kantner and Zelnick 1972). It was estimated that about eleven million of the 21 million young Americans between the ages of fifteen and nineteen were sexually active. Of these eleven million, four million were young women (Lincoln et al. 1976). Approximately 420,00 females under the age of fifteen and ten percent of the female population at age thirteen are sexually active. This rises to 51 percent at age nineteen. Overall, the prevalence of sexual acivity in adolescents has increased over the last 25-30 years. The consequence of this increased sexual experience among adolescents has been a remarkable increase in teenage pregnancy throughout the population of the United States, but especially in the suburban areas (Moore and Wilson 1976).

Approximately one million females 15-19 years old become pregnant each year (Lincoln et al. 1976). About 600,000 of these pregnancies end in births, 33 percent of which are out of wedlock. Twenty-seven percent of the million pregnancies were terminated by voluntary abortion; fourteen percent experienced spontaneous abortions.

Complications and adverse effects of teenage pregnancies include higher infant mortality rates (2-3 times greater than for adult pregnancies), growth-retarded newborns (twice as frequent), anemia and toxemia of pregnancy (30% greater) and higher maternal mortality. In addition to the health risks, school dropout rates are twice as high for pregnant teenagers as for nonpregnant females (Tyrer and Josimorich 1977).

Contraceptive practice among unmarried teenagers has interesting correlations with socioeconomic status, race, residency status, and education. Adequate sex education, as well as availability of contraceptive facilities, are two important factors in the control of undesired teenage pregnancies. White teenagers are more likely to have access to a private physician, whereas black teenagers depend more on clinic services. In general, poverty increases the dependence on clinics for contraception. Residents of city centres and suburban areas prefer different methods of contraception. The most conscientious users of contraceptives among unmarried sexually active teenagers are black women living in the suburbs of large cities – 98 percent – (Lyle and -Segal 1979).

A study by the Department of Population Dynamics at Johns Hopkins University (Zelnick and Kartner 1972) indicated that teenage women were fairly well informed about contraceptive methods but knew little about the biology of the reproductive system. Half of the sexually active unmarried 15-19-year-old females in their study had used no form of contraception during their last sexual intercourse; half of those not using contraceptives felt they were too young to conceive or that it was the wrong time of the menstrual cycle for conception to occur.

I. FACTORS CONTRIBUTING TO TEENAGE PREGNANCY

Although a great deal has been written suggesting that teenage girls who become pregnant are rebels against their families or the product of poor or broken homes, several studies indicate that the subject is much more complex. One has to take into consideration the biological, psychological, social and cultural changes of the past few decades (Cobliner 1970). These changes are:

- puberty occurs at an earlier age;
- the sexes mingle much earlier;
- controls exerted by families and schools have relaxed;
- leisure time is less structured;
- values governing intimacy have been liberated;
- the age of economic independence has been delayed, so decisions regarding marriage and so on are delayed;
- an additional influence is exerted by the news and entertainment media.

These factors are reflected in the results of a study done at the University of Kentucky from 1971 to 1974 involving 417 unmarried pregnant teenagers. This study clearly indicates that a fair number have a strong desire to have a baby and suggests that out-of-wedlock pregnancies are not purely accidental and may stem from subconscious wishes in a setting of close interpersonal relationships with firm sexual bonds. Nevertheless, a survey of a large group of unmarried, sexually active teenage women between fifteen and nineteen years of age who were not using contraception clearly indicated that unavailability of contraception and lack of sex education are the two main factors for not contracepting (Shah et al. 1975).

Many teenage women are reluctant to request contraceptive advice or prescriptions from private physicians because they fear a lecture on morality as well as a refusal of their request. Some visit a gynecologist or clinic with some minor complaint with the actual purpose of gaining access to the health care system and to gauge the attitude of the physician regarding contraception for minors. Contraception information should be offered, and if the parents are present the patient should be consulted privately about her interest in contraceptive methods. Surprisingly, many admit their willingness to use a contraceptive method. The teenager should be given the method she prefers providing that no contraindications to that particular method exist for her.

The intrauterine device might be the contraceptive of choice (Kreutner 1978) for a number of reasons:

- the only motivation required is for the initial insertion;
- once the IUD is in place it is hidden, and there is no possibility of parental discovery of contraceptives;
- the sporadic nature of adolescent sex makes this method desirable;
- the Cu-7 and Progestasert are small and easy to insert in a nulliparous female;
- an IUD has a pregnancy rate of 2-4 percent/100 women-years and is the second most effective temporary contraceptive method.

II. SUMMARY AND CONCLUSION

The teenage population in the United States is rising. The age of onset of sexual activity is declining, and the population experiencing undesired pregnancy is increasing. The necessity for providing proper sex education, contraceptive advice, and supply is strongly emphasized.

A 100-percent effective, safe, and practical contraceptive is still to be discovered. Most contraceptives available today have some undesirable side effects. Of course, these are far less serious than the complications of teenage pregnancy.

The Cu-7 and Progestasert may be the methods of choice for an unmarried teenage woman with sporadic, unplanned sexual activity.

Preservation of confidentiality is very important, and the physician caring for the contraceptive needs of adolescents is to take special precautions to assure the privacy of care.

Contraception should be encouraged in the sexually active adolescent to prevent undesired teenage pregnancies and unwanted babies with all the related complications and unfavourable social consequences.

REFERENCES

Dobliner WG: Teenage out-of-wedlock pregnancy. Bull NY Acad Med 46: 438, 1970.

Kantner J, Zelnick M: Sexual experience of young unmarried women in the United States. Fam Plann Perspect 4: 9, 1972.

Kreutner AK: Contraception. In: Adolescents obstetrics and gynecology, Kreutner AKK, Hollingsworth DR (eds), Yearbook Medical Publishers, Chicago, 1978.

Lincoln R, Jaffe, FS, Ambrose A: 11 million teenagers, New York, Alan Guttmacher Institute (Planned Parenthood of America), 1976.

Lyle KC, Segal SJ: Contraceptive use-effectiveness and the American adolescent. J Reprod Med 22: 5, 1979.

Moore EC, Wilson H: Children rearing children: youthful pregnancy in a suburban community, New York, Adelphi University Institute for Suburban Studies, 1976.

Shah F, Zelnick M, Kantner J: Unprotected intercourse among unwed teenagers. Fam Plann Perspect 7: 39, 1975.

Tyrer LB, Josimovich J: Contraception in teenagers. Clin Obstet Gynecol 20: 3, 1977.

United States Department of Health, Education, and Welfare National Center for Health Statistics: Vital statistics of the US, 1968, vol 1, Washington DC, Government Printing Office, 1974, tables 1-16.

Zelnick M, Kantner J: Sexuality, contraception and pregnancy among young unwed females in the United States. In: Demographic and social consequences of population growth, Westoff CF Parke R Jr (eds) Washington DC, Government Printing Office, 1972.

20. THE USE OF IUDs IN ADDICTED WOMEN

J.C. Stryker

A women with a long-standing addiction to heroin is usually infertile, as heroin prevents the anterior pituitary gland from producing follicle-stimulating hormones (FSH) by inhibiting the hypothalamic surge of LH-RH-/FSH-RH. The subsequent decrease of FSH in the female creates an anovulatory state with frequent amenorrhea (Santen 1973; Schally et al. 1972; Bai et al. 1974). On enrollment in a methadone therapy clinic, however, the lifestyle of the heroin addict undergoes a change, and within a six-month period following the institution of methadone therapy, either methadone maintenance or gradual detoxification, the menstrual cycle and ovulation are usually restored with a subsequent return of fertility. The majority of addicts are unaware of this return of fertility (Wallach et al. 1968) and continue unprotected coitus. It is important at this time in the life of an addict to explore her attitude toward a wanted pregnancy.

This group of patients has a higher incidence of all varieties of infection, thromboembolic disease and hypertension than the female population not abusing drugs (Stryker 1979). In addition to their physical pathology, the basic psychological differences between drug-abusing women and other women are a lack of self-discipline and the inability to observe a set health routine continuously.

Women who have a lifestyle that leads to drug abuse must be considered first as an entity and then individually for contraceptive counselling. These women do have a need for family planning counselling and the major areas of concern are what currently available family planning methods should be considered, and what guidelines should be followed.

The present paper is directed to the physician who is caring for these women while they are in methadone therapy.

I. MATERIAL AND METHOD

The patients who form the basis of the present analysis were all postgestational, therefore their return of fertility had been exemplarily demonstrated. The women in the drug-addicted group were enrolled in the Hutzel Hospital Pregnant Drug Addict Program under the auspices of Wayne State University School of Medicine Department of Gynecology and Obstetrics.

From the Pregnant Drug Addict Clinic population of 1,700, 440 case histories were selected for the present study. The medical histories, physical examination results, laboratory data, prenatal course, labour and delivery notes, and postpartum diagnoses of the study group were compiled, computerized and analyzed. Ninety-two patients from the Hutzel Hospital Prenatal Clinic were selected as matched drug-free controls.

As an index of the responsibility and reliability of the drug-addicted group, the number of patients who kept their prenatal appointments and the number of patients who returned for their postpartum examinations were calculated. It was revealed that the drug addicted group kept an average of only six of the possible thirteen prenatal appointments, while the control group had an average of ten prenatal visits. Sixty-five percent of the addicted group returned for their postpartum examinations: 38-percent at the time of the six-week checkup and 27-percent who eventually returned. Seventy-four percent of the control group returned at six weeks for their postpartum examinations. It would thus seem that the patient who abuses drugs is not responsible for her own health needs and therefore requires a family planning method that does not demand motivation (Stryker 1979).

II. CONTRAINDICATIONS

The necessity for many of these patients to resort to prostitution in order to support their habit requires that the method of contraception be separated from the sexual act. This eliminates the use of contraceptive methods such as foam, which must be inserted just prior to the sexual act.

With regard to the other methods of contraception that are currently available, very definite absolute contraindications are indicated for the use of ovulatory control pills (Table 1).

The incidence of pathologies that contraindicate the use of ovulatory control pills in the drug population is demonstrated in Table 2. The absolute contraindications for the use of intrauterine devices are shown in Table 3. The incidence of pathologies found in the drug addict group that contraindicate the use of intrauterine devices are shown in Table 4. The figures for a history of gonococcus are not available at this time.

The high percentages of absolute contraindications found in the drug addict population for the use of ovulatory control pills and/or intrauterine devices are shown in Table 5.

Table 1. Absolute contraindications for ovulatory control pills.

History or presence of
Thromboembolic disease
Thrombophlebitis)
Subacute bacterial endocarditis
Hypertension
Hepatitis

Table 2. Incidence of pathologies that contraindicated the use of ovulatory control pills in the subject drug addicts.

Pathology	%
History of skin infections	7.3
History of thromboembolus	1.3
Developing thromboembolus	1.3
Acute abscess	9.1
Developing thrombophlebitis	3.0
History of hypertension	3.0
Developing hypertension	5.6
History of bacterial endocarditis	2.2
Developing bacterial endocarditis	1.0

Table 3. Contraindications for IUD use.

Pregnancy
Active pelvic inflammatory disease
History of pelvic inflammatory disease in past six months
Fibroid uterus
Menorrhagia
Gonorrhea
Vaginitis

Table 4. Incidence of pathologies that contraindicated the use of IUDs in the subject drug addicts.

Pathology	%
History of pelvic inflammatory disease	9.5
Developing pelvic inflammatory disease	1.0
History of gonococcus	n.a.
Developing gonococcus during pregnancy	3.0

Table 5. Patients with contraindications to ovulatory control pills and/or IUDs.

	%
No contraindications to pill or IUD	49.5
Contraindications to pill and IUD	3.6
Contraindications to pill	33.8
Contraindications to IUD	16.7

III. GUIDELINES

In consideration of the contraindication statistics, guidelines may be established for contraceptive requirements of patients who abuse drugs (Table 6).

IV. METHODS OF CONTRACEPTION ACCEPTED FOLLOWING DELIVERY

Table 7 lists the various methods of contraception accepted by the patients at the time of discharge from the hospital. It should be noted that the intrauterine device was not offered immediately postgestation. The 7.7 percent receiving a hysterectomy had a prenatal diagnosis made of either severe cervical dysplasia or carcinoma in situ, following appropriate colposcopy, biopsy, or cold-knife conization. Because of the difficulty in retrieving these patients postgestionally for definitive

Table 6. Guidelines for contraceptive requirements of drug abusers.

Requirements
1. A method that does not require patient motivation or responsibility
2. A method that does not interfere with the sexual act
3. A method with a low complication risk index
4. A method with a high baby-proof effectiveness

Table 7. Contraception at postgestational discharge from hospital.

Type of contraception	*Treatment patients* (%)	*Control patients* (%)
Tubal ligation	2.9	0.0
DepoProvera (medroxy-progesterone acetate)	31.6	0.0
Ovulatory control pills	36.8	65.9
Barrier		
Diaphragm	0.4	0.0
Foam and condoms	19.5	33.3
Refused	1.0	0.0
Cesarean section hysterectomy	7.7	1.0

surgery, the heroic Cesarean hysterectomy has been employed in this clinic as a safeguard against any extension of the malignancy. Other patients eventually received hysterectomies for the following disorders: fibroid uterus, relaxed pelvic floor, persistent cervical dysplasia or carcinoma in situ (Blinick 1973: Eschenback et al. 1977), a pelvic 'cleanout' for severe chronic pelvic inflammatory disease, and ovarian malignancy.

At the six-week postgestional checkup, the IUD was offered as a family planning method and was accepted by nine percent of the patients formerly using ovulatory control pills and by 25 percent of the patients formerly using the barrier types of contraception, to make a total of 3.9 percent of the entire drug addict population (54 patients). Table 8 illustrates the contraceptive methods accepted at discharge from the hospital and the methods selected at the six-week postgestational checkup.

In contrast to the 3.9 percent acceptance of the IUD by the drug population, 6.7 percent of the nondrug patients attending the hospital's general family planning clinic accepted the IUD as their family planning method of choice. Acceptance of the intrauterine device by the general population of the United States rose to 12.5 percent in 1978 due to the Federal Drug Administration's ban on the use of DepoProvera as a contraceptive.

V. DISCUSSION

What were the reasons for such a low percentage of acceptance of the insertion of an IUD by the drug addicts? Was this low percentage due to the clinic physician's prejudice in not prescribing an IUD? Did the drug addict just not accept the IUD, or were contraindications present to its use?

A review was made of five epidemiological studies that associated the presence or the suspected presence of pelvic inflammatory disease and the use of an IUD (Eschenback et al. 1977; Neri et al. 1977; Niebyl et al. 1978; Ory 1978; Weiland et al. 1978). A premise was made that the presence of an IUD in a

Table 8. Contraception acceptance and continuance.

Type of contraception	*Acceptance at discharge from hospital* (%)	*Postgestational checkup: continuance* (%) *Tubal ligation*	*DepoProvera*	*Ovulatory control pills*	*Barrier*	*Refused*	*IUD*	*Hysterectomy*
Tubal ligation	2.9	100	—	—	—	—	—	—
DepoProvera	31.6	0	80.0	0	4.5	4.5	0	9.1
Ovulatory control pills	36.8	0	6.1	63.6	12.1	0	9.0	9.1
Barrier	20.0	0	0	41.7	16.6	0	25.0	16.7
Refused	1.0	0	0	0	0	0	0	0
IUD	—							
Cesarean hysterectomy	7.7	100	—	—	—	—	—	—

patient whose lifestyle may be associated with the development of acute inflammatory disease brings about a three to fivefold increase in its incidence. Is the physician then justified in making the assumption that this patient population is more prone to pelvic inflammatory disease or systemic infections? To substantiate this assumption, the history, physical examination findings and hospital course of our patients were analyzed from the data in the computer. The proportion of patients who had a history of pelvic inflammatory disease, a history of bacterial endocarditis, current pelvic inflammatory disease, or a positive culture for gonorrhea was 16.7 percent. The remaining 83.3 percent of these patients had no contraindications for the insertion of an IUD, however only 3.9 percent accepted this method.

In contrast, noting the absolute contraindications to ovulatory control pills, it was found that 37.8 percent of this population were not candidates for ovulatory control pills due either to a past history or present history of thromboembolic phenomena, thrombophlebitis, moderately severe tissue infections, or hypertension. Of the remaining 63 percent who were eligible for ovulatory control pills, 36.8 percent of the population accepted this method of contraception. In other words, a larger number of our women had contraindications to ovulatory control pills, yet approximately nine times the number accepted ovulatory control pills as their method of family planning.

The computer was then asked for the identification of the 54 patients in whom IUDs had been inserted. The charts were then subjected to a retrospective search regarding the history of the continued use or outcome of the IUDs.

Six patients were classified as lost to follow-up as no further clinic contact had been made. Of the 48 patients involved in the retrospective chart search, none had retained their IUDs for over eight months: eight intrauterine devices had been removed in emergency rooms for signs and symptoms of pelvic inflammatory disease; twelve patients had antibiotics prescribed and their IUDs were removed at a later date for persistent signs and symptoms of pelvic inflammatory disease. The remaining 28 patients had their IUDs removed for signs and symptoms of bleeding or cramps, due, undoubtedly, to a variety of reasons including malnutrition or smoking (Table 9). Of the twenty patients (37%) who developed pelvic inflammatory disease, five were hospitalized and two required definitive surgery for tubo-ovarian abscesses (Golde et al. 1977). Our experience is not quite similar to that of Dashow and Llorens (1977), in that only two patients demonstrated a positive culture for gonorrhea.

Table 9. Follow-up on IUDs.

Number of patients	54
Emergency room pullout for pelvic inflammatory disease	8
Antibiotics and later pullout for pelvic inflammatory disease	12
Pullout; bleeding and cramps	28
Lost to follow-up	6

Therefore, patients with increased risk of pelvic inflammatory disease, such as the addicted patients with a 16.7 percent pelvic infection rate, multiplied by the three to fivefold increased incidence of pelvic infection from the use of an IUD, will have a 50 percent chance of developing the disease. The theoretical percentage of 50.1 percent compares with the actual known pelvic inflammatory disease rate of 41 percent. Is this high risk percentage for pelvic inflammatory disease due to the drug addict's lifestyle, with the potential for multiple sexual partners, or is it due to their poor nutrition and the decrease in their autoimmune globulins?

To test the second offered reason for nonacceptance of the intrauterine device by the addicted woman, the present pregnant drug addict population was surveyed on the preferred type of contraception following delivery and if they would consider an IUD. The conclusion of the survey was: in the drug world, the IUD is in disfavor because of the street 'folklore' that it will always cause pain and bleeding. Due to the economic necessity of maintaining their habit, many of our women resort to prostitution. Pelvic pain and vaginal bleeding are counterproductive to the coital act, therefore an IUD was unacceptable, regardless of the possible complications of IUD use.

VI. CONCLUSION

Even with the small number of 54 IUD insertions,

there were 48 patients (six lost to follow-up) with documented symptoms of pain and bleeding or pelvic inflammatory disease; the pullout rate was 88 percent, which is more than the theoretical rate of 36 percent. Thus the physician's reluctance against inserting an IUD in a patient who is a chronic drug abuser is justified, even if her past history or current physical condition would not contraindicate the insertion of a device.

Because of our experience, an IUD is rarely inserted in a known drug addict at the family planning clinic. The present methods prescribed are ovulatory control pills and the barrier type methods. In the United States we are unable to prescribe a long-lasting injectable progesterone due to the Federal Drug Administration ban on this method of contraception. In Europe, this method is available and data have been presented which strongly support its prescription for a patient population that is socially unreliable and at risk for a pelvic infectious disease.

Both our practical experience over the years and corroboration from the literature agree that patients who have pelvic inflammatory disease or have a predisposition for developing pelvic inflammatory disease are not ideal candidates for an IUD.

REFERENCES

Bai J, Greenwald E, Caterini H, Kaminetzky HA: Drug related menstrual aberrations.) Obstet Gynecol 44: 713-719, 1974

Blinick G: Menstrual function and pregnancy in narcotics addicts treated with methadone. Nature 219: 180, 1973.

Dashow EE, Llorens AS: Resistant gonococcal infection from an intrauterine contraceptive device. Am J Obstet Gynecol 129: 230, 1977.

Eschenback DA, Harnisch JP, Holmes KK: Pathogenesis of acute pelvic inflammatory disease: role of contraception and other risk factors. Am J Obstet Gynecol 128: 838-850, 1977.

Golde SH, Israel R, Ledger WJ: Unilateral tubo-ovarian abscess: a distinct entity. Am J Obstet Gynecol 127: 807-810, 1977.

Hofer U, Hochuli E: Severe infections in our obstetric-gynecologic case material including non-social infections (1972-1976). Geburtshilfe Frauenheilkd 37: 268-277,1977.

Neri A, Joel-Cohen SJ, Ovadia J: Ovarian abscess associated with incomplete abortion and intrauterine contraceptive device. Isr J Med Sci 13: 305-308, 1977.

Niebyl JR, Parmley TH, Spence MR, Woodruff, JD: Unilateral ovarian abscess associated with the intrauterine device. Obstet Gynecol 52: 165-168, 1978.

Ory HW: A review of the association between intrauterine devices and acute pelvic inflammatory disease. J Reprod Med 20: 200-204, 1978.

Rosenfeld A: Oral and intrauterine contraception: a 1978 risk assessment. Am J Obstet Gynecol 132: 92-106,1978.

Santen RJ: How narcotics addiction affects reproductive function in women. Contemp Obstet Gynecol 3: 93-96. 1973.

Schally AV, Kastin AJ, Arimura A: The hypothalmus and reproduction. Am J Obstet Gynecol 114: 423-441, 1972.

Wallach RC, Jerez E, Blinick G: Pregnancy and menstrual function in narcotics addicts treated with methadone: the methadone maintenance treatment program. Am J Obstet Gynecol 105: 1226-1229, 1968.

Weiland RJ, Rarzy BJ, Young PE: Ligneous cellulitis associated with an IUD. Obstet Gynecol 51: 48-51, 1978.

Stryker JC: Drug dependence in pregnancy: clinical management of mother and child, National institute on drug abuse services research monograph series, Rockville, Maryland, US Department of Health, Education, and Welfare, 1979.

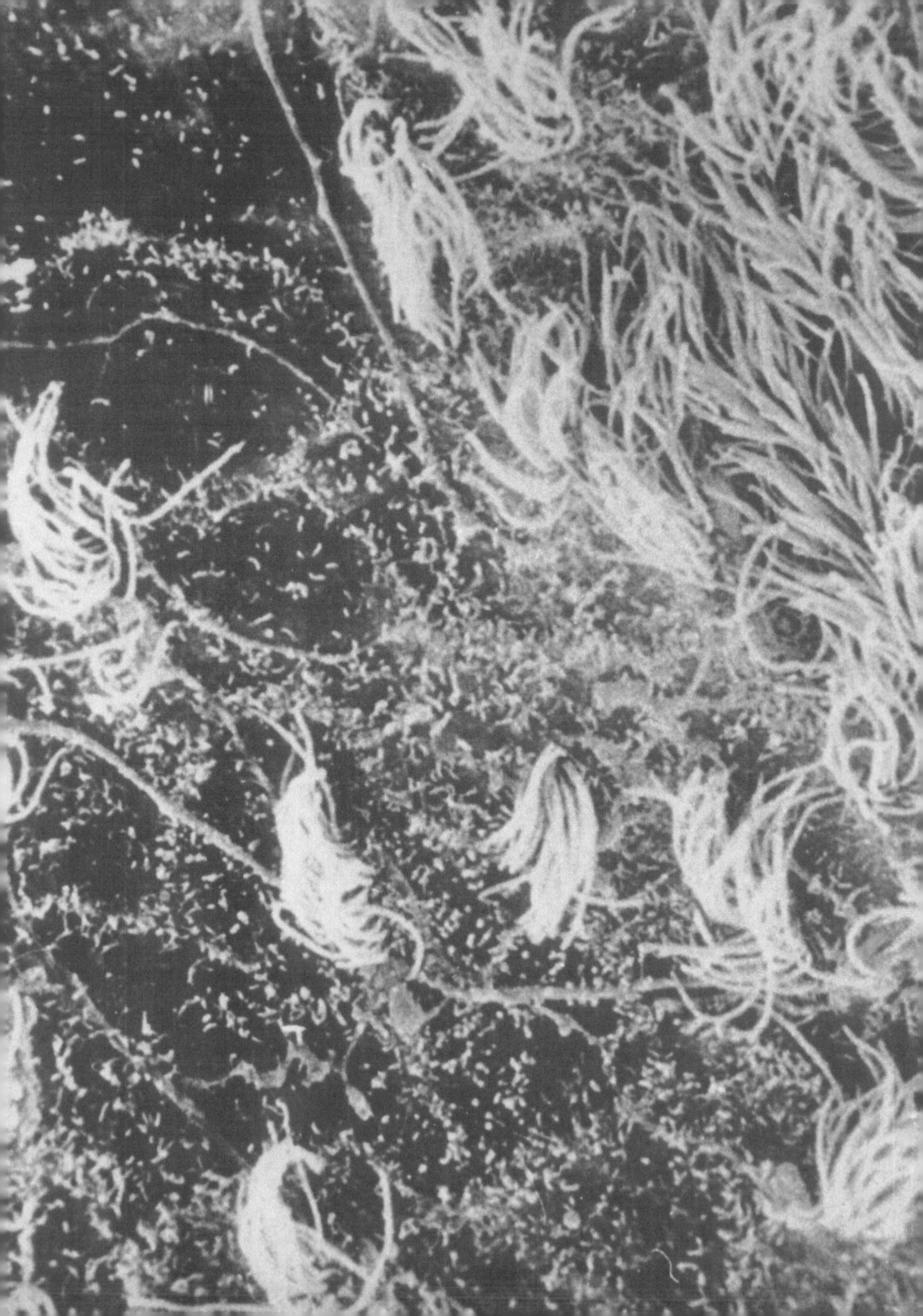

III. FUTURE DEVELOPMENT

21. FUTURE DEVELOPMENTS IN INTRAUTERINE CONTRACEPTION

G.I. Zatuchni and J.J. Sciarra

In 1909, Dr. Richard Richter, a Polish gynecologist published his experience with the first intrauterine device, which was made of silkworm gut in the form of a ring (Richter 1909). The insertion technique was described and Dr. Richter's results are best summarized in a translation of his own words:

> After many years of testing and improving I am able to offer to my colleagues a simple, safe contraceptive. This is a silkworm gut suture which is inserted into the uterus. Irritation of the endometrium by the thread is so that the majority of women never feel it, yet it does prevent pregnancy. In some of my cases, women have used the device for almost four years. Insertion is easy... minor bleeding stops after a few days... Removal is easy as the thread can be pulled out of the uterus with a forceps. Following removal, fertility is restored.

Unfortunately, Dr. Richter's device met with scientific negativism, and it was not until 1923 that Dr. Karl Pust published his results with a similar ring made of silkworm gut (Pust 1923). Pust's device included a tail of similar material fixed to a cervical button made of glass. This button was thought to serve the function of closing the cervical os, thereby forming a mechanical barrier to the ascent of spermatozoa and bacteria.

During the late 1920s, Dr. Ernst Gräfenberg published his results with his own intrauterine rings, and presented his findings at several international conferences. Other physicians also reported favorable results with similar intrauterine rings, including Ota (Japan), Luenbach (Denmark), Manes (Germany) and Heire (England). After a series of clinical trials, Gräfenberg finally evolved his intrauterine ring composed entirely of silver coils. In 1930, among 600 women fitted with the silver ring, he reported a 1.6-percent pregnancy rate, and a four-percent expulsion rate. Gräfenberg frowned upon the use of any IUD having a connecting bridge (thread or tail) from the uterus to the vagina, because of his great fear of the increased possibilities of ascending pelvic infection.

Except for a few gynecologists, mostly in the United States and Japan, no enthusiasm existed for this method of birth control for the next 25 years.

Several developments occurring more or less simultaneously took place in the early 1960s which jointly led to the reemergence of intrauterine contraception and, more importantly, to the use of IUDs by millions of women in almost every country of the world. The favourable reports published from Israel by Oppenheimer (1959) and from Japan by Ishihama (1959) on intrauterine rings made of silkworm gut prompted others to investigate the use of modern plastics, metal and other materials manufactured or moulded into a variety of shapes and sizes. During that period, many world leaders developed an acute awareness of population growth rates, and researchers began thinking of appropriate contraceptive technology that could be used by the millions of women in need. It seemed that the establishment of national family planning programmes coupled with the promotion and use of intrauterine contraception could provide the solution to the problem of ever-increasing numbers of people. Indeed, by 1965, approximately six million women worldwide had had an IUD insertion, making this medical procedure one of the most commonly performed. Unfortunately, intrauterine contraception has not provided the mass solution because of several disturbing side effects, and a potential for adverse health situations directly or indirectly attributable to intrauterine contraception. In 1970, approximately twelve million women were using IUDs, but by 1978 estimated users had increased to only 15 million, the vast majority of them in developing countries (United States Agency for International Development, 1978). In the United States IUD use has remained more or less stationary for several years at a level of nine percent of all contraceptors.

Intrauterine contraception, despite its low levels of acceptance and use and the fact that it has not provided *the* answer to the world's population problems, still maintains an important role in fertility control. Certainly, the appeal of a contraceptive method that requires only one act of motivation, a simple insertion procedure, that subsequently provides years of safe protection from pregnancy, continues to be strong. No other reversible method of contraception has these excellent attributes. Accordingly, it is fully appropriate that clinicians, scientists and researchers continue to seek improvements in this wonderfully simple contraceptive technology.

I. IS IMPROVEMENT IN INTRAUTERINE CONTRACEPTION POSSIBLE?

Table 1 indicates, in an acrostic fashion, the major concerns with intrauterine contraception. These concerns exist for both nonmedicated and medicated IUDs, although certain of the concerns, for example development of neoplastic change and congenital anomalies, are more closely linked with devices medicated with such compounds as copper, other metals or steroid hormones. Each of these areas of concern will be discussed with the objective of trying to answer the question, 'Is improvement possible?'

I.A. Contraceptive effectiveness

There is no question that IUDs are potent inhibitors of intrauterine pregnancies in all animal species, including the human female. Most types of devices, in clinical situations, provide an effectiveness rate of about 1-3 pregnancies per hundred woman-years. It is remarkable that intrauterine contraceptive devices achieved this effectiveness despite the fact that the precise mechanism of action is as yet unknown.

Table 1. Areas of concern for IUDs.

I nfection
U nwanted effects (bleeding, pain, discharge)
D uration of action (expulsion)

C ontraceptive effectiveness
O ther effects (for example anemia, perforation)
N eoplastic change
C ongenital anomalies
E ctopic pregnancy
R estoration of fertility
N onmedical concerns (cost, manufacture, acceptability)
S pontaneous (Septic?) abortion

Because nonmedicated IUDs exert different biological effects in different species conclusions regarding the possible mode of action in humans cannot be drawn on the basis of research in animals. What seems certain is that IUDs are effective via their local action in the uterus and that there are no systemic mechanisms in operation. These local effects include the continued presence of large numbers of macrophages and polymorphonuclear leukocytes in both the endometrium and uterine fluid; mononuclear cells, plasma cells and foreign body giant cells may also be present. It is presumed that these inflammatory response cells provide the contraceptive action of IUDs, perhaps by prevention of blastocystic implantation, or by phagocytosis of the spermatozoa or blastocyst (Morese et al. 1971). Other mechanisms have been suggested; prostaglandin-E and F levels are increased in several animal species and in humans in the presence of an IUD. The increase in prostaglandin levels may be an important factor in preventing blastocyst implantation (Chaudhuri 1971). Additionally, there are changes in various endometrial enzymes in the presence of an IUD, although none have been specifically implicated as a possible explanation for the IUD contraceptive action.

Copper-bearing IUDs elicit uterine responses similar to those of conventional IUDs, but the added copper release exerts its own effects. Copper interferes with uterine hormone receptors for estrogen and progesterone. Copper increases the fibrinolytic activity of the endometrium in rabbits. Copper ions may interfere with enzymatic activity in the endometrium, which may in turn affect blastocyst implantation (Tatum 1977). These additional effects may explain the greater contraceptive effectiveness with such devices.

Progesterone-releasing devices exert their main contraceptive effect by progestogenic changes in the endometrium resulting in endometrial repression and glandular atrophy, in addition to the changes caused by the carrier IUD. Although there is uterine adsorption of progesterone with consequent systemic effects, the daily dosage released is so small that ovulation continues to occur regularly. Other devices utilizing a variety of progestagens, however, may suppress ovulation if the release rate of the steroid and the consequent blood levels of hormones are sufficient.

As the mechanism of contraceptive action is incompletely understood, a completely effective device cannot be designed except by trial and error. It is in this way that devices have been developed to the extent that only a small margin remains for improvement. Recent data indicate that copper-bearing IUDs provide somewhat better contraceptive efficacy than do nonmedicated IUDs (Tatum 1977). On the other hand, progesterone-releasing IUDs are associated with higher pregnancy rates. Considering the effectiveness of the large array of devices in use and in clinical research, it appears unlikely that any new device will be developed that could provide hundred-percent contraception over many years duration and still have the potential for reversibility.

The situation is somewhat different with regard to ectopic pregnancies in IUD wearers. The issue of whether nonmedicated IUDs are causal in the statistically observed increased rate of ectopic (tubal) pregnancies among all IUD pregnancies is still controversial. There is no question, however, that an abnormally high proportion of ectopic pregnancies does occur in women becoming pregnant with an IUD in situ. It is also obvious that an IUD in the endometrial cavity does not prevent fertilization from occurring in the tube, with possible subsequent development of a tubal or even an ovarian pregnancy. Fortunately, the number of ectopic pregnancies is not as high with nonmedicated devices. Recent data suggest a greater proportion of ectopic pregnancies among pregnancies occurring in women wearing copper devices (Tatum and Schmidt 1977). But here again, the issue of causation is controversial. More clear is the statistically increased incidence of ectopic pregnancies occurring with progesterone-releasing IUDs, perhaps because of the progesterone effect on tubal motility. A similar effect has been noted with the use of progestin-only contraceptive pills. Obviously there is great concern about the increased rates of ectopic pregnancy among certain IUD users, especially those women who have little or no access to appropriate medical care.

Although we know little about intrauterine pregnancy deterrence, we know even less about ectopic pregnancies, and their causation and their relationship, if any, to IUDs. The only insights we can offer for reducing the occurrence of ectopic pregnancies are based upon the clinical observation that wearers of certain types of IUDs seem to experience fewer of them. Certainly, this provides us with a less than optimum developmental approach.

Many of the empirical observations noted above have played an important role in the design and improvement of IUDs. It is well-known that the contraceptive effectiveness of an IUD is directly related to its total surface area, for example the larger Lippes Loop D is far superior to the small Lippes Loop A. Other device design features are not as clear-cut in their implications, but there seems to be some relationship between contraceptive effectiveness and the shape, geometry, material and rigidity of the IUD. It appears unlikely, however, that future design changes of these characteristics alone will result in more effective contraception with nonmedicated IUDs.

An important consideration in contraceptive effectiveness is the duration of action. With nonmedicated IUDs, experience has indicated virtually lifelong reproductive protection with a single IUD. This is not the case with medicated IUDs, either copper-bearing or hormone-releasing types. With the presently available copper-bearing IUDs, the copper wire erodes and fragments and a calcific layer develops, generally after some years, perhaps three to six, of use. To obtain longer periods of action copper sleeves have been substituted for copper wire and theoretically provide longer durations of contraceptive action. On the other hand, the duration of action of a hormone-releasing IUD is dependent upon the steroid itself, the reservoir, and the type of carrier. The use of potent progestins, for example levonorgestrel, in IUDs in a suitable carrier providing minimal daily release rates can result in longer action than the presently available progesterone-releasing IUD, which must be changed annually. Unlike the prospect for many years of contraceptive action offered by IUDs with copper sleeves, it is unlikely that sufficient quantities of steroid hormones can be mounted on an IUD to provide more than three to five years of use.

I.B. Bleeding

The major unwanted side effect of IUD contraception is bleeding, probably accounting for over half the IUD discontinuance rate. The bleeding is rarely sufficient to cause anemia, except in malnourished women where the additional blood loss can aggravate the symptoms associated with an underlying anemia. The cause of the increased menstrual bleeding associated with IUD use is unknown. There is some evidence of an increase in endometrial prostaglandin-E and in fibrinolysis among IUD users, but some studies have suggested that IUD-induced menorrhagia may in fact be due to early abortion. Other causative factors have also been suggested.

The major problem in comparing blood loss associated with one or another IUD is the lack of precision in blood loss measurement. Only within the past three years have accurate measurements of menstrual blood loss been attempted, using either the alkaline hematin method or atomic absorption spectrophotometry.

At first IUD comparison studies were done by merely noting the number of women terminating their IUD experience because of bleeding. Obviously this statistical parameter is subject to great variation depending upon the clinic, the health worker, and the patient herself. Despite these shortcomings, certain empirical observations have been made which seem to be true: (1) the smaller the device, the less bleeding that occurs; (2) the shape of the device, exclusive of size, is not related to menorrhagia and; (3) device thickness and stiffness do seem to exert an influence on the amount of bleeding. Copper IUDs cause increased menstrual bleeding, but the amounts are usually less than in women with noncopper devices. Progesterone-releasing IUDs cause the least amount of abnormal bleeding, and in fact may be therapeutic for women having menometrorrhagia. To add to the confusion, J. Lippes and L. Jacobs found that when copper sleeves were added to the Lippes Loop D, the amount of bleeding, as measured by IUD terminations, was significantly increased (unpublished data).

P. Tauber and L.D. Zaneveld have attempted to decrease IUD-induced bleeding by the addition of Silastic capsules containing one of several antifibrinolytic agents (unpublished data). The rationale behind this development is that increased fibrinolytic activity has been noted among IUD wearers, hence the addition of an antifibrinolytic agent should decrease the amount of fibrinolysis occurring in the endometrium. Whether this fibrinolytic mechanism is the major cause of increased bleeding, and whether the addition of locally acting antifibrinolytic agents can reverse the effect remains to be demonstrated.

Another type of uterine bleeding, metrorrhagia or irregular spotting, is commonly seen among IUD wearers. This bleeding, although insignificant in amounts, may be even more responsible for discontinuation of the method than is menorrhagia. Usually the spotting occurs during the first two to three months following IUD insertion, and with appropriate encouragement, most women continue with the method. However, in some women, metrorrhagia begins again toward the end of the first or second year of IUD use. It is easier to explain the initial spotting following IUD insertion (on the basis of pressure on the endometrial vessels causing erosion and vascular leaking) than the irregular bleeding that suddenly recurs after months of IUD use. In these situations, capillary and small vessel fragility has been observed and may be related to hormonal or enzymatic changes subsequent to the prolonged use of an IUD. Calcification of the IUD creates sharp edges that may be responsible for traumatically induced uterine bleeding.

We are convinced that the future development and increasing use of intrauterine contraception hinges on the bleeding problem. When modern IUDs were introduced in the early 1960s there was great optimism that they were the answer to uncontrolled fertility; in India, in 1964, over four million women had an IUD, the Lippes Loop, inserted. It soon became obvious that women would not and could not tolerate the abnormal bleeding that occurred. Consequently, after two years more than half of the women had the devices removed, in most cases because of the bleeding and associated cramping pain. Perhaps even more significant were the detrimental effects of the reports about the numerous removals on the motivation and acceptance of potential IUD users. Such reports have resulted in low levels of IUD acceptance in India and in many other countries, both developed and developing. It behooves us then, as persons interested in research and development in intrauterine contraception, to explore and support every possible avenue that could lead to the design of an IUD causing little or no abnormal bleeding.

I.C. Expulsion

The major factor influencing retention of an IUD is the geometry of the device, its size, shape and configuration, with respect to the geometry of the intrauterine cavity. Several writers have indicated that the efficiency of this relationship is summarized in the measurement of rates of expulsion. Many subfactors influence this important relationship: uterine size varies according to the parity; the shape of the uterine cavity may be distorted; there are significant racial differences with regard to uterine cavity size regardless of parity; the size of the device in relation to the given uterine cavity; the device itself may possess characteristics which increase or decrease its retention – projections may result in better retention due to embedment; 'fundal-seeking' devices, when properly placed, seem to exhibit lower expulsion rates; and rigidity of the device and its composite material may lessen the likelihood of expulsion.

The importance of fundal placement of an intrauterine device has been long recognized. Regardless of the geometry of the device and its inherent mechanical characteristics, improper insertion in the lower uterine segment will result in high rates of expulsion. This is especially true immediately postpartum (Zatuchni 1970). If the device is assured a fundal placement, even postplacental insertion can be done with expulsion rates similar to those among women having insertions done outside the postpartum period. Correct fundal placement is directly related to the experience and technique of the person performing the insertion. Most IUDs are inserted through a tube in a push-retract mechanism. This poor insertion technique can lead to perforation, particularly with a severely anteflexed or retroflexed uterus, as well as insertion in the lower uterine segment or even the cervical canal. A preferable insertion technique would utilize the newer T-shaped devices; with these, the device inside the cannula is brought to the top of the uterine cavity, and the cannula is then pulled out of the uterus, leaving the device in situ.

H. Hasson (personal communication, 1979) has studied the relationships between uterine cavity and device lengths and has developed a prototype instrument, capable of measuring the total length of the uterine cavity, the length of the intracervical portion (external os to internal os), and the greatest and least widths of the uterine cavity. Using this type of measuring device exact dimensions of the uterine cavity can be obtained, hence a better fit of device to cavity may be expected with consequent improvement in expulsion rates, and perhaps improvement in discontinuance due to cramping pain or bleeding. Unquestionably, the capability to measure accurately the size and shape of the uterine cavity will be a major improvement in IUD technology.

The material from which an IUD is made bears a distinct relationship to expulsion rates and also to discontinuation rates due to bleeding or pain. Rigid devices tend to be less frequently expelled, but have higher probability of discontinuation because of the associated bleeding or cramping. On the other hand, more flexible devices tend to have higher rates of expulsion, but exhibit better continuation rates due to lower incidence of bleeding and pain. From a developmental point of view, however, it has been difficult to demonstrate clinical improvement simply by varying the material from which the device is made. It seems more likely that improvements in expulsion characteristics may come about due to the addition of certain medications.

Progesterone-loaded IUDs exhibit low rates of expulsion as well as a low incidence of bleeding and/or pain. These low rates are due to the smallness of the device, its shape and flexibility and most importantly, the effects of low doses of progesterone – prostaglandin antagonism? – on uterine contractility. The addition of copper wire does not significantly improve expulsion characteristics – the lower rates of expulsion noticed with copper-bearing IUDs are mostly related to the size of the carrier. In a recent unpublished study, Lippes and Jacobs noted that the addition of copper sleeves to a loop did not reduce expulsion rates.

In many species, including humans, the presence of an IUD causes an increase in endometrial prostaglandins. The role of prostaglandins with respect to uterine contractility and IUD expulsion remains unknown, although there is a strong suggestion that the uterine cramping – attempted expulsion? – is directly related. Accordingly, J. Biggers (personal communication, 1979) has suggested incorporating prostaglandin synthetase inhibitors in an IUD to provide better device characteristics with regard to expulsion and pain and perhaps greater effectiveness. He postulates this on the basis of small-animal studies showing the necessity for prostaglandins in the process of implantation. On the other hand, some researchers have indicated the important role that prostaglandins might play in disturbing implantation, and they would argue that the use of prostaglandin inhibitors might lead to lower rates of IUD effectiveness.

I.D. Pelvic infection

The threat of pelvic inflammatory disease (PID) to IUD wearers has been recognized for over fifty years. How much risk is present seems to depend more upon the woman herself and her sexual habits than upon the type of device she wears. The disease occurs in all socioeconomic classes but is much more common among women having frequent sexual intercourse with many partners. The use of an IUD by such women may be especially hazardous. An IUD cannot cause infection, but the presence of an IUD can alter the host's response to invading bacteria or viruses with resulting more severe or more extensive pelvic infection. A history of pelvic inflammatory disease has rightly been a contraindication to IUD insertion.

The relationship of PID to IUD use is difficult to measure. In susceptible groups, for example nulliparous women under 25, women with a previous history of pelvic infection, prostitutes, and certain other groups having a higher prevalence of pelvic inflammatory disease, the frequency of PID occurring with an IUD in situ obviously will be greater. It is also known that PID can occur with any IUD, regardless of size, shape, added medication, material, or tail configuration. Regarding the latter, Tatum (1977) demonstrated that a multifilament tail can transport bacteria from the vagina to the uterine cavity given certain prerequisites. However, pelvic infection occurs even more commonly among wearers of devices with monofilament tails. Gräfenberg, in his early publications, indicated the potential hazards of pelvic infection with any device having an appendage that could serve as a bridge between the vagina and the uterine cavity.

A major unanswered question is the potential loss of fertility due to subclinical pelvic infection occurring after prolonged use of an IUD. Data provided through the cooperative statistical IUD study indicated no loss of fertility among IUD discontinuers, but these were based on women who had discontinued IUD use after periods of one to three years (Tietze and Lewit 1970). At Zatuchni's suggestion that certain studies might be carried out to determine the relative risk of infertility secondary to long-term IUD use, Jain and Moots (1977) reexamined IUD data from Taiwan and found an unexplained loss of fertility among those having used IUDs for over four years. This loss of anticipated fertility might have been due to unreported abortion, use of another unreported contraceptive, or to subclinical PID resulting in certain disturbances in tubal function leading to infertility. The aging factor was discounted. In Thailand, Phaosavasdi et al. (1975) noted unsuspected pelvic infection in IUD users desiring tubal sterilization. Indeed the incidence and extent of pelvic infection was sufficiently high that a third of these women did not need the intended sterilization procedure.

Concern about fertility restoration is particularly great in the case of young women with no children, or with only one child, who desire prolonged IUD use. Clinical research studies similar to Smith and Soderstrom's work (1976) are needed; these investigators, like the Thais, noted unsuspected pelvic tubal infection among former IUD wearers undergoing laparoscopic sterilization. Epidemiologic studies are also indicated, with a focus on long-term IUD wearers seeking later additional fertility. These studies are difficult and expensive to accomplish in a prospective manner, but may be severely biased if done retrospectively. Nevertheless, the concern is of sufficient importance that funding support should be provided to determine the relative risks.

In the postpartum or post-abortal period, it has been conclusively demonstrated that the introduction of an IUD does not interfere with uterine involution, nor is the incidence of endometritis or similar infection increased (Zatuchni 1970).

An IUD that is not associated with any increased risk of pelvic infection following short-term or long-term use is needed. Perhaps Gräfenberg's basic principles should be reemphasized, and devices developed without appendages that might serve as bridges for bacterial invasion. The true importance and necessity of a device tail must be questioned, since it is doubtful that most women check the cervical strings for the presence of the device. Devices can be relatively easily removed by trained persons even when the strings are drawn up into the uterine cavity, and the presence of intracervical strings does not necessarily indicate intrauterine presence of the device. Indeed, beyond the first three months of IUD use the tail serves little functional purpose and offers little convenience for removal. At the same time, the tail may be the factor responsible for the increased risk of PID among IUD users. Accordingly, development of a biodegradable suture destined to dissolve and disappear three months after insertion could be an important addition to intrauterine contraception.

I.E. Neoplasia

There have been a number of studies of exfoliative cytology, both endometrial and cervical, among IUD users. In none of these studies has there been any demonstration of increased risk of dysplasia or neoplasia. For the most part these studies have dealt with nonmedicated IUDs made of polyethylene or polypropylene materials, almost all having minute quantities of barium sulphate added for radiologic location. The tails of devices are made from either nylon or plastic materials similar to those used in the device. About ten years ago several studies in animals indicated a lack of carcinogenic effect of these materials.

On the other hand, the clinical experience with medicated IUDs containing copper or progestational steroid is limited, both in the number of studies that have been done and the length of time of observation. In animal studies, neither copper nor progesterone exhibit any carcinogenic effects in the reproductive organs or elsewhere. Nevertheless, new studies are needed among long-term wearers of copper-bearing IUDs. As the presently available progesterone-releasing IUD has sufficient reservoir for only one year of use, it is highly unlikely that this use would result in neoplastic changes. However, certain steroid-releasing devices in which the steroid loading is sufficient to last for several years are in clinical trials. In this situation, prospective studies are needed to establish the lack of neoplastic potential.

Certainly, any new IUD should undergo testing of its various materials for mutagenic and carcinogenic properties. These studies are carried out in vivo and in vitro and do provide a limited screen for such potential. Whether or not such results apply to humans is unknown. Nevertheless, in the development of future IUDs those materials that cannot pass these studies will not gain approval of drug regulatory agencies.

I.F. Congenital anomalies

We have long been assured that IUDs, either nonmedicated or copper-bearing, exhibit no teratologic effects in laboratory animals or in humans (Guillebaud 1976). Several large international series of pregnancies occurring with IUDs in situ demonstrated only a normal, or less than normal, incidence of malformations.

The recently unearthed diethylstilbestrol (DES) story regarding the relationship between DES administration to pregnant women and subsequent development of reproductive organ changes in significant numbers of male and female offspring has led to parallel concerns with regard to women who become pregnant in the presence of a steroid-releasing IUD. This concern is relevant to all steroids, even natural ones like estradiol and progesterone itself. Thus far, animal studies have not indicated anomalous developments or carcinogenic potential of these steroids in the minute low doses provided by the steroid-releasing IUDs. However, with much larger doses, in certain animal species, developmental anomalies, particularly of the reproductive tracts, do occur among fetuses so exposed. The relevance of these studies to the human is unknown, but caution must be exercised, and continuing animal and human research is needed in order to determine with certainty the potential risks involved with steroid-releasing IUDs.

An ever-increasing number of drugs and chemical compounds is being examined as potential components of a medicated intrauterine delivery system: these include heavy metals, quinicrine, prostaglandins, prostaglandin synthetase inhibitors, and enzyme inhibitors. The development of any such IUD must include studies to rule out the potential for neoplasia in the female and in her offspring, and the teratogenic potential in the offspring. It is likely that when such studies are done, some of the above compounds will be eliminated from consideration in the development of intrauterine delivery systems. These studies will supplement standard drug toxicology studies required by drug regulatory agencies. As the studies are not inexpensive, the impact on the development of new material-releasing IUDs is expected to be substantial. The appropriate sequence of testing for toxicology, carcinogenicity, mutagenicity, and clinical effectiveness is the subject of debate within the United States Food and Drug Administration (FDA) and among researchers. Obviously, no one wishes to pour money into a new development for elaborate and complex testing for safety, prior to determining the actual effectiveness and side effects of the new development. If the FDA insists that such testing must precede large-scale human investigations for effectiveness and acceptability, development of new IUDs will be unlikely in the United States. A more rational approach to the dual concerns of safety and effectiveness would involve preliminary studies in limited, but large, numbers of humans with close monitoring and follow-up, followed by long-term and more elaborate safety testing in animals and in humans.

Surveillance studies of an epidemiologic nature, when properly done, can provide answers to long-term safety concerns. In fact, many suspected but undefined relationships have been uncovered by such studies. These studies are expensive but necessary and drug regulatory agencies support limited numbers of them. Unfortunately, in the area of intrauterine contraception support for such studies has been virtually zero. It is unlikely that research institutions or pharmaceutical companies could support these long-term surveillance studies without funding from government sources.

II. NEW CONCEPTS IN INTRAUTERINE DELIVERY SYSTEMS

Dissatisfaction with metallic or plastic IUDs, from the points of view of both the user and the contraceptive provider, has led to an increasing interest in the development of IUDs containing one or another agent in an attempt to do the following:

1. Decrease the incidence and amount of abnormal uterine bleeding;
2. Decrease the incidence of spontaneous expulsion;
3. Decrease the incidence of pregnancy;
4. Develop new approaches in fertility regulation; and
5. Provide certain therapeutic effects in addition to contraceptive effects.

The addition of copper wire or sleeves has been a step in the right direction with regard to all of these objectives. However, problems have arisen: for example the duration of action of a copper-bearing IUD of the wire type is not fully known and it may be as short as three to five years; the incidence of tubal ectopic pregnancy may be increased; and due to the lack of long-term data the safety risks among long-term users are unknown.

The addition of steroids housed in a capsule affixed to an IUD has also led to certain improvements in device characteristics, especially the decreased incidence and amount of IUD-associated bleeding and a lowering of the IUD expulsion incidence. One may speculate that the progesterone or progestin may be exerting an antiprostaglandin effect at the endometrial level, thereby causing improvement in these parameters. Despite the improvements, other problems have been noted: among them the relatively high failure rates with progesterone-loaded IUDs; a worrisome increase in tubal ectopic pregnancies; and the debated possibilities of abnormal embryonal developments in the presence of steroids, even in the microdose quantities that are released by the IUD.

Accordingly, the search continues for an intrauterine delivery system that would be capable of providing all the wanted characteristics of an IUD without any of the unwanted characteristics that have thus far been associated with every one invented. Undoubtedly, over the next decade, new types of IUDs will be marketed, but given restraints of government regulations regarding safety and the attendant cost of development it is unlikely that radically different intrauterine delivery systems will come into general use. More likely, newer devices will embody variations in design, such as shape, size, or geometry; copper configurations; or quantities and types of loaded steroids.

Tables 2, 3 and 4 list possible opportunities for intrauterine delivery systems that go beyond present-day thinking about intrauterine contraception. Preliminary research efforts are under way to develop IUDs for special users during various times of the female reproductive life cycle. For example, a Lippes Loop has been redesigned to provide excellent retention characteristics when inserted in a postpartum uterus immediately following delivery of the placenta. Copper devices have been inserted in women having had unprotected intercourse at midcycle in order to interfere with the process of implantation, assuming that fertilization has occurred. Biodegradable devices are being considered for short-term use extending over a period of months.

Table 2. Special uses of IUDs.

Nulligravida
Postpartum
Post-abortion
Postcoital
Premenopausal
'Honeymoon' IUD
Abortion IUD
Sterilization IUD

Table 3. Intrauterine delivery systems for fertility regulation.

Tubal closure substances
Tubal motility activators
Follicle maturation inhibitors
Luteolytic substances
Progesterone-receptor blocking agents
Decidualization inhibitors
Immunological agents (local) against:
zona pellucida
sperm acrosin
sperm membrane
trophoblast
Sperm enzyme inhibitors
Placental enzyme inhibitors
Cervical mucous rheologic disturbers

Table 4. Examples of medical conditions amenable to therapeutic intrauterine delivery systems.

Dysfunctional uterine bleeding
Dysmenorrhea
Endometriosis
Uterine synechia
Endometrial hyperplasia
Endometrial carcinoma in situ
Radiation therapy of endometrial carcinoma
Pelvic inflammatory disease
Chronic pelvic infection (for example granulomatous)
Preventive treatment against certain bacteria/viruses

Future systems may include agents or drugs that would exert fertility-inhibiting effects beyond those of present-day IUDs. For example, certain substances could be loaded onto an IUD that might cause tubal sclerosis at the site of entry of the fallopian tube into the endometrial cavity. Taking advantage of the uterine-tubal-ovarian local circulation, it is possible to conceive of certain substances, for example luteolytic substances and inhibitors of endometrial decidualization, exerting tubal or ovarian effects when released from a carrier IUD. More effective intrauterine contraception may be provided by the incorporation into an IUD of various immunological agents, for example sperm acrosin inhibitors and sperm enzyme inhibitors, that interfere with sperm motility or capacity for fertilization. Finally, advantages may be forthcoming in developing intrauterine delivery systems capable of providing local immunological changes that would be incompatible with implantation for example of antitrophoblastic or antiplacental agents.

Future developments must address the annoying side effects that occur with IUDs, especially bleeding, cramping pain and expulsion. To circumvent these problems, research work is ongoing to determine the beneficial effects, if any, of the incorporation of such drugs as antifibrinolytic agents, for example epsilon aminocaproic acid (EACA) or trasylol, or inhibitors of prostaglandin synthetase. Preliminary animal and human studies with EACA are favourable insofar as decreasing the incidence of IUD-associated bleeding.

The addition of certain agents, for example copper or zinc, to an IUD may be effective in the establishment of a milieu unfavourable to the growth and multiplication of bacteria and viruses. It has recently been demonstrated that zinc ions can destroy the Herpes virus. As the type-II Herpes virus appears to be related to cervical carcinoma, a zinc-containing IUD might interfere with this relationship, thereby eliminating or at least decreasing the incidence of this pathology.

Intrauterine delivery systems can be developed to release microquantities of drugs that are not necessarily intended for the control of fertility; examples are progesterone-releasing systems which exhibit a marked amelioration of hypermenorrhea and dysmenorrhea. Indeed, many gynecologists use the only available progesterone-releasing system as therapy for these clinical conditions rather than for its antifertility effect. It is probable that in the future local intrauterine therapy may be utilized in the treatment of a wide spectrum of gynecological conditions, such as endometriosis, pelvic infection, Asherman's syndrome, chronic granulomatous infection, actinomycosis, endometrial hyperplasia, endometrial carcinoma in situ, and other female reproductive organ diseases. An intrauterine delivery system capable of releasing daily small quantities of active agent over a long period of time could be an important therapeutic alternative for drugs that are not effective when administered orally, or for drugs having a short duration of action, hence requiring frequent or even continuous administration.

In conclusion, fertility regulation provided by a nonmedicated intrauterine device represents merely the initial step in the ultimate development of entirely new modalities of contraceptive and medical therapy. More than fifty years passed before physicians and researchers recognized the potential for intrauterine delivery systems of contraception. This potential is limited only by the imagination; preliminary results of research and clinical experience already indicate the feasibility and usefulness of a wide variety of intrauterine delivery systems applications for enhanced fertility regulation. Beyond these antifertility effects future developments should provide new means of gynecological therapy.

REFERENCES

Chaudhuri G: Intrauterine device: possible role of prostaglandins. Lancet 1: 480, 1971.

Guillebaud J: IUD and congenital malformation. Br Med J 1: 1016, 1976.

Ishihama A: Clinical studies on intrauterine rings. Yokohama Med J 10: 89, 1959.

Jain AK, Moots B: Fecundability following the discontinuation of IUD use among Taiwanese women. J Biosoc Sci 9: 137-151, 1977.

Morese DN, Peterson WF, Allan ST: Endometrial effects of an intrauterine contraceptive device. Obstet Gynecol 111: 66-80, 1971.

Oppenheimer W: Prevention of pregnancy by the Gräfenberg ring method. Am J Obstet Gynecol 78: 446-454, 1959.

Phaosavasdi S, Israngkun C, et al.: In: Analysis of intrauterine contraception, Hefnawi F, Segal S (eds), Amsterdam, North-Holland Publishing, 1975.

Pust K: Ein brauchbarer Frauenschutz. Dtsch Med Wochenschr 49: 952-953, 1923.

Richter R: Ein Mittel zur Verhütung der Konzeption. Dtsch Med Wochenschr 35: 1525-1527, 1909.

Smith MR, Soderstrom R: Salpingitis: a frequent response to intrauterine contraception. J Reprod Med 16: 159-162, 1976.

Tatum HJ: Clinical aspects of intrauterine contraception. Fertil Steril 28: 3-28, 1977.

Tatum HJ, Schmidt FH: Contraception and sterilization practices and extrauterine pregnancy. Fertil Steril 28: 407-421, 1977.

Tietze C, Lewit S: Evaluation of IUDs: ninth progress report. Stud Fam Plann 55, 1970.

United States Agency for International Development: Family planning service statistics, Office of Population, 1978.

Zatuchni GI (ed): International postpartum family planning program, McGraw-Hill, New York, 1970.

22. IUD DECISION GUIDE: DETERMINANTS OF IUD CONTINUATION

R.G. WHEELER

I. DETERMINANTS OF SATISFACTION AND EVENT RATES

Ideally, an IUD should provide contraception, free of side effects, until it is removed at the request of the user. In practice, occasional pregnancy, expulsion or any of a number of side effects are possible. Because of the dramatic variation in the ways women respond to an IUD, it would be beneficial to predict in advance which women are most likely to experience a given side effect.

The use of a decision guide based on each individual woman's answers to selected questions asked before insertion would enable the service provider to:

- select the IUD type or size with the best combination of expected results;
- advise women predicted to have a high risk of early discontinuation to use a more effective method;
- compare results from IUD studies in different populations under conditions that standardize results for differences in acceptor characteristics;
- use empirically derived relationships between predictor variables* and outcome of discover physiologic cause-and-effect relationships.

Numerous authors have looked for correlations between IUD respondents' characteristics and outcome, but there have been few attempts to use multidimensional methods to see how the predictor variables interact. Potter et al. (1966) conducted a careful follow-up of 7295 acceptors form Taiwan and found that pregnancy, expulsion and side-effect event rates, calculated by the multiple decrement lifetable method, were dependent on a number of predictor variables. Total termination rate at the end of twelve months was 34.4 per 100 women. In descending order of their importance, age, education, geographic location, prior contraception, last pregnancy outcome, last pregnancy interval and type of device correlated with continuation.

In a sociodemographic analysis of IUD users (Morehead 1975), the following characteristics of respondents were found to be predictors of continuation rates:

- sexuality images (attitudes about menstruation);
- contraceptive attitude (approval of contraception and child desire);
- side effects and somatization (perceived change in menstrual flow);
- conjugal interaction (who makes decisions).

A number of notable studies (Peng et al. 1970; Tietze and Lewit et al. 1970; Chi et al. 1978), including a casebook (Wishik and Hulka 1969) that provides preinsertion case histories and makes recommendations regarding IUD insertion, have been useful in establishing the individual correlation of predictor variables with outcome.

Although a general consensus prevails on the patient characteristics that may be useful, there is a dearth of information on the interactions of the various predictors. Controlling for age and parity is a common practice in comparative clinical studies of IUD performance, but these and the other predictor variables are treated as if their effects act independently on event rates. By implication, age and parity are considered to be among the important predictors of outcome. This work is concerned

* The term predictor variables is used to describe those patient characteristics that correlate with IUD event rates and side effects.

with both the relative importance of predictor variables and their interactions.

I.A. Ranking of predictor variables

A system that predicts the outcome of IUD contraception could be developed by simulating, with a computer program, the logic of someone having proven expertise in making such predictions. Although records of the outcome of IUD use are plentiful, there are no records of predictions. However, a predicting model can be developed correlating the information on admission forms with results recorded on follow-up records.

As a first step in the empirical development of a decision guide, it is informative to see how individual predictor variables correlate with duration of IUD use and to see how subjective impressions correspond with statistical data.

To get a qualitative impression of the importance that gynecologists and other IUD researchers assign to the different variables, five gynecologists and seven researchers were given a deck of cards with the name of one predictor variable on each card. They were asked to sort the cards in descending order of the importance of each variable as a predictor of continuation. Their average ranking is listed alongside the first ten variables of the computer ranking in Table 1 which is based on actual data from 2000 cases. Also, in a column of Table 1, there is a listing of references in which an author on IUDs has correlated the corresponding variable with IUD events.

With some exceptions, the rankings by gynecologists and IUD reseachers are not too different from those produced by the computer. Since most of the variables interact with others, it is somewhat misleading to rank them according to their separate effects on continuation. These ranks of predictor variables may indicate which ones to include in a multivariate analysis, but rankings tell nothing about the interaction of variables.

At best, all of the predictor variables are weak predictors of duration of IUD use. A measure of their predicting power is the amount of variance accounted for or the square of the Pearson correlation coefficient. By this measure, age and total live births account for about one percent of the variance in duration of IUD use. Since they are individually weak predictors, they need to be combined in a way that will strengthen their predicting power.

Since the physicians' rankings of predictor vari-

Table 1. A comparison of the ranking of IUD acceptor characteristics according to their effect on continuation rates.

Predictor of continuation	*Variables* Computer Ranking*	*Gynecologist's Ranking*	*IUD Researcher's Ranking*	*Typical References*
Total live births	1	2	10	Bernard (1970), Tietze and Lewit (1970), Snowden et al. (1977).
Length of cervix	2	7	11	Tejuja and Malkani (1969), Hasson et al. (1976)
Distance: external os to fundus	3	3	5	Davis and Israel (1964), Hasson et al. (1976)
Interval since last pregnancy	4	14	9	Potter et al. (1966), Ratnam and Tow (1970),Tatun (1973)
Length of cycle	5	15	15	Muranatsu (1973), Rodriguez et al. (1976)
Previous contraceptive method	6	17	20	Morehead (1975), Vessey et al. (1978)
Age	7	1	4	Tietze and Lewit (1970), Muranatsu (1973), Jain (1975)
Total number of abortions	8	13	19	Bernard (1970), Muranatsu (1973) Chi et al. (1978)
Additional children wanted	9	16	16	Chi et al. (1978)
Flow duration	10	8	7	Guttorm (1971), Rodriguez et al. (1976)

* The computer ranking was based on duration of IUD use by 2000 women.

ables are subjective, nonreproducible values, a Searching For Structure (SFS) technique (Sonquest et al. 1971; Hartigan 1975) was used to obtain quantitative results from the data bank of 2000 cases. The first step of this SFS program ranks predictor variables according to their individual power to account for variance of the dependent variable, duration of IUD use. An example of these results is the computer ranking presented in Table 1.

I.B. Importance of uterine measurements

The high SFS program ranking of uterine measurements as predictors of IUD continuation (Table 1) is in accord with studies of the effect of uterine cavity size on IUD continuation (Burnhill and Birnberg 1966; Hasson et al. 1976; Kamal et al. 1971; Davis and Israel 1964). Unexpectedly, the study revealed that the length of the cervix had a greater positive effect on IUD continuation rates than the length of the uterine cavity. Dimensions obtained by sounding the uterus before IUD insertion are generally as important as age and parity in determining duration of IUD use.

II. DEVELOPMENT OF A DECISION GUIDE

The term *decision guide* is intended to describe a procedure for using the answers to a few questions to determine if a woman is likely to have fewer or more than the average number of events that lead to termination of IUD use. The decision guide defines several subgroups of the original population that have different average durations of IUD use. Each woman falls into one, and only one, of these subgroups depending on her *age*, *total live births*, *length of cervix* and *distance from outer os to fundus.*

The predictive power of the decision guide increases as each subgroup is split into two new ones, providing there are enough cases remaining in each of the two parts to meet statistical criteria for sample size. By choosing to compare Lippes Loop D results with those of copper IUDs, the sample size available was 1469 women. Because of this limitation to splitting, the model decision guide presented here requires the answer to no more than four questions to classify a woman into a risk group.

II.A. Source of data

Studies from several European countries were pooled to provide the data set. Lippes Loop D, Cu-T and Cu-7 IUDs were evenly represented. Another set of IUD data consisted of 400 randomly allocated insertions of Lippes Loop D and Cu-T IUDs. This latter data set was used to determine if the prediction model developed with one data set would predict the event rates of another consisting of 400 cases.

II.B. SFS program

The SFS computer program is one of a variety of cluster analysis methods for dealing with multidimensional problems (Hartigan 1975). For the purpose of illustrating how the SFS program works, it was used to classify the women into clusters having similar durations on the basis of their *age* and *total live births*. In this case the variable *total live births* was found to explain more variance than age and to explain the most variance when the split was made between one or less and two or more children (Figure 1). The original group of 1469 women was split into Group 2 consisting of 518 women and Group 3 consisting of 951 women

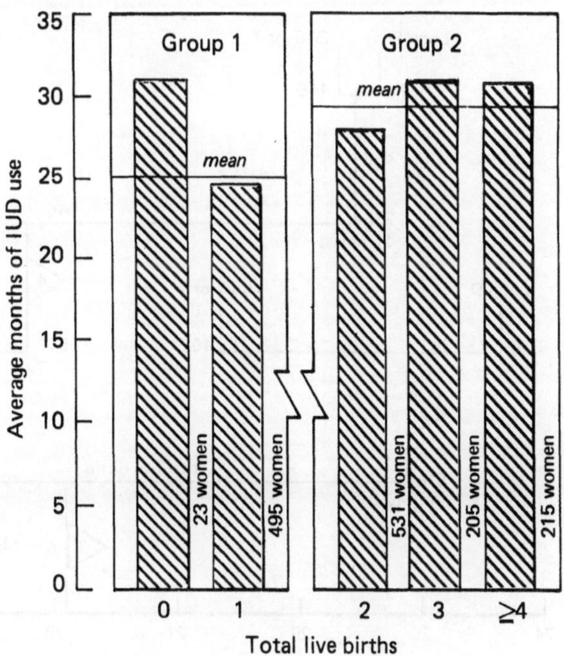

Figure 1. The most variance in months of IUD use is explained when the split in total live births is between one and two.

(Figure 2). As shown in Figure 2, the program chooses to split either Group 2 or Group 3 by selecting the one with the greatest sum of the squared variances, that is, the one with the greatest potential for explaining variance.

Note that in Figure 2 the variable *total live births* was better than *age* for splitting Group 3 into two groups consisting of 531 women (Group 4) and of 420 women (Group 5). The next split of Group 4 on the variable *age* completes the splitting of the population into four clusters using two predictor variables. In reality, the population has been separated into only two clusters because Group 5 and Group 7 both have an average duration of IUD use near 31 months and Group 2 and Group 6 are close to 25 months. The mean duration of IUD use of Group 5 and Group 7 combined is statistically much different from the mean of Group 2 and Group 6 combined. Use of the predictor variables *total live births* and *age* properly combined explains more of the variance in duration of IUD use than either of these variables alone.

There are three criteria that are set by the analyst for halting the splitting process. These are the minimum number of women in a group after a split, the minimum amount of variance explained or the maximum number of groups created. In this case the program was halted at four nondivided groups or clusters.

Both separation of risk categories and accounting for variance can be improved by including additional predictor variables such as uterine measurements. Figure 3 schematically illustrates the further clustering of the women into risk categories. Creating Risk Group 2 with an average duration of 25 months and Risk Group 3 with an average duration of 29.5 months (see Figure 3) explains one percent of the variance in duration of IUD use. If the entire prediction model of Figure 3 is used to create separate risk groups out of branches 8, 9 and 10, 7 and 11, and 5, these four risk groups will explain three percent of the variance or three times that of *total live births* alone.

III. APPLICATION OF THE DECISION GUIDE

The tree representation of a decision guide for

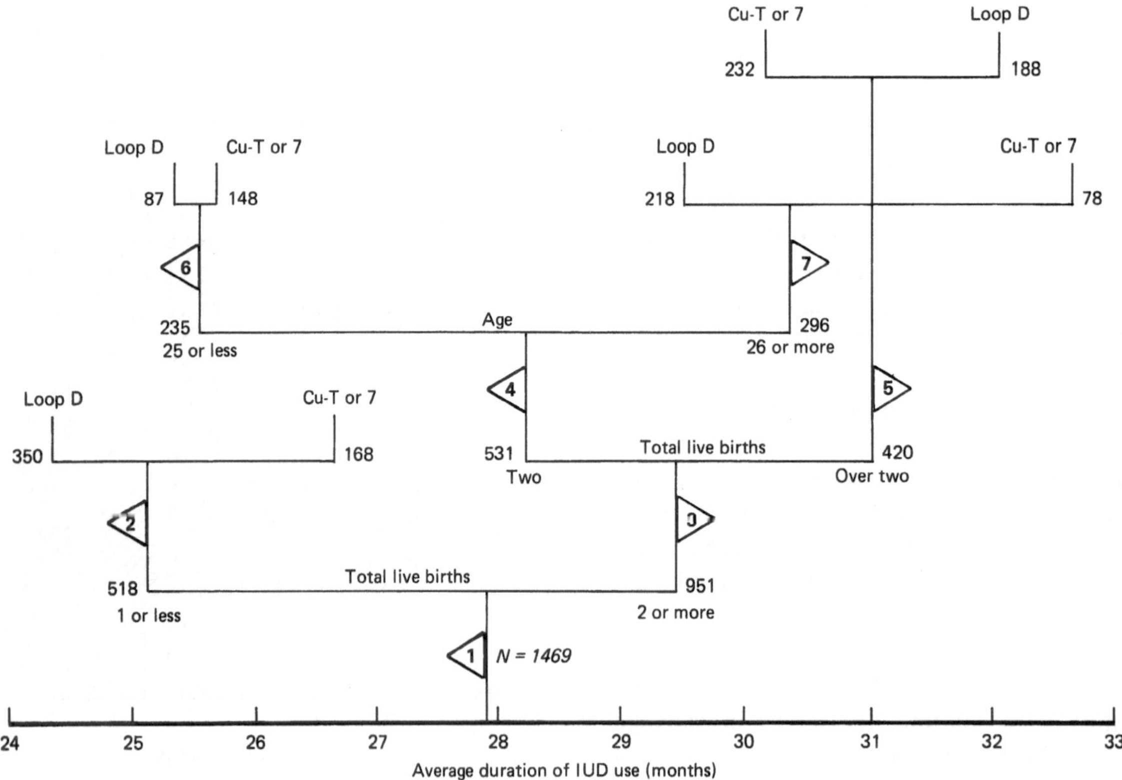

Figure 2. IUD continuation by IUD type, age and total living children.

predicting duration of IUD use (Figure 3) has six terminal branches numbered 5,7,8,9,10 and 11. The same logic represented by the tree is presented in Figure 4 as pages of a booklet, a form more suited for use in a clinic than a tree diagram. Terminal branches of the tree of Figure 3 correspond with risk groups in the booklet (Figure 4) as follows: branch 8 is Risk Group 1, with an average duration of 22.7 months; branches 9 and 10 are combined as Risk Group 2; branches 7 and 11 are combined as Risk Group 3; and branch 5 is Risk Group 4, with an average duration of 33.7 months.

Not many of the available predictor variables were used in the decision guide because the sample size of 1469 cases was too small to justify much more splitting. Even so, the guide should produce some of the expected benefits. These expectations are discussed below.

III. A. IUD selection

Of the 1469 women represented in Figure 3, 904 used a Lippes Loop D and 565 used copper IUDs. In Figure 2 and Figure 3, each of the terminal branches has been split into Lippes Loop D and copper IUD users. Notice that there is no significant trend for one type of IUD to have a longer duration of use than the other. In most cases the separation between the two classes of IUDs is about one standard error of estimation. All other things being equal, one could justify preference for a copper device for a woman with one or less live births and a length from external os to fundus less than 71mm (branch 8 of Figure 3). For a woman with two or more live births and a cervical length of 31 mm or more (branch 5), the Lippes Loop D appears to have a longer duration of IUD use. Important factors such as availability, cost, access to medical facilities and ease of insertion are not considered here.

III.B. Identification of high-risk cases

A data set, representing 400 cases evenly divided between Lippes Loop D and Cu-T users, was split into four risk groups with the decision guide. Lifetable results for this test sample are listed in Table 2, from which it can be seen that the average pregnancy rate of Group 1 is about three times the average for the whole sample. Expulsion rates and bleeding/pain removal rates for Group 1 and Group 2 are both about 1.3 times the overall average. Knowing what average event rate to expect for a given woman should influence clinical decisions and advice to the patient.

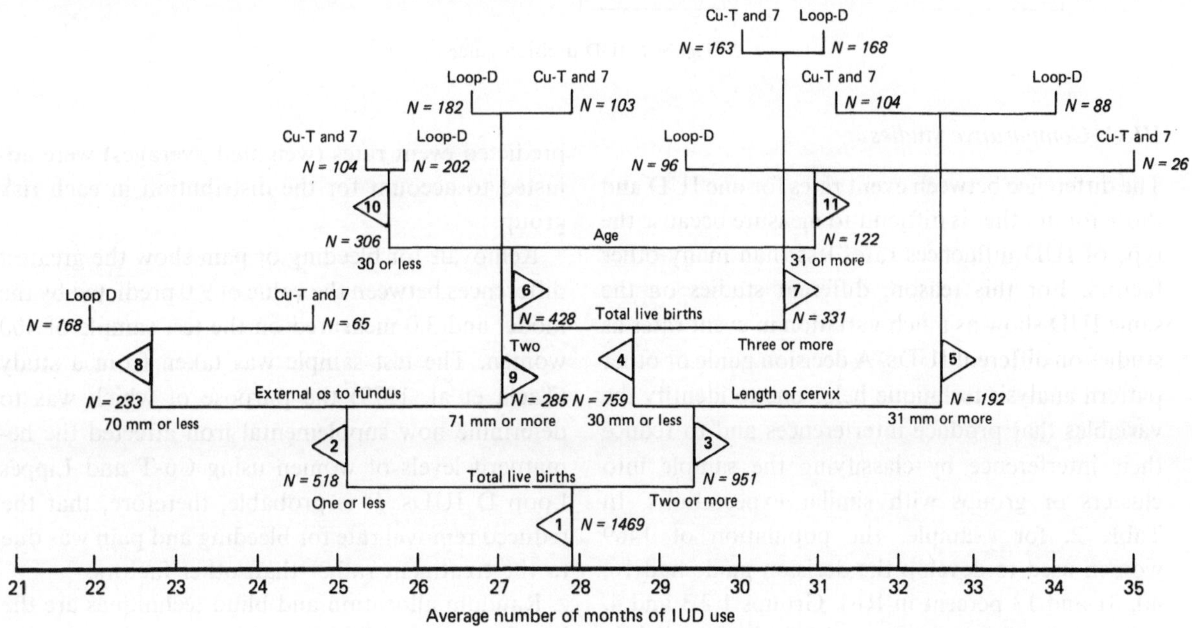

Figure 3. IUD continuation by IUD type, age, total living children and uterine soundings.

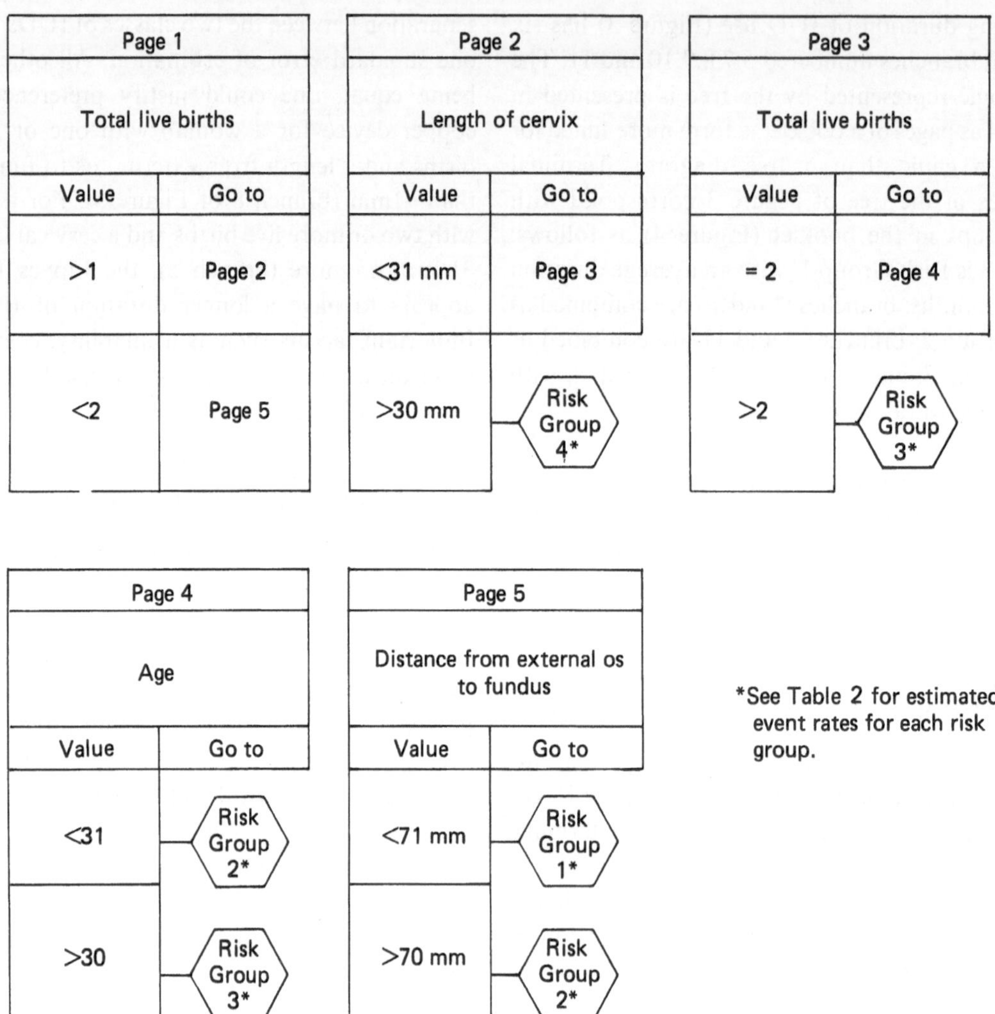

Figure 4. IUD decision guide.

III.C. Comparative studies

The difference between event rates for one IUD and those for another is difficult to measure because the type of IUD influences rates less than many other factors. For this reason, different studies on the same IUD show as much variation in event rates as studies on different IUDs. A decision guide or other pattern analysis technique helps one to identify the variables that produce interferences and to reduce their interference by classifying the sample into clusters or groups with similar expectations. In Table 2, for example, the population of 1469 women used to develop the decision guide had 16, 40, 31 and 13 percent in Risk Groups 1,2,3 and 4, respectively. Since the test sample had a slightly different distribution of 6, 58, 26 and 13 percent, the predicted event rates (weighted averages) were adjusted to account for the distribution in each risk group.

Removals for bleeding or pain show the greatest differences between the value of 9.0 predicted by the model and 3.0 measured on the test sample of 400 women. The test sample was taken from a study (Tacla et al. 1979) the purpose of which was to determine how supplemental iron affected the hematocrit levels of women using Cu-T and Lippes Loop D IUDs. It is probable, therefore, that the reduced removal rate for bleeding and pain was due to the treatment rather than other factors.

Random allocation and blind techniques are the best but not infallible ways to control interfering variables because random partitioning of a few of

Table 2. Gross termination rates per 100 users.

	Groups ranked by increasing probability of continuation					
	Risk Group 1	*Risk Group 2*	*Risk Group 3*	*Risk Group 4*	*Total weighted average*	*Test rates*
Number of insertions	25	229	105	41	400	400
Fraction of total	0.062	0.58	0.26	0.10	1.00	
Rates	Estimated	Estimated	Estimated	Estimated	Estimated	Measured
Pregnancy	5.2	1.0	1.4	2.0	1.5	3.1
Expulsion	16.0	13.0	3.0	5.0	11.0	10.0
Removal						
Bleeding/pain	13.0	12.0	5.0	3.0	9.0	3.0
Other medical	2.0	3.0	2.0	1.0	3.0	6.0
Planned pregnancy	4.0	2.0	1.0	0.0	3.0	6.0
Other personal	5.0	4.0	4.0	2.0	4.0	3.0
Lost to follow-up	23.0	18.0	24.0	13.0	19.0	11.0
Continuation (12 months)	61.0	69.0	80.0	33.0	73.4	74.0

the more important predictor variables can produce an unexpected bias. Showing the case and control distributions in each of the various risk groups provide a way to determine when random allocation has failed to proportion the cases evenly in each of the risk groups.

III.D. Cause- and-effect relationships

Although the investigator plays a crucial role in determining what and how information goes into the SFS program, producing the results is a computerized application of statistical processes. Critical examination of the results, however, can lead to discovery of sociologic and physiologic causes of the patterns disclosed. Often the results present a question that demands an answer. For example, in the original population of 2196 women, there was one group in which each woman had two living children and a cervix less than 31 mm long and had previously used either no contraception or something other than a barrier method. Those women in this group who experienced moderate or severe dysmenorrhea before IUD insertion had a longer average duration of IUD use than those who experienced only mild dysmenorrhea or no dysmenorrhea during the cycles preceding IUD insertion. This observation points out how, for some women, severe dysmenorrhea may have an effect that is the opposite of intuitive expectations. If further investigation confirms these preliminary results, the cause of the relationship should be explored because of the resulting clinical benefits.

IV. CONCLUSION

There are considerable dividends for the added effort needed to apply multidimensional scaling-cluster analysis techniques to IUD study data. The technique could, of course, also be applied to any prescriptive therapy with a measurable end point. Researchers on IUDs are usually concerned with the effect of the type of IUD, clinical procedure or type of patient on event rates. More efficient studies will result if variance in event rates and side-effect rates are reduced. Accounting for some of the individuality of women by cluster analysis reduces the large variance in the outcome of IUD use.

In the process of quantifying the power of predictor variables on admission and follow-up forms, those that have trivial predicting power can be eliminated from the record-keeping and analysis process and thus reduce work and expense in the clinic and study centre without loss of research value.

If a system for classifying women of all races and nationalities according to their expected outcome of

IUD contraception is to work well, the data base should be large and should be taken from a representative sample of the whole population. All of these criteria were not met in this analysis of a data set of less than 2000 insertions from a few countries. Fortunately, there are numerous IUD data bases large enough to evaluate the interactions of predictor variables by cluster analysis techniques. These valuable data sets should be utilized to pursue the concept of classifying women according to their risk of experiencing IUD side effects and events. It is possible to foresee application of this approach through easy-to-use clinic guides that could be especially useful to auxiliary medical workers (Figure 4).

ACKNOWLEDGEMENT

The author wishes to thank the many professionals who contributed the data used in the preparation of this chapter. This work was supported in part by the International Fertility Research Program and the Office of Population, United States Agency for International Development (AID/pha-C-1111).

REFERENCES

Bernard RP: IUD performance patterns: a 1970 world review. Int J Gynaecol Obstet 8: 926, 1970.

Blake J: Income and reproductive motivation. Popul Stud 21(3) : 185, 1967.

Burnhill MS, Birnberg CH: The size and shape of the uterine cavity determined by hysterography with an intrauterine contraceptive device as a marker. Int J Fertil 11 : 187, 1966.

Campenhout JV, Blanchet P, Beauregard H, Papas S: Amenorrhea following the use of oral contraceptives. Fertil Steril 28(7) : 718, 1977.

Chi I, Kessel E, Mitra M: An epidemiologic study of intrauterine contraceptive devices; a preliminary report. In: Risks, benefits and controversies in fertility control, Sciarra JJ, Zatuchni GI, Speidel JJ (eds), Hagerstown, Harper and Row, 1978, p 478ff.

Davis HJ, Israel R: Uterine cavity measurements in relation to design of intrauterine contraceptive devices. In: Intrauterine contraception, Segal S, Southam A, Shafer KD (eds), International congress series 86, Amsterdam, Excerpta Medica, 1964, p 135ff.

Guttorm E: Menstrual bleeding with intrauterine contraceptive devices. Acta Obstet Gynecol Scand 50 : 9, 1971.

Hartigan JA: Clustering algorithms, New York, John Wiley and Sons, 1975.

Hasson HM, Berger GS, Edelman DA: Factors affecting intrauterine contraceptive device performance. Am J Obstet Gynecol 126 : 973, 1976.

Jain AK: Safety and effectiveness of intrauterine devices. Contraception 11(3) : 243, 1975.

Kamal I, Hefnawi F, Ghoneim M, Talaat M, Abdalla M: Dimensional and architectural disproportion between the intrauterine device and uterine cavity: a cause of bleeding. Fertil Steril 22 : 514, 1971.

Morehead JE: Intrauterine device retention, a study of selected social-psychological aspects. Am J Public Health 6(7): 720, 1975.

Muramatsu M: Statistical analysis of long-term wearers of Ota Ring, Tokyo, Institute of Public Health, Department of Public Demography, 1973.

Peng JY, Chow LP, Corsa L: Medical correlates of termination of use of intrauterine contraceptive devices in Taichung. Int J Fertil 15 : 120, 1970.

Potter RG, Chow LP, Jain AK, Lee CH: Social and demographic correlates of IUCD effectiveness: the Taichung IUCD medical follow-up study. In: Proceedings of the American Statistical Association, Washington DC, 1966.

Ratnam SS, Tow SS: Translocation of the loop. In: Post-partum intrauterine contraception in Singapore, Wolfers D (ed) Amsterdam, Excerpta Medica, 1970, p 134ff.

Rodriguez G, Faundes-Latham A, Atkinson LE: An approach to the analysis of menstrual patterns in the critical evaluation of contraceptives. Stud Fam Plann 7(2) : 42, 1976.

Snowden R, Williams M, Hawkins D: The IUD: a practical guide, London, Croom Helm, 1977.

Sonquest JA, Baker LE, Morgan JN: Searching for structure (alias, AID-111), Ann Arbor, Survey Research Center, Institute for Social Research, University of Michigan, 1971.

Tacla X, Baeza R, Colven C: La T de cobre y el Lippes Loop: Cual es mejor para la mujer chilena? Rev Colomb Obstet Ginecol, 1979.

Tatum HJ: Metallic Cu as an intrauterine contraceptive agent. Am J Obstet Gynecol 117(5) : 602, 1973.

Tejuja S, Malkani PK: Clinical significance of correlation between size of the uterine cavity and IUCD. Am J Obstet Gynecol 105 : 620, 1969.

Tietze C, Lewit S: Evaluation of intrauterine devices: ninth progress report of the cooperative statistical program. Stud Fam Plann 55, 1970.

Vessey MP, Wright NH, McPherson K, Wiggins P: Fertility after stopping different methods of contraception. Br Med J 1: 265, 1978.

Wishik SM, Hulka JF: Casebook for the intrauterine contraceptive device, Chapel Hill, Carolina Population Center, University of North Carolina, 1969.

23. TESTING THE CLINICAL PERFORMANCE OF AN IUD

T. LUUKKAINEN

The results of clinical trials with the same IUD show great variations. In a multiclinic study in Finland with Cu-T200 the pregnancy rate at twelve months varied between 0.0 and 5.5 in different clinics (Luukkainen et al. 1975). A collaborative study (Sivin 1973) performed in five countries reported pregnancy rates from 0.3 to 2.9 and removal rates from 6.9 to 21.0 for Cu-T200. Both studies were carefully planned to minimize the clinical effect. The same instructions for insertion technique and for the patients were used. The clinical records were the same in the different clinics and data were collected and analyzed in one unit. It is evident that the results of various investigators on the performance of the same IUD, using different insertion techniques and data collection, are more variable than the results in these studies, where guidelines were kept similar by the central team.

I. FACTORS AFFECTING IUD TRIALS

The factors affecting the results of the IUD trials have been identified by Mishell (1975). He reported that the following factors may be responsible for great variation in IUD performance among different clinics: patient population, physician experience, tolerance of side effects in the population, clinic attitude and additional contraceptives available.

The patient population varies. The age distribution should always be reported. Very low pregnancy rates were observed in trials with an experimental IUD using an older population selected for ethical or safety reasons. The results then may reflect only the age structure of the subjects, not the design of the new IUD. The age of subjects at insertion clearly affects not only the pregnancy rates but also the expulsion rates (Table 1). The termination rates are also influenced by the parity of the subjects. The pregnancy, expulsion and removal rates usually decline with increasing parity (Tietze and Lewit 1970; Timonen and Luukkainen 1974). It is surprising that recent reports do not describe the age and parity distribution of their patient population (van Os et al. 1978).

The physician's experience and skill may influence event rates, as stated by Mishell (1975). The results of a highly trained small team (Thiery et al. 1978a, 1978b) may not be reproducible by less trained personnel; the results then rather reflect the training of the team than the performance of the experimental device. The physician's experience could influence results also in the opposite direction. A single physician could repeat the same incorrect insertion and have, for example, a high expulsion rate (Fylling and Fagerhol 1979). It

Table 1. The influence of age at insertion on net cumulative pregnancy and expulsion rates of loops (Tietze and Lewit 1970) and Cu-T devices (Jain 1975) at two years.

Age	*Loop C* *Pregnancy*	*Expulsion*	*Loop D* *Pregnancy*	*Expulsion*	*Cu-T* *Pregnancy*	*Expulsion*
15-19 20-24	6.0	38.0	5.8	24.9	5.7	14.9
25-29	5.2	22.6	4.7	13.9	5.4	9.3
30-34	3.9	14.8	2.8	9.6	2.5	6.4
35-39	1.7	7.4	1.5	6.1	0.5	3.0

should be realized that correct insertion is one of the main factors affecting the performance of an IUD. Misplacements cannot be corrected after the insertion.

The tolerance of the patients to the side effects varies from country to country. It may be different in rural and urban populations in the same country. The lower removal rate for bleeding and pain in women of high parity or in women who have accomplished their desired family size could be attributed to high tolerance of side effects (Timonen and Luukkainen 1974).

The clinic's attitude can explain extremely low removal rates of devices which are known to produce bleeding (Table 2) or, on the other hand a very high removal rate of a device which in the same study was well tolerated in another clinic (Table 3).Additional contraceptives used with an IUD will greatly reduce the pregnancy rate. This was clearly demonstrated by Thiery et al. (1978a), who observed the following pregnancy rates at one year and at two years with Cu-T220 C: without a spermicide 1.4 and 3.1 and with spermicide 0.0 and 0.0, respectively. The use of an additional spermicide cannot be recommended in the trials for testing an experimental IUD but their use in family planning programs could greatly increase the protection. A vaginal contraceptive with a demonstrated protective action against venereal diseases could be used by an IUD patient with high risks of infection (Osser et al. 1978; Luukkainen et al. 1978).

In addition to these factors it has been found that the time of insertion is important. The expulsion rate is lower if the insertion is performed between days 1-7 than 8-14 of the menstrual cycle. The removal rate for bleeding is higher if the insertion is performed during the luteal phase of the cycle; the removal rate for infection is lowest when the insertion is performed on days 1-3 of the cycle (Timonen 1976). The stability of the sexual relations as reflected by the marital status seems to be of great importance among IUD users under 25 years of age (Luukkainen et al. 1979c). Women in the age group below 25 years had a high rate of infection, whereas the age group 25-29 had a very low rate of infection. Nulliparous and primiparous women had equally high rates of removal due to infection.

II. TESTING METHOD FOR CLINICAL PERFORMANCE

For these reasons the only valid method of testing

Table 2. Cumulative event rates and women-months of use at 17 ordinal months of use per 100 users of Lippes Loop D, Cu-T200, Cu-T220C and ML Cu 250 (van Os et al. 1978).

Event	*Lippes Loop D*	*Cu T200*	*Cu-T220C*	*ML Cu-250*
Pregnancy	2.0	0	1.2	0.4
Expulsion	3.5	3.4	3.7	0.8
Bleeding or pain removal	2.3	3.4	2.5	2.6
Continuation	88.1	85.9	83.8	91.3
Lost to follow-up	0.8	0	0.7	0
Woman-months of use	12,562	3,587	11,636	6,356

Table 3. Postmenstrual series: termination rates (± standard error) and number of events by clinics (Luukkainen 1979a).

Rates	*Denmark*				*Finland*			
	Nova-T	*n*	*Copper-T*	*n*	*Nova-T*	*n*	*Copper-T*	*n*
Accidental pregnancy	0.68±0.78	1	1.29±1.01	2	0.67±0.49	2	2.95±1.00	9
Expulsion	4.01±1.73	6	8.43±2.87	12	3.33±1.06	10	2.66±0.96	8
Removals								
bleeding and/or pain	17.72±3.95	25	24.49±5.41	31	3.37±1.09	10	2.63±0.95	8
infection	2.69±1.46	4	2.77±2.08	3	0.66±0.47	2	1.38±0.89	3
other medical	2.80±1.58	4	3.22±1.60	5	1.06±0.83	5	0±0	0
planning pregnancy	3.74±2.41	4	3.49±2.26	4	1.73±0.81	5	1.70±0.95	4
other personal	1.36±1.07	2	1.87±1.16	3	0±0	0	0±0	0
All terminations	33.02±3.39	46	45.56±5.00	60	10.82±1.88	31	11.33±1.96	32
Continuation rate	67.0		54.4		89.2		88.7	

an experimental IUD is to perform randomized insertions of the experimental IUD and the standard IUD, which recently has been Cu-T200. These studies should be carried out using a multiclinic approach with a great number of persons inserting the devices. If possible, the training of persons who perform the insertion should be representative for a usual family planning clinic and the trial could be carried out simultaneously in different countries using the same instructions and protocols and a centralized data collection. The testing of Nova-T was conducted recently using Cu-T200 as a standard control IUD in the randomized comparative trial (Luukkainen et al. 1979a). The pregnancy rate of Nova-T was a third of that of Copper-T-200 (Luukkainen et al. 1979b).

It is important that the rate of those lost to follow-up (LFU) is as low as possible. Thiery et al. (1978a) have reported LFU rates as low as 0.0 percent for one year. This would be ideal and may be possible with a very stable population. It is difficult to explain why the same team reports an LFU rate of 36.7 percent at three years. However the last insertion was done only one month earlier than the data were computed (Thiery et al. 1978b). We have found it difficult, but not impossible, to reach an LFU rate less than seven percent at one year. Then a patient, who was seen at eleven months but not at twelve months was taken as LFU at one year. Some reports have taken the LFU rate as if it were an event rate and calculated all subjects lost to follow-up as though they had terminated use of the device (Tejuja et al. 1974). This procedure is over-conservative and should not be recommended. A high LFU rate is not evenly distributed through the age groups. It may be that a moderate LFU rate completely eliminates the young and fertile part of the patient population and makes the results distorted. It seems important that in all IUD studies an effort be made to contact all subjects at one year, to take the last menstrual period after one year as an individual cutoff date (Timonen and Luukkainen 1974), and to analyze the results when the subject who has had the latest insertion has completed one year. Therefore, in the reports the number of women completing the year should be given. The analysis of the data is performed by the lifetable method according to Potter (1966) or Tietze and Lewit (1973), but these methods will not give adequate results if they are applied to clinical data during the course of study when the whole cohort has not completed X years of experience. People who use the Tietze method of computation without the individual cutoff date at one year may report a very low LFU during the first year of the study when, in fact, quite high percentages have not been observed beyond the sixth month. For example, if 1000 women accept an IUD in May 1978 and are last observed in December 1978, and if a cutoff date of 31 May 1979 is used, all women continuing in December 1978 will be credited with use through to May 1979 (one year) if the data are processed in July 1979. None seen in December will be classified as LFU by August 1979 according to Tietze (I. Sivin, personal communication, 1979). This critical definition has played a central, and at times pernicious role in reports of rates which are used to promote new IUDs. The analysis and the recommendations of the use of life table methods have been recently reported (Jain and Sivin 1977). Hopefully the editors of scientific journals will change the policy and only accept studies with the correct use of the lifetable analysis. For the statistical comparison of the individual event rates in a randomized study one could use the Azen et al. (1977) procedure, but it seems that the final event rates should be reported according to Tietze and Lewit (1973) to avoid confusion.

Because factors other than the IUD itself greatly affect the clinical performance of an IUD, as has already been discussed in detail, it seems that studies should be directed to learn how these problems may and should be solved in an actual practical situation. Complete instructions for the insertion, honest information on the real performance of the IUD and a training program for personnel may be more important than modification in the design of an IUD or change in the surface area of, for instance, the copper wire around the device. Zipper et al. (1974) concluded that the copper surface placed on the devices is a determining factor in expulsion and pregnancy rates. The optimal surface area of copper needed to minimize expulsions is 120 mm^2 but to minimize pregnancy it is 200 mm^2. Any increase in this surface area increases expulsions without significantly decreasing the rate of pregnancy.

REFERENCES

Azen SP, S Roy, Pike MC, Casagrande J, Mishell DR: A new procedure for the statistical evaluation of intrauterine contraception. Am J Obstet Gynecol 128 : 329, (1977).

Fylling P, Fagerhol M: Experience with two different medicated intrauterine devices: a comparative study of the Progestasert and Nova-T. Fertil Steril 31 : 138, (1979).

Jain AK: Comparative performance of three types of IUDs in the United States. In: Analysis of intrauterine contraception, Hefnawi F, Segal S, (eds), Amsterdam, North-Holland Publishing, 1975, pp 3-16.

Jain AK, Sivin I: Life-table analysis of IUDs: Problems and recommendations. Stud Fam Plann 8 : 25, 1977.

Luukkainen T, Timonen H, Sivin I: Multiclinic copper-T studies in Finland. In: Analysis of intrauterine contraception, Hefnawi F, Segal S, (eds), Amsterdam, North-Holland Publishing, 1975, pp 243-248.

Luukkainen T, Nielsen N-C, Nygren K-G, Pyörälä T: Combined and national experience of postmenstrual insertions of Nova-T and copper-T in a randomized study. Contraception 19 : 11, 1979a.

Luukkainen T, Nielsen N-C, Nygren K-G, Pyörälä T, Kosonen A: Randomized comparison of clinical performance of two copper-releasing IUDs, Nova-T and copper-T, in Denmark, Finland and Sweden. Contraception 19 : 1, 1979b.

LuukkainenT, Nielsen N-C, Nygren K-G, Pyörälä T, Nulliparous women, IUD and pelvic infection. Ann Clin Res, 1979c.

Mishell DR Jr: The clinic factor in evaluating IUDs. In: Analysis of intrauterine contraception, Hefnawi F, Segal S, (eds), Amsterdam, North-Holland Publishing, 1975, pp 27-36.

Os WAA van, de Nooyer CCA, Bakker S, Bomert L, Rhemrev PER, Loendersloot EW: Evaluation of the combined Multiload copper IUD ML Cu-250 and MC Cu-375. Int J Fertil 23 : 152, 1978.

Osser S, Gullberg B, Liedholm P, Sjöberg N-O: Is development of a pelvic inflammatory disease in women using intrauterine device equal regardless of parity?: one-year follow-up study. Contraception 17 : 563, 1978.

Potter RG Jr: Application of life-table techniques to measurement of contraceptive effectiveness. Demography 3 : 297, 1966.

Sivin I: The effectiveness of the copper-T intrauterine device: a collaborative study in five countries. Stud Fam Plann 4 : 162, 1973.

Thiery M, van der Pas H, van Os WAA, van Kets H: Clinical experience with two newer copper-loaded IUDs (T-Cu220C and ML Cu-250; simultaneous use of an IUD and a spermicide; postplacental insertion of the ML Cu-250. In: Human fertilization, Ludwig H, Tauber PF, (eds), Stuttgart Thieme, 1978a, pp 253-260.

Thiery M, van der Pas H, van Os WAA Tauber PF, Dombrowicz N, MacDonald JS, Haspels AA, Drogendijk AC, van Kets H, Boogers W: Three years experience with the ML Cu-250, a new copper-wired intrauterine contraceptive device. Adv Planned Parenthood 13 : 35, 1978b.

Tietze C, Lewit S: Evaluation of intrauterine devices: ninth progress report of the cooperative statistical program. Stud Fam Plann 55 : 1, 1970.

Tietze C, Lewit S: Recommended procedures for the statistical evaluation of intrauterine contraception. Stud Fam Plann 4 : 35, 1973.

TimonenH: Intrauterine contraception with copper-T, Helsinki, Kirjapaino OY Tieto Ab, 1976.

Timonen H, Luukkainen T: The use-effectiveness of the copper-T200 in a simulated field trial. Contraception 9 : 1, 1974.

Zipper J, Medel M, Pastene L, Rivera M: Factors that limit the efficiency of copper-carrying IUDs. IN: Intrauterine devices, Wheeler RG, Duncan GW, Speidel JJ, (eds), New York, Academic Press, 1974, pp 235-242.

24. SOME LEGAL AND ETHICAL ASPECTS OF IUD USE

M.T. Cooper

There are many differences in the way IUDs are controlled in different countries around the world. The decision to use contraception and in particular an IUD is one which is subject to many influences. Customs, aims and objectives vary; the patient is only one of the people involved in the decision-making process. The attitude of those involved varies: patient, physician, lawyer, politician, spouse and priest they all have their points of view, which are often different and often opposed to one another. This diversity in the attitudes to contraceptives and IUDs results in equally diverse legal and priest all have their points of view, which those involved, particularly the physicians and the regulatory agencies.

I. INAPPROPRIATE REGULATIONS

One of the major problems in IUD use around the world is that the countries where their use is desired for population control often do not have any regulations for IUDs, nor do they have the resource to implement an IUD program. The results are quite predictable: an agency with the necessary resources steps in and offers to help; this agency is usually from a country which does have IUD regulations and therefore abides by those regulations. We now have a situation where regulations developed in one country and hopefully relevant in that country are forcefully imposed on another where their relevance is at best questionable. This problem is very real. The agencies which take an interest in this kind of work are naturally answerable to their contributors and therefore feel that they must use only approved devices. When the basis on which the device approved is not applicable to the conditions of use to which it will be subject, then we have the ridiculous situation where the approval is merely an inappropriate sop to the conscience of the donors.

The problems: regulatory, legal and ethical, have been arbitrarily divided into four groups as indicated in Figure 1, in order to address some of the concerns more lucidly.

I.A. Canadian regulation

In Canada, more so than in many other countries, the device itself – its manufacture and sale – is

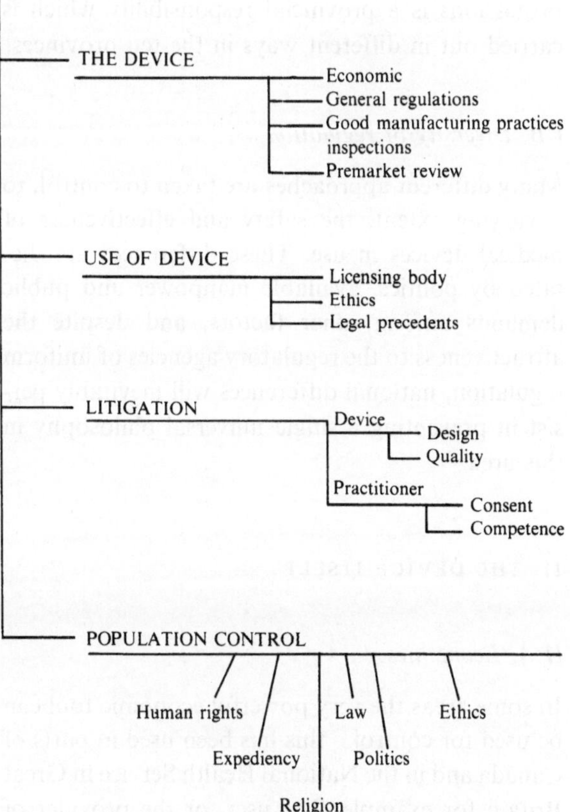

Figure 1. Intrauterine devices: regulatory and legal problems.

regulated by an authority different from that which regulates the use of the device. There is an area in between which is very difficult to define, and which can result in a division of authority; the division between federal and provincial governments is clearly stated in the British North America Act, but gives rise to much argument because of the very different interpretations which can be put on different parts and the different inferences which can be made. There is always a problem of overlapping jurisdiction in these cases and this can lead to problems, but a far more serious situation occurs when an area is ignored by both. This is something which must be carefully guarded against and it is a very good reason to have all the interface areas very clearly spelled out, written down and agreed upon.

In Canada the safety and efficacy of a device is subject to federal jurisdiction under the Food and Drugs Act, administered by the Bureau of Medical Devices of the Health Protection Branch. The use of the device by the medical profession is regulated provincially through the appropriate licensing body, the jurisdiction of which is limited to its own province. Health and the regulation of the health professions is a provincial responsibility which is carried out in different ways in the ten provinces.

I.B. Diversity of regulation

Many different approaches are taken to control, to a varying extent, the safety and effectiveness of medical devices in use. These differences are dictated by politics, available manpower and public demands among other factors, and despite the attractiveness to the regulatory agencies of uniform regulation, national differences will inevitably persist in preventing a single universal philosophy in this area.

II. THE DEVICE ITSELF

II.A. Economics

In some areas the very powerful economic tool can be used for control – this has been used in parts of Canada and in the National Health Service in Great Britain for example. The user, or the provider of funds, can insist on his specifications for a device by writing them into his purchase order. There are problems in this approach: a compromise must be demanded; it requires that someone have sufficient expert knowledge to make the specifications acceptable and attainable.

This is not an easy task, and the method has been seen to fail for this very reason. Within limits however this is a very persuasive and useful form of control, but because of the expertise required to make it workable it is really only applicable to large organizations and even here there is a tendency for individual preferences rather than basic principles to determine the stated requirements. The benefits therefore of this approach are minimal to the user in general and tend to be negative as far as the manufacturer is concerned.

II.B. General regulations

There are various general regulations in different countries to which IUDs are required to conform: medical device regulations in some, drug regulations in others, but plastic products regulations and general packaging requirements are the only applicable ones in some countries. These regulations range all the way from nothing at all, through simple notification of intent to sell a product, to full disclosure of materials, methods and test results with certification of the manufacturing plant and procedures.

II.C. Good manufacturing practices inspection

Good manufacturing practices requirements with the inevitable plant inspections are onerous and by no means foolproof in assuring an acceptable manufacturing facility, but they can be very useful in assessing the quality of the product and the probability that this quality will be consistent. An inspection programme of this type requires enormous amounts of expert manpower in order to monitor the manufacturing facilities adequately. The time involved and the costs both to the regulatory agency and to the manufacturer are large, and the costs of this of course are eventually passed to the consumer. Many countries do not have available either the manpower or the finances to carry out this kind of programme.

II.D. Premarket review

Canada has taken an intermediate route with IUDs: premarket review. This requires that all the information concerning materials, design, methods of manufacture, quality control and the evidence to support the claims made for the device be submitted for evaluation in the requested format – this is an important point to ensure an efficient review and an economical use of resources. Permission to sell an IUD is dependent on the acceptability of the information provided in the submission and in any subsequent supplement that may be requested by the Bureau. There are occasions with certain products where close familiarization is required and it should be made quite clear that the approach described does not exclude plant inspection, independent testing, or any other method that may be thought to be useful or necessary at any time in the future.

III. USE OF THE DEVICE

In many countries, including most Western countries, the use of the device is controlled by the physician even though he may not in some instances actually insert the IUD. There are however areas of the world where people other than physicians take the responsibility for the insertion of IUDs. This is often the situation where the programme is one of population control rather than individual birth control.

III.A. Licensing body

Where the use of the device is controlled by the physician, he is, as always in medical practice, ultimately responsible for the results, but this liability is strongly influenced and modified by the extent to which his patterns of practice conform to the attitude of his licensing body; in any situation where his judgement or decision is called into question it is much simpler to justify a position with which the licensing body agrees. This usually means an opinion which is the consensus of the senior practitioners in that jurisdiction. It is quite clear that this state of affairs, while being a protection against renegades, also tends to inhibit innovation. The path to be followed is narrow; perhaps all innovators are renegades but without question not all renegades are innovators and these are the ones from whom the licensing bodies should protect us.

III.B. Ethics

The accepted medical ethic in his medical environment is a considerable factor in determining a physician's ultimate fate in any conflict of opinion, and here we have many factors with which to contend. Medical ethics are no longer a static thing to which we can refer for an absolute judgement, for they are coloured and shaped by many factors: age. religion, time and place all have their modifying effect on basic medical ethics.

III.C. Legal precedents

The law and legal precedents are of course of fundamental importance when a physician's use of an IUD, or the results obtained from its use, are called into question.

IV. CHANGING ETHICS

Which of these three factors will be more important in any specific instance is very difficult to predict. There was a time when ethics and the attitude of the licensing authority were identical – this is no longer so, since the licensing bodies are subject to many pressures, the political and economic ones now being ascendant. This is perhaps because of changes in attitudes in general, but certainly it is influenced to some extent by the more widespread availability of government-controlled medical services. Wherever government or its agencies pay for medical care, irrespective of the mechanism used, it has control of medical practice by virtue of that most basic of influences – economics.

Medical ethics were relatively static for a very long time but changes have been many, rapid and basic in the last decades. The attitude to ethics is bound to be influenced by the fundamental changes which have occurred in medical technology. The very final event of death is now difficult to recognize without some arbitrary definition; the viability of an arm, a person or a fetus can be defined quite differently from that which was the case thirty years ago, and these changes are all due to advances in medical knowledge and in technology.

IV.A. Ethics and law

It is now very difficult to decide whether professional ethics influence legal judgements, or legal precedents alter medical ethics. This may sound rather cynical, but consider what modern abortion laws have done to the basic, fundamental medical ethic to preserve life. On this point rationalization is rampant and the medical profession is suddenly full of apologists.

IV.B. Written codes

Written medical ethics have perhaps impeded progress. The code of laws of Hammurabi and the later oath of Hippocrates both concern themselves with money and of course we have two parts of the oath, no poisoning and no abortion, on which is based the basic preservation of life. This oath of Hippocrates was so long taken as 'gospel' that it was most traumatic for the profession to change it; the part which required one to support one's teachers was ignored, but the rest was treated as unchangeable. In some medical schools graduates actually 'swore' the oath on graduation. If one then ignores the basic ethic, what is left? How can one justify adherence to one part and rejection of another part? This is why writing medical ethics is about as useful as writing about how to ride a bicycle.

IV.C. Theory and practice

To practice medicine ethically requires, first of all, that one practices medicine. This may sound obvious but if one looks at most of the writings, pronouncements and edicts concerning medical ethics one finds that few of these authors have been involved in real medicine: they are theorists – they are by and large philosophers, theologists, medical historians, medical technicians and university teachers. Their opinions are suspect because medical ethics concerns real people and actual situations, not 'patients' and hypothetical cases. People have homes and families and jobs and friends and hopes and fears, only someone in tune with the person, his environment, and the interaction between the two can know how to make an ethical medical decision. Here again we have a grey area and perhaps a conflict: How large is the environment that must be considered in making this ethical medical decision? Do we always favour the individual whatever the effects on his environment? This is why the size of the environment to be taken into account is so important and also why real answers can only be given in response to a real specific question. An interesting point in this respect is the difference between the titles *consultant* and *specialist* in medicine:both sometimes refer to the same thing, but they indicate a very different attitude.

V. LITIGATION

Litigation is, of course, an ever-present possibility where patient procedures are concerned. This is particularly a problem in the United States, where lawyers are allowed to make their charge a percentage of the awards, but it is present everywhere. The possibility is a safeguard to the patient and a modifying factor affecting all activities where people interact, but the spiral of increasing awards, increasing liability insurance premiums and eager lawyers is frightening on the medical scene. It seems to be difficult for the courts to accept that risk is acceptable and inevitable; in many medical procedures progress would be impossible without it. One of the bizarre effects of this in North America, now largely corrected by so-called Good Samaritan laws, was that the victims of accidents were treated by a passing physician only at great financial risk to himself. That financial ruin could result from doing one's best led to physicians passing accidents on the other side. A loophole in the breathalyser laws in Canada was also produced in effect by the threat of litigation. If a driver was stopped and suspected of being in violation of the law in driving with a blood alcohol level above an arbitrary limit he was obliged to submit to a breathalyser test, but he could legally avoid this by giving permission for a blood test. The catch here was that a physician needs the patient's permission to take blood, and if the level was too high the patient could claim that he was not competent to give permission and then sue the doctor.

V.A. The device

Litigation may be aimed at the device itself – the two aspects for attack being firstly design, including the concept and the engineering of the device, this being an attack which requires considerable technical expertise but one which has been used successfully against some aspects of car design and is therefore a possibility which cannot be ignored. Secondly, quality as influenced by the manufacturing process itself, and by the quality control procedures and the packing and shipping arrangements, is the more usual approach, sterility being perhaps the most frequently questioned aspect.

V.B. The practitioner

Usually, the main target for litigation is the practitioner, including his assistants and the hospital, clinic, or office in which the procedure was performed. One area for attack concerns informed consent, an area of widely differing interpretations where any precaution taken may turn out to be inadequate. This is definitely a field where the physician is in difficulty, since books have been written on the subject, and decisions in court have been reversed.Some judgements suggest that the patient must understand as much about a procedure and its possible side effects as the physician performing it. The implications of this attitude are ridiculous, and yet it is logically deduced from the meaning of *informed consent.*Hospitals have great trouble with this problem and at the moment it seems that adequate insurance is essential however careful one is in explanations, having permissions signed and all the other preventive measures that can be taken.

Competence is the second area for litigation. This area is more straightforward; in general good medical practice with good record-keeping is a good defence. No one is expected to be perfect and the physician is judged against the accepted norm rather than against excellence.

VI. POPULATION CONTROL

Population control with IUDs poses much more severe ethical and legal problems. The influence of the many factors to be taken into account is not constant and the relative importance of the different factors varies according to the actual case being discussed. The differences in political philosophy, in geography, in religion and in wealth will ensure that decisions about population control can only be properly made from within the population in question.

REFERENCES

Annas GJ: Beyond the Good Smaritan, should doctors be required to provide essential services. Hasting Cent Re 8(2): 16-7, 1978.

Blanquist CD: From the oath of Hippocrates to the declaration of Hawaii Ethics Sci Med 4(3-4): 139-49, 1977.

Burns CR: Richard Clark Cabot and reformation in American medical ethics. Bull 41st Med 51(3):353-68, 1978.

Curran WH: Setting the medicolegal issues concerning brain death statutes: matters of legal ethics and judicial precedent. N Engl J Med 299(1): 31-2, 1978.

Davies IJ: Clinical responsibility: Br Med J 1 (6105): 104-105, 1978.

Gellharn A: Medical ethics, so what's the story? In Vitro 13(10): 588-594, 1977.

Journal of medical ethics: Editorial: conflict of loyalties: Hippocratic or hypocritical? J Med Ethics 4(1): 42-4, 1978.

Lancet: Editorial: applications for ethical approval: Lancet 1 (8055): 87-89, 1978.

Rolt LTC: Red for danger, Bodley Head, 1957.

Shumiateher MC: Medical heroics and the good death. Can Med Assoc J 117 (5): 520-522, 1977.

Shapo M: Legal responsibility at issue: emphasis on informed consent. In Vitro 13 (10); 612-631, 1977.

Wildawsky A: No risk is the highest risk of all. Am Sci 32-37, Jan-Feb, 1979.

DISCLAIMER

This article represents the views of the author. It does not necessarily represent the views or policies of the Department of National Health and Welfare of Canada.

25. THE CONSULTANT AND FUTURE DEVELOPMENT

E.S.E. Hafez, P.E.R. Rhemrev and W.A.A. van Os

The future control of human reproduction depends on further development of contraceptive methods. So far only two principles are available in an employable state: ovulation-inhibitory methods and intrauterine devices, but development of a nonsystemic contraceptive device has grown to be one of the principal objectives at present. Based on already acquired knowledge and practical experience a body of experts who are able to give professional or technical advice in relation to such development has come into existence.

The longer the history of contraceptives the more dependent the design group or discoverers will be on these consultants; what results is exchange of still secret plans and knowledge. At this moment ethical and legal aspects arise regarding the relationship of the designers with the interested industry and the consultant. This relationship can only gain the desired result if satisfactorily defined agreements are made in advance between the two partners. These agreements have to settle questions in relation to (1) the development of the project and (2) financial settlements. Before starting to approach this question a distinction has first to be made between the two existing principal different kinds of consultant: (1) the scientific consultant, dealing with experimental laboratory research; and (2) the practical consultant, dealing with investigations in clinical trials.

Although much resemblance can be found between these two as specialists operating in different ways, the latter is confronted with the question of who is responsible in the event of calamities in testing the device in human beings.

I. THE RESEARCH PROJECT.

A written research project including its title; an abstract of the whole proposal; detailed information on intended experiments, such as in-vitro studies or in-vivo studies in animals or in a standardized human population; a description of proposed clinical trials; a tabular plan of experiments; and specific aims and method of procedure must be prepared.

II. EMPLOYMENT OF METHODS AND RESULTS

In the negotiations on the agreement a clear description of investigation methods must be outlined: this should include the equipment to be used, and methods of determination such as ultrasonic technique, radioimmunoassay, or microbiological methods. Methods of recording of compiled data and criteria of statistical evaluation shall be stated; they may be based on previous literature studies or existing computer data methods like life table analysis.

III. RESPONSIBILITIES

An agreement can only succeed if the responsibilities of persons involved are laid down. Therefore a written research project must also include not only the names, duties and responsibilities of principal and coprincipal investigators – the consultants – but also of the executive technicians, postdoctoral associates, secretarial help and all other personnel involved. Who is responsible in the event of disagreements or in sufficient progress in experiments should again be made clear. A more delicate matter is the delineation of the responsibility of the practical consultant, dealing with clinical trials, regarding what the law requires this consultant to do in relation to those who might be affected by his action. Such jurisprudence can differ greatly between countries where clinical studies are planned. Who is responsible in case of an unwanted pregnancy or in case of an infection possibly due to this contraceptive device? To what extent is it necessary to inform and come to an agreement with the subject of the experiment, in this case the woman, since it is she who has to suffer the consequences of a practical trial?

IV. BUDGETING

An estimated proposed budget should include allowances for the time and effort of key investigators and senior personnel and all costs of experiments including laboratory equipment and needed materials, including the devices to be tested. Also payments for using outpatient departments; costs of physical examinations, including laboratory tests; and, eventually, payment of patient volunteers, should be taken into account. Of course family planning programmes already contribute in most of these clinical trials.

V. THE RESULTS

Publishing of results of experiments in scientific journals and scientific meetings is a normal end for any scientific worker, to give the principal certainty that this strife will be fulfilled in a proper time. This way of collaboration can only lead to a positive development if both parties agree to proposals about progress reports at regular intervals. These progress reports should be evaluated among the various concerned parties.

Various arrangements i.e., travel, should be agreed upon in advance to avoid any legal implications. Forms usually used by granting agencies such as the National Institute of Health and the National Science Foundation can be modified to apply to such ends.

After achieving the definitive form of the contraceptive device the consultant and the investigator should provide specific information for the practical application of the findings and their improvement. A good agreement can guarantee the collaboration of different scientific workers to achieve the substantial development of a new contraceptive device without the eventuality that important ideas break down on increasing difficulties between the investigator and designer resulting in useless delay of development of future contraception.

26. EPILOGUE

E.S.E. Hafez

I. INERT AND MEDICATED INTRAUTERINE DEVICES

The historical descriptions of contraceptive IUDs made of flexible rings of silkworm gut or silk wire were made by Richard Richter (1909), Ernst Gräfenberg (1929), Oppenheimer (1959) and Ishihama (1959). Year 2000 may witness a wide application of slow steady-releasing biodegradables, computerized and custom-made IUDs, as well as sophisticated family planning clinics for the preservation of 'quality of life'. Several sizes, shapes and configurations have been designed in an attempt to improve the effectiveness and acceptability of inert IUDs. Modifications of device geometry to reduce the side effect of bleeding result in lower efficacy and high expulsion rates. Thus, the performance of inert IUDs can be expected to be improved over only by the development of bioactive and medicated IUDs.

Several instruments have been developed to evaluate the geometry of the uterine lumen (Figure 1). The geometric factors which reduce IUD performance are due to unfavourable geometric relationships between the IUD and the endometrial cavity (length, greatest transverse dimensions, anteroposterior dimension surface area and volume). Changes in uterine shape and dimensions occur throughout the menstrual cycle. Conditions at the time of menstruation produce a generally negative effect on IUD-uterine relationships. Unfavourable uterine characteristics include reduced luminal space, congenital fundal anomalies and uterine space-occupying lesions. An IUD with a small lower end diameter, a dependent vertical arm with a pointed tip or sharp edges may perform poorly regardless of other geometric parameters and relations.

Because of their intrinsic limitations, inert IUDs have failed to give continuation rates which differ significantly. An IUD with a greater surface area would always offer a low pregnancy rate and a higher removal rate because of metrorrhagia. The expulsion rate of IUDs has been inversely related to their stiffness. When stiffness is increased, expulsion rate decreases but metrorrhagia increases. Thus the physical and biological properties required to obtain an optimal contraceptive result with low metrorrhagia and low expulsion rates are intrinsically opposed (Zipper et al. 1972).

Extensive multicentre clinical trials were conducted on the progestin-releasing IUD, Cu-T, Cu-7 and combined Multiload Cu-250 and Cu-375. A copper wire 0.2 mm in diameter provides an antifertility effect for some 3.5 years, when 40 percent of the original amount of copper is released. Neither calcium carbonate deposits nor wire corrosion prevents copper release. Using life table and computer programming for the ML Cu-250 involving 55,000 women, the net cumulative event rates per 100 women at three years of use were: pregnancy 1.3, expulsion 3.2, removal for bleeding or pain and other medical reasons 7.0 and 2.3, respectively; and a continuation rate of 71 percent at three years. Women over 30 tend to have a lower pregnancy rate. The Nova-T furnished with silver-cored copper wire has an effective lifetime of five years.

Progesterone-releasing IUDs improve contraceptive efficiency and alter menstrual bleeding patterns. The progestin-releasing IUD caused various histological and cytological changes: chronic nonspecific inflammation and irregular arrested shedding of endometrium; decrease in number of endometrial granulocytes; suppression of nucleolar channel systems and endometrial glycogen; decrease in number of ciliated cells in the endometrium; and increased lysosomal aggregates in the oviductal

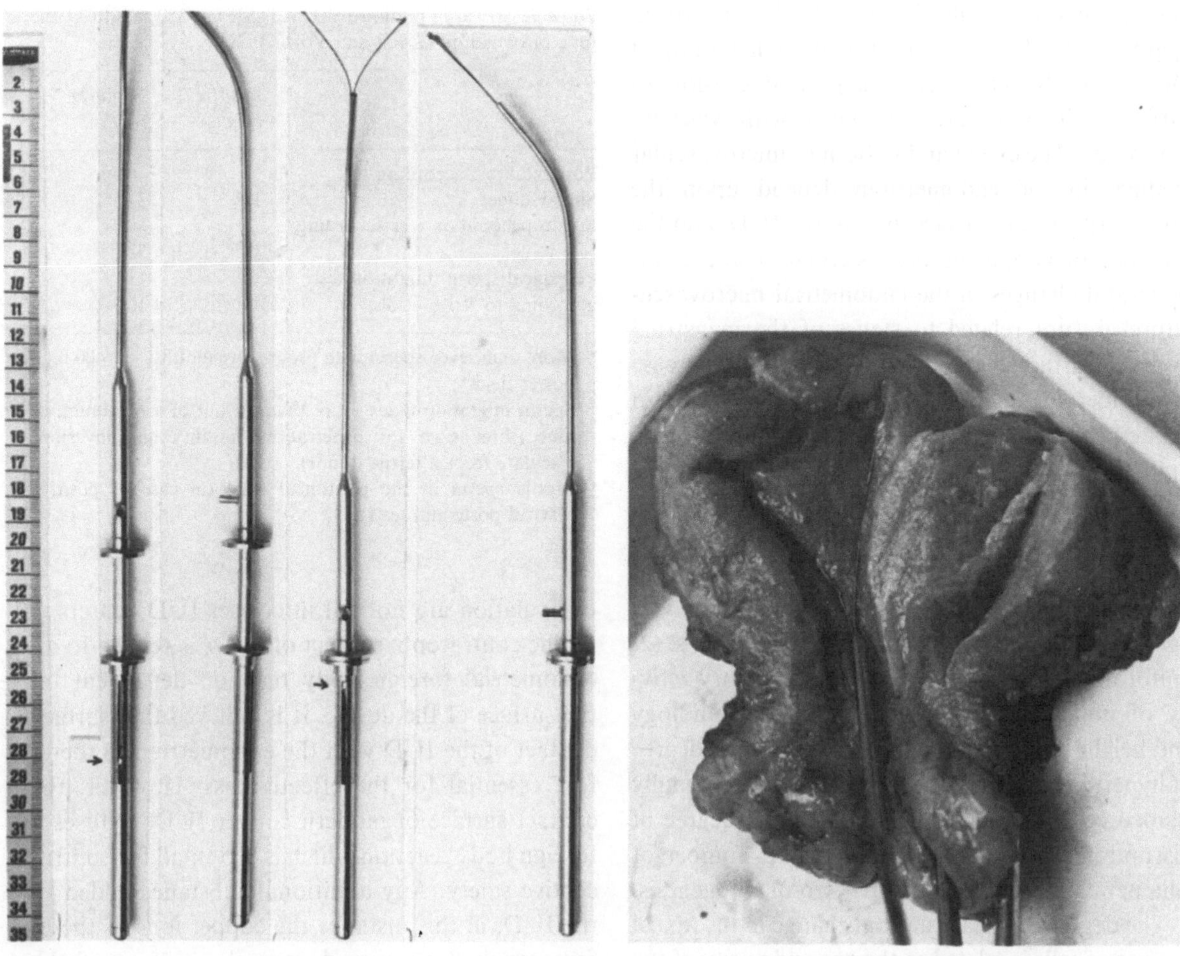

Figure 1. Left: the Cavimeter developed by Dr. K.H. Kurz to measure dimensions and geometry of the uterus before placing an IUD. *Right:* the Cavimenter in utero (Kurz 1979).

epithelium typical of first trimester pregnancy. Physiological responses with this device include decreased prostaglandin concentration in endometrium and menstrual blood, reduced myometrial activity, reduced menstrual blood loss and reduced dysmenorrhea.

The effectiveness of intrauterine progestins is related to their ability to induce decidual and suppressive changes in the endometrium. Endometrial changes may play a significant role in the mechanism of contraceptive action of intrauterine progestins. Pregnancy rates with progesterone-releasing IUDs are less than two per 100 women per year for parous women and slightly more for nulliparous. The ectopic pregnancy rate is about 0.4 per 100 woman-years with regional variations as a result of variations in user characteristics and tubal damage due to previous pelvic inflammatory disease. The rate of spontaneous abortions with the IUD in utero is ten percent. The levonorgestrel-releasing IUD caused a significant decrease in menstrual blood loss from 21 ml during treatment to 52 ml before treatment. The decrease in blood loss is associated with a significant increase in peripheral blood hemoglobin concentrations.

II. PHYSIOLOGICAL MECHANISMS OF IUDS

Endometrial stromal capillaries below the IUD

undergo microthrombosis with platelet and fibrin aggregations filling gaps in the endothelial lining of the vessels. Stromal hemorrhage and erosion of surface epithelium are associated with vascular pathology. The extent and pattern of microvascular changes in the endometrium depend upon the proximity and the surface area of the IUD, and the presence of copper or progesterone. These ultrastructural changes in the endometrial microvasculature are not related to stages of the menstrual cycle. In surface endometrial epithelium, a decrease in numbers of microvilli and a scarcity of cilia in ciliated cells occur. Accumulation of glycogen and lipids and dilation of endoplasmic reticulum are noted in the endometrial glands. The physiological and clinical significance of changes in cell organelles is not known. In the endometrial areas adjacent to the IUD there are remarkable changes and individual variations in: (1) percentage of ciliated cells; (2) uniformity in size, morphology, and secretory activity of nonciliated cells; (3) number, morphology and height of microvilli of secretory cells; (4) degree of hyperplasia of cells; (5) percentage of abnormally shaped cells; (6) intercellular spaces and degree of disruption among cells; (7) height and number of cilia per ciliated cell; and (8) pattern of ciliogenesis.

The degree of ultrastructural change in the apical surface of cells is related to the age and parity of the patient, duration of period with the IUD in situ, and type of side effect and complaint associated with the IUD. Fewer ultrastructural changes are noted in areas not adjacent to the IUD. The effect of the IUD per se on the endometrium is not known since some of the endometrial changes may be due to certain side effects or other gynecological problems not associated with the presence of the IUD.

Several physiological mechanisms have been implicated in the contraceptive action of IUDs: (1) disruption of the egg or sperm transport pattern (Table 1); (2) changes in biophysical and biochemical characteristics of the endometrial fluid with subsequent inhibition of implantation of the blastocyst; and (3) qualitative and quantitative alteration of oviductal and myometrial contractivity. The mode of action of copper IUDs seems to involve more than one of these effects. There is no evidence of any inhibition of ovarian functions and luteal activity through the hypothalamo-hypophyseal-ovarian axis; follicular maturation and the time of ovulation are normal in copper IUD bearers.

Table 1. Sperm migration tests with Ml Cu-250 in situ at the time of ovulation (Koch and Vogel 1979).

	Positive results	*Negative results*
Postcoital test according to Sims-Huhner	13[a]	37
Sperm penetration test according to Kremer	18[b]	32
Peritoneal sperm migration test according to Koch et al.	0[c]	10

[a] More than seven sperm with progressive motility per 400 high power field.
[b] Sperm migration index more than six out of a maximum of nine (three each for penetration, motility and invasion-ejaculate from a fertile donor).
[c] Motile sperm in the peritoneal fluid (in case of positive cervical postcoital tests).

The contraceptive effect of IUDs is related to an endometrial foreign body reaction dependent on the surface of the device. It is believed that surface contact of the IUD with the endometrium is therefore essential for the effectiveness. However, the contact surface of modern copper IUDs induces a foreign body reaction which is too small for contraceptive safety. Any additional substance added to the IUD, in this instance the copper ions, is therefore required to spread over the surface of the endometrium distant from the device. It is therefore the copper that modifies the surface epithelium sufficiently to prevent implantation.

There is a negative influence on sperm migration, but the migration is not completely blocked (Table 1). When there is a large number of leukocytes in the cervical mucus, there is excellent migration in some cases in the Kremer sperm penetration test. The peritoneal sperm migration test is alway negative. The increase in the proportion of granulocytes, plasma cells, lymphocytes and macrophages in the endometrium and in the uterine secretion, with no pathological bacterial invasion, demonstrates a reaction of the endometrium to the foreign body and not an inflammation caused by an infection (Koch and Vogel 1979). The sperm migration disturbances can be considered as a partial effect in the multifactorial mode of action of IUDs.

In animal experiments, prostaglandin biosynthesis inhibitors can interfere with the antifertility effect of IUDs. It would appear that the absolute production rates and the delicate balance between the different prostaglandins may be crucial elements in the development of side effects and in the antifertility action of IUDs. There are remarkable changes in enzyme and metal contents of cervical mucus in patients with copper IUDs. A depression of amylase activity may interfere with the availability of monosaccharides necessary for sperm survival. Alkaline phosphatase involvement in energy production for the sperm may also be implicated in copper device users.

Cupric ions in solution form copper oxide which is removed by aminoacids. The copper released from the IUD binds with uterine protein, is taken up by the endometrial tissue or is excreted in the uterine secretions and menstrual flow. The chemical state and the release rate of copper from the IUD are influenced by pH, O_2 tension, amount of blood loss, and protein components of the endometrial secretions. Copper serum levels of IUD users are normal, and the endometrium of copper IUD users does not contain copper, as is shown by X-ray dispersive analysis. The contraceptive action of inert and medicated IUDs depends on their ability to evoke inflammatory responses in the endometrium. The degree of inflammatory response evoked by copper IUDs is conflictingly reported in animal experimentation. Leukocytes are noted in the uterine fluid of users of copper IUDs but not in the same numbers as with the larger inert IUDs. This difference may be due in part to variation in IUD shape. Inert and copper IUDs cause an increased fibrinolytic activity in the endometrium. Qualitative and quantitative alterations in the biochemical responses in the endometrial cells are evident during the secretory phase, coinciding with the time of implantation of the blastocyst. There is evidence that the secretory activity of the endometrial cells may be impaired. Myometrial contractivity is influenced by inert and copper IUDs, whereas the addition of copper to in-vitro systems alters the contractile activity of myometrial strips. Copper ions have also an effect on the myometrial steroid receptors. In-vitro copper interferes with the specific progesterone-binding capacity of human endometrial cytosol, suggesting that one mode of action of copper IUDs is to interfere with progesterone at its target sites.

Copper IUDs do not seem to inhibit sperm motility and metabolism except during the first months after IUD insertion when the copper levels are high in cervical mucus and endometrial secretions. In a few cases there is normal pregnancy and healthy babies are born with copper IUDs in situ, indicating little effect on implantation of the blastocyst. Failure rate with copper IUDs decrease with increasing surface area of copper in the device up to 200 mm^2 and more. Pregnancy with a copper IUD in situ may be due to certain specific characteristics in: (1) the geometry of the uterine cavity, (2) contractile activity of the myometrium causing displacement of the device; (3) biochemical and biophysical characteristics of the endometrial fluid and menstrual blood (Figure 2); (4) impaired or diminished immunologic response of an individual to a foreign body; (5) the use of drugs such as prostaglandin antagonists; or (6) the rate of deposit of calcium and other coating material on the copper.

III. MANAGEMENT OF INTRAUTERINE DEVICES

In the absence of contraindications, small models of IUDs are used in adolescent girls. The correct model should be chosen and adapted individually to the sometimes underdeveloped uterine cavity. Devices too small or too large tend either to be expelled or to increase the risk of unwanted pregnancies. However, IUDs are not recommended for drug abusers. Unconscious motives for or against contraception can exist side by side in the same individual. On the one hand, resentment of parental responsibilities may favour the use of the IUD while at the same time realization that IUD is a hostile act directed toward the unborn infant produces guilt and rejection of birth control. Compliance in the use of the IUD and acceptance of side effects is directly related to the amount and intensity of counselling and the degree of motivation of patient and physician.

There are several advantages for IUD insertion immediately after placental expulsion, for example immediate protection without additional motivation for repeat contraception or postnatal follow-up, ease of insertion through a dilated cervix under sterile conditions, and masking of postinsertion symptoms by lochia and afterbirth pains. A pos-

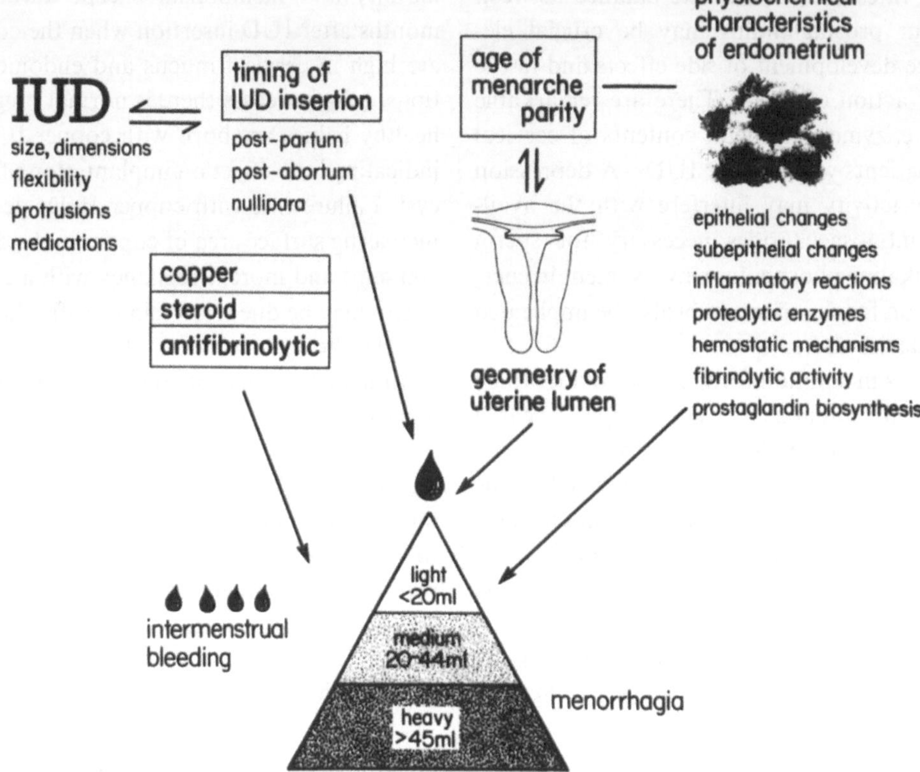

Figure 2. Maternal factors affecting IUD-induced blood loss.

sible theoretical risk is intrauterine translocation of the device, which could lead to erosion and subsequent uterine perforation. Randomized comparative trial of postplacental IUD insertion shows that Cu-T200 had a lower pregnancy rate but a higher expulsion rate than ML Cu-250.

Efforts to improve the inserter, the insertion technique or the device design have not solved the problem of postpartum expulsion. It is possible that the use of biodegradables may create temporary architectural configurations which will improve IUD retention. Several maternal factors may be correlated, in descending order, with continued use of IUDs, for example parity, length of cervix, length of uterus, time from last menstrual period to insertion, length of menstrual cycle, previous contraceptive method used, age, total number of abortions, additional children wanted and duration of menstrual flow.

The counsel and opinion of physicians are sought with as much or greater frequency than their diagnostic or therapeutic skills. Concern over potential side effects, subsequent fertility and the use of IUDs is significant as information is received from the patient's physician, peers and news media. The provision of information regarding all aspects of contraception is a prerequisite for optimal decision making. Future investigations are needed to evaluate the social and psychological characteristics of (1) women primarily using IUDs, and of women using different contraceptives, especially the pill; (2) the decision for or against the use of this contraceptive method; (3) psychological resistance against IUD use; and (4) the male partner's and the physician's attitude towards the IUD when compared with other contraceptive methods. The role of the physician's counselling on this attitude; factors which determine the degree and frequency of side effects and the desire for IUD removal; and optimal contraceptive counselling, which takes into account medical, psychological and social aspects of the woman, all are important areas for investigation (Frick-Bruder 1979).

IV. SIDE EFFECTS AND COMPLICATIONS

Side effects and complications of IUDs include uterine pain, dysfunctional uterine bleeding, expulsions, perforations, pelvic inflammatory disease (PID), accidental intrauterine pregnancy, and ectopic pregnancy (Hafez and van Os 1980). It seems that geometrical parameters of IUD-uterine lumen relationships are implicated in most IUD pathologies; these parameters include low IUD position in the uterine cavity, with the device being present in the isthmus or cervix; geometric factors not related to IUD position that result in an inadequate contraceptive effect; endometrial or myometrial injury due to penetration or excessive compression; and myometrial distension sufficient to trigger increased myometrial activity.

Pregnancy can result from low positions of IUDs and inadequate contraceptive effects not related to position. Expulsion is caused by low IUD positions or excessive myometrial distension, whereas bleeding is provoked by endometrial injury. A definite relationship exists between pain and excessive myometrial distension. Pelvic infections may occur if the IUD is in a low position or there is endometrial injury. Uterine perforations result from certain myometrial injuries. Prostaglandin biosynthesis inhibitors have been used with success to alleviate uterine pain and bleeding problems due to IUDs; this implicates prostaglandin overproduction in the pathogenesis. Since the presence of an IUD is thought to be associated with increased endometrial levels of prostaglandins and since prostaglandins increase uterine contractions, local administration of prostaglandin synthetase inhibitors might be expected to inhibit this activity.

Several factors are involved in uterine perforation and displacement of the IUD: intra-abdominally various physiological or pathological uterine conditions weakening the uterine wall or hampering the access to the uterine cavity; size, shape, design and components of IUDs; and the insertion technique of some devices. Migration and subsequent visceral perforation depends upon the shape of the device and peritoneal irritation; severe tissue reactions occur with copper IUDs.

Clinical symptoms associated with intra-abdominal IUDs are variable. There are various diagnostic and therapeutic possibilities for the management of lost IUDs. Ultrasonography has been reliable for detection of IUDs in close proximity to the uterus. The sonographic recognition of lost IUDs however can be difficult beyond the eighth week of pregnancy because of the interfering fetal echo patterns. Closed devices (bow and ring), rarely used, should be removed because of risk of intestinal obstruction. Most patients prefer to have the device removed once they are informed of its location. Laparotomy is not always necessary; the devices frequently can be removed by laparoscopy or colpotomy.

The uterine lumen is normally maintained in a bacteria-free state, but the tail of the IUD interferes with the protective mechanism of the cervix and allows bacteria to ascend from the vagina. The higher rate of *Staphylococcus aureus* and *Staphylococcus epidermidis* on IUDs drawn transcervically seem to result from secondary contamination during the removal of the device. In cases of PID, IUDs have intense growth of pathogenic microorganisms, for example hemolytic streptococci β-coli and *Staphylococcus aureus* with no anaerobic bacteria. There is a great correlation between bacterial flora on the IUD and PID. The majority of salpingitis develops within the first month after insertion; the development of salpingitis is regardless of parity. The risk for removal because of infection of an IUD is dependent on age and not on parity. In cases of suspected PID the device is removed and adequate therapy is initiated. To prevent these complications, patients should be carefully selected before insertion, and strict aseptic techniques of IUD insertion should be employed in the immediate postmenstrual period. Sterile salpingitis occurs less frequently with progesterone-releasing IUDs. Intrauterine pregnancy with a device in situ is terminated particularly if the tail of a copper IUD is completely withdrawn into the gravid uterus. Aspirotomy, a modified surgical mid-trimester abortion, combining dilation, aspiration and evacuation, and immediate post-abortum IUD insertion did not increase the incidence of bleeding or pain.

The incidence of ectopic pregnancy among IUD users is not related to age, gravidity, race, socioeconomic status or prior induced abortion. However, prior infectious salpingitis, prior ectopic pregnancy and tubal reconstructive surgery predispose to ectopic pregnancy. The majority of ectopic pregnancies are tubal, but the proportion of ovarian pregnancies is higher than in the general population. The ectopic pregnancy rate is higher for Progestasert and lower for copper IUDs than it is for nonmedicated IUDs. Women who become pregnant with any type of IUD in situ are at a higher risk of ectopic pregnancy than those women who do not use an IUD and become pregnant. Unfortunately, some of the published data did not utilize life-table analysis, and the diagnosis of ectopic pregnancy was not confirmed by histological criteria. During early menstruation, pieces of the functional layer are shed. Extravasation of blood occurs in the superficial layers of the functional layer. The depth of this infiltration with blood increases with time and the vessels ending on the shedding area and in the extravasation zone are plugged by thrombi containing variable amounts of platelets and fibrin. The relative amount of fibrin and the degree of platelet degranulation increases with time. Few thrombi of platelets occur at the transition of the basal to the functional layer. During late menstruation, almost all functional endometrium is shed with no extravasation of blood or intravascular thrombi. Menstruation starts two days earlier in IUD wearers than in controls, with slowing down of the tissue shedding process together with a relatively diminished hemostatic reaction. Hemostatic plugs have hemostatic purposes and promote tissue shedding.

Device- induced dysfunctional bleeding involves: (1) increased menstrual blood loss, (2) intermenstrual bleeding (spotting) and, (3) prolonged duration of the menstrual period for 1-2 days. Blood loss increases after insertion of inert IUDs and copper IUDs, but decreases after insertion of progesterone IUDs. The blood loss, roughly the same one year after insertion as during the cycles closer to insertion, may cause discomfort and a negative iron balance. In Sweden, the upper tolerance limit of blood loss is 80 ml.

Increased blood loss in the IUD wearer seems to be due to increased fibrinolytic activity of the endometrium as a result of the presence of a urokinaselike plasminogen activator. The fibrinolytic activity of the endometrium, not related to the stage of the menstrual cycle, is apparent in cases of dysfunctional bleeding. The inhibition of fibrinolytic activity explains the reduction of menstrual loss with the use of the progesterone IUD. Inert and copper IUDs increase fibrinolytic activity at the superficial layer of the endometrium in contact with the device. The uterine fluid contains a proteolytic enzyme, probably an activator of plasminogen.

Progesterone-releasing IUDs give the endometrium a decidualike appearance, and do not cause any increase in fibrinolytic activity in the endometrium. Intermenstrual bleeding during the first cycles, with frequent gradual decrease, is very small and does not cause a negative iron balance. This dysfunctional bleeding is probably due to mechanical damage to the endometrium. Device-induced dysfunctional bleeding can be treated by oral administration of synthetic antifibrinolytic agents, that is, proteinase inhibitors: epsilon aminocapronic acid (EACA), tranexamic acid (AMCA) and aprotonin (Trasylol). The disadvantage of oral application of these inhibitors is the occurrence of unwarranted side effects due to the large quantities that have to be given.

V. ETHICAL AND LEGAL ASPECTS

Ethical aspects of IUDs should be considered in relation to religion, ethnic groups, cultural patterns, role of gynecologists, government regulations, family planning centres, marketing promotions, package inserts and prevention of teenage pregnancies. There are great variations among countries in the certification required for clinical trials, licensing for manufacture and marketing and regulations of labelling, advertising and sale of IUDs. Government regulation of IUDs affects the worldwide availability of these contraceptives. Different countries have different risk-benefit ratios and demographic considerations. The impact of developed countries' regulations may be expressed in several ways: (1) in delaying the process of research and development presently being undertaken, (2) in discouraging future research by individuals or corporations who feel the investment needed is not justified by the return, (3) in increasing the cost of contraceptives, and (4) in placing local administrators in the politically difficult position of using contraceptive products not approved by regulatory agencies in the developed world (Duncan 1979). Guidelines for marketing of IUDs include (1) manufacture and quality control, (2) toxicological testing, and (3) clinical evaluation of the device.

The ethical and legal aspects concerning the insertion of IUDs differ from the mere prescription or distribution of oral or other contraceptives since IUDs cannot be self-administered, and must be inserted by trained physicians and paramedical personnel. There are certain legal parameters which should be considered. Laws and regulations do not specifically regulate IUD insertions. However, historically, IUDs have been inserted primarily by trained physicians. In most countries the situation is merely ambiguous and there is no specific prohibition on IUD insertions by paramedical personnel. Many countries do not frown on nondoctor insertions, as long as those who do it are properly trained (Paxman and Cook 1979).

France in one of the few countries with a detailed law on the insertion of IUDs. Since 1967, IUDs may be inserted by a physician only in a hospital establishment, an approved treatment centre, or in conformity with conditions to be determined by public administrative regulations.

It is of interest to report that a thirty-year-old housewife in Denver, Colorado, was awarded a $6.8 million judgement when a jury found that a Dalkon Shield IUD brought about a miscarriage that nearly caused her death in 1973. This was the largest award in Denver's legal history and one of the largest personal injury awards ever, bringing to about $42 million, in approximately 2,400 cases, the claims made on the A.H. Robins Co. by women who suffered septic abortions while the device was in place. Robins, which marketed the Dalkon Shield, suspended its sales in mid-1974 at the request of the Federal Drug Administration when the association between the shield and the abortions, including several fatal to women, first became known. Attorneys for the drug company argued that factors other than the IUD could have caused the septic abortion. A gynecologist acknowledged under questioning by Robins's attorneys that he was uncertain whether the IUD was in place at the time of his patient's miscarriage. Some 480 Dalkon Shield cases were pending in various state and federal courts, and an additional 245 claims that had not yet resulted in litigation were being evaluated by the company. Regulations of marketing of new contraceptive delivery systems including medicated IUDs should cover clinical requirements, design, materials, drugs delivered and performance. Contraceptive devices are subject to varying degrees of legal constraint during manufacture and sale, ranging from full premarket review of the product and inspection of the manufacturing facilities by government agencies to merely buying a licence. Several aspects should be considered: informed consent prior to application and methods of documentation for later proof; legal influence on the physician of literature written on the subject generally as well as manufacturers' package inserts for both physician and patients; legal hazards at time of insertion as they relate to patient selection, applied technique of insertion and evaluation of suitable placement; advice and cautionary considerations during initial period after a successfull insertion and methods of documentation; legal exposure on a continuing basis during long-term usage, including evaluation of continuing proper placement, which should be considered when there is a pregnancy with a device in place; legal factors as they relate to proper time for removal; and imposition of standards on physicians – what the standards are and how compliance with such standards can be shown.

Several ethical and legal aspects should be considered in the consultant's relationship with the pharmaceutical industry dealing with contraceptive agents. Written agreements have to include detailed information on basic animal experimentation as well as anticipated clinical trials. A written research project should include its title, an abstract of the whole proposal; names, duties and responsibilities of principal and coprincipal investigators, technicians, postdoctoral associates, graduate students and secretarial help; and objectives of study, previous research on the subject, summary of progress conducted, tabular plan of experiments, rationale of experiments, specific aims, methods of procedure, equipment used, method of determination, experimental design, statistical analysis and significance of results.

REFERENCES

Duncan GW: Impact of regulations on availability. Presented at the symposium: Medicated IUDs and polymeric delivery systems, Amsterdam, 1979.

Frick-Bruder V: Psychological implications in current IUD studies. Presented at the symposium: Medicated IUDs and polymeric delivery systems, Amsterdam, 1979.

Hafez ESE, van Os WAA (eds): *IUD pathology and management*, Lancaster, MTP Press, 1980.

Kurz KH: Das Cavimeter. Presented at the symposium: Medicated IUDs and polymeric delivery systems, Amsterdam, 1979.

Koch UJ, Vogel M: Effects of ML Cu-250 on endometrium and sperm migration. Presented at the symposium: Medicated IUDs and polymeric delivery systems, Amsterdam, 1979.

Paxman J, Cook P: Law and planned parenthood. In: *Birth control: an international assessment*, Potts M, Bhiwandiwala P (eds), Lancaster, MTP Press, 1979.

Zipper J, Şegura R, Medel M, Torres L: Development of a new type of intrauterine contraceptive. In: New concepts in contraception, Potts M, Wood C (eds), Oxford: MTP Press, 1972.

27. INVENTORY OF QUESTIONS AND ANSWERS

E.S.E. Hafez, editor

I. The intrauterine device and uterine geometry

Drs. Beerthuizen, El-Badrawi, Hafez, Haspels, Hasson, van Os, Ros and Thiery

Q: (1) The surface area of inert IUDs must be proportional to that of the uterine lumen. What of the stainless steel Hall-Stone ring which, after all, covers only a tiny part of the endometrial surface? (2) Has it been proven that the expulsion rate is increased in women having a history of an incompetent os syndrome?
A: (1) Data on the use-effectiveness of the Hall-Stone stainless steel ring show a relatively high pregnancy rate and relatively low bleeding and pain.
(2) I have preliminary data collected through the use of the wing sound for the assessment of cervical competence in IUD users that show a greater tendency for IUD expulsion with an incompetent cervix. The number of cases. however, is not large enough to reach statistical significance. I am not aware of other studies on the subject.

Q: Do you really believe that the endometrial damage is responsible for the infection? Do you then agree that we should avoid stretching the projected uterine cavity with IUD models?
A: Yes I do.

Q: Do IUDs cause growth of the uterus? Do you change smaller IUDs for larger IUDs after three or six months?
A: The uterine cavity remains the same. However, the uterine weight increases, as has been shown in rats, therefore, an IUD may be used in patients with an infantile uterus for three months. We observed four pregnancies in these cases after removal of the IUD.

Q: The spring force, that is to say the lateral extension properties, of your device are rather strong in comparison to other devices. Have you ever tried to record the contractions caused by stirring the Caldeiro Barcia trigger points?
A: The lateral spring force is similar to that of the copper-T lateral arms when they are bent. Dysmenorrheic women fitted with No-Gravid have less algomenorrhea after insertion.

Q: Are you not afraid of damaging the ostium of the tubes with the Cu-V with consequences to subsequent fertility?
A: After the use of this IUD the fertility is equal to that in a normal woman (see Ros et al. 1979).
Q: In the radiographic slide, how could you be sure that the different shape you found was due to an abnormal position of the uterine cavity with the X-ray projector and not due to the IUD?

A: The hysterosalpingography was performed under X-ray scope and the uterine cavity was filled slowly; it was always easy to see the geometry of the IUD in the uterine cavity.

II. Copper intrauterine devices

Dr. Agoestina, Barwin, Bromwich, Delbeke Jarvela, van Kets, Kosonen, Nohlen, van Os, Peer Hoevik, Ros, Smith and Wilson

Q: Do you have any experience on the fertility pattern in your multiparous women after they used the IUD as compared with the nulliparous women who have not used IUDs?
A: Our experience has been that there is no difference in the pregnancy rates with either of the IUDs. There is no increase in the tubal factor in infertility, probably as a result of stringent rules regarding: (1)

observing the contraindications, and (2) removing the IUD at the first signs of infection. This however, will require long-term follow-up.

Q: What is the basis for advocating routine antibiotic coverage when withdrawing an IUD?
A: You cannot be too careful to avoid tubo-ovarial abscesses. Those patients who developed a tubo-ovarian abscess following removal of an IUD elected sterilization.

Q: What happens when the sliver core of the Nova-T is exposed within the uterine environment, as the copper covering the core corrodes and disintegrates, in terms of reactivity and contraceptive effect.
A: There is dissolution of silver, consequently when the copper is dissolved the IUD behaves like an inert one.

Q: Explain precisely the two methods you use to insert the IUDs.
A: The push-in technique which gave the worst results uses the insertion tube to push in the IUD without bending the arms, that is, without 'loading' the device in the tube, the plunger is not used. The retraction method, as described by Tatum requires bending the arms in the tube and introducing it in the uterus up to the fundus, after which the outer tube is retracted over the plunger, thereby ejecting the device.

Q: Why do you apparently not apply intracervical or paracervical block analgesis when IUD insertion (or sounding of the uterus) is difficult or painful?
A: At the time of this study, we did not consider it necessary. The three cases of syncope occurred within two weeks toward the end of the study; this made us begin to use an intracervical block.

Q: What is your definition of pelvic inflammatory disease?
A: Endometritis, salpingitis or tubo-ovarian infection. However PID is a clinical state which should be treated early and the accuracy of this clinical diagnosis is poor.

Q: (1) Does the copper ion produce negative effects on the embryo or fetus?
(2) Could you please explain the reason for the increasing percentage reporting bleeding or pain after the first year of use?
A: (1) With the potential danger of intrauterine infection in mind our policy is to remove the IUD as soon as pregnancy is proven by radioimmunoassay and providing no ill effect on the fetus has been found. Chromosome cultures were normal in all cases. If the pregnancy is too far advanced, abortion for medical reasons is a possibility.
(2) Removal for bleeding and pain increases for a human reason rather than a medical reason. A number of women are willing to give the IUD a try, but after bleeding for over one year they just have had enough of it.

Q: Was each of the patients followed up for 36 months?
A: I regret to say, no. Our oldest insertions were performed four years ago and these people have already been fitted with a new IUD, but this study also includes women who have had their IUD only for one year. But we continue.

Q: Have you compared the average copper release (μg/day) between surface areas of 200 and 250 mm^2. The Population Council reports less release with 300 mm^2 than with 200 mm^2 because the active surface area is smaller when the winding is tight.
A: No studies have been done on this subject.

Q: How many times, in nulliparous women, has the lower extremity of the IUD been contained in the endocervical canal?
A: Our computer program reads these as 'expulsions' in a personal series of 300 ML Cu over 6,600 cycles. I have seen four partial expulsions in nulliparous women.

Q: How do you choose the particular type of Multiload to use? What parameters govern the use of each particular size?
A: Our study is made exclusively with one type of IUD, the standard size ML Cu-250. The small Multiload was developed for small uterine cavities, whatever that may mean and however one is going to determine this. The short Multiload was designed when the sounding of the uterus gave a depth of less than 6 cm. I see some use for this last one, but personally I do not feel a great need for size changes in the large majority of cases.

Q: In how many cases (percent) did you have to give up insertion, in (1) nulliparous and (2) in

parous women (because of pain, narrow cervix, and so on)?
A: The computer program does not list the 'giving up' when encountering difficulties. I must limit my answer to my own experience of about 300 insertions and some 6,600 cycles of use. I recorded eight nullipara in which I preferred not to insist; I do not report any parous women.

Q: Your data shows a higher expulsion rate in older and nulliparous women. What is your explanation for this fact?
A: My answer to this is purely tentative. In nulliparous women it appears to me that the size of the uterine cavity and the tonus of the myometrium is involved. In older women we find a number of multiparae with a possibly damaged cervix or developing myomata.

Q: In some IUDs of the 'sleeve' type (Cu-T220C) all the copper metal appears to be covered with a deposit. By what mechanism do you suppose copper is still released?
A: Copper diffuses through the deposit.

Q: On what is based your contention that there is no correlation between coating (calcium carbonate) of the copper surface and the rate of copper release?
A: Because the calcium carbonate is not present in every device removed from patients, we have not had sufficient material to indicate that there is a correlation between the thickness of calcium carbonate and the corrosion. There have been some cases with heavy calcium deposit where the corrosion has been smaller than expected. However, the copper release in those cases has been sufficient for those patients because they have not had any pregnancies. Further, we have examined IUDs removed from patients which have had a pregnancy and have not found any calcium carbonate deposit to them. The conclusion is that the calcium carbonate may reduce the copper release, but it is better to suggest that the dissolving medium in those cases is not capable of dissolving more copper than has been corroded.

Q: Does corrosion increase the surface area of ionizable copper?
A: The corrosion causes a rough surface on the metal; thereby, at least in the beginning, the surface area is increased. At the same time, however, the corrosion products and deposit cover the surface, increasing the length of the path the copper atoms have to pass along to be diffused through consequently reducing the dissolution. At the later stage of use the diameter of the wire is also reduced and the total surface area is correspondingly decreased.

Q: How were IUDs randomly inserted?
A: By random number tables.

Q: Did you see any effect of surface area of copper on pregnancy rate?
A: The pregnancy rate and the surface of copper are still to be ascertained. It is too early to tell, as this is a preliminary study.

Q: You found no difference between ML Cu 375 and Cu-7 at one year in either multiparae or nulliparae, however, your results are exceptionally good. The questions are (1) What was the age distribution? (2) What was the follow-up rate at one year? and (3) Type of women? Private practice?
A: (1) Age distribution: 16-32 years of age; (2) eighty percent in multiparae and eighty percent in nulliparae and (3) both clinic and private practice in Ottawa. The major difference is in the expulsion rate.

Q: Is it possible that localized impurities in the wire or surface contamination of faults (for example scratches or nicks) may provide centres of more rapid corrosion?
A: Such particles of foreign material normally initiate corrosion. However, in wire production such particles cannot be formed and mechanical faults like scratches have no effect on the corrosion.

Q: Does the silver case of your IUD influence the Pearl index? If so, how?
A: Because the silver is practically insoluble, it has no chemical effect like copper and when after long use age the silver is visible, it has the same effect as an inert IUD with a rough surface; in short the silver has no effect on pregnancy rate.

III. PROGESTERONE-RELEASING INTRAUTERINE DEVICES

Aznar, Bonnar, Hafez, Hanita, Lincoln, Ludwig, Drs. Mack, Massouras, Nilsson, van Os, Rybo, Sapire, Scommegna, Spornitz and Thiery

Q: Does the relatively high expulsion rate of the Progestasert have anything to do with the Progesterone effect on the model, which needs greater lateral extension properties to stay in situ?
A: I am not aware of the fact that progesterone-T has a high expulsion rate. The expulsion rate of the progesterone IUD has been reported by various investigators to be between three and seven percent, which compares favourably with the expulsion experience obtained with other IUDs, whether medicated or unmedicated (Population Reports 1979). I have no personal experience with the Multiload Cu-250, whose expulsion rate has been reported to be lower. However, we must remember that there is likely to be a greater variation in event rates among different clinics using the same IUD than among different types of IUDs in the same clinic.

Q: Were ovulation cycles documented in women for several months before progesterone IUD placement? Were they documented with the same accuracy employed after the insertion of the progesterone IUD?
A: Yes, they were documented by determination of serum concentration of FSH, LH prostaglandin-E_2 and progesterone in the pretreatment cycle from 5-8 samples taken from the same patients.

Q: How would you delineate the indications for progesterone IUDs?
A: We recommend the Progestasert IUD mainly for women suffering from dysmenorrhea and hypermenorrhea and also for the rare cases of women who are allergic to copper.

Q: Could you compare the endometrial effects of the Progestasert with that of luteal supplementation (mini-pill)?
A: (1) Under the mini-pill the effects on the glandular cells are much more pronounced than the effects on the stromal cells.
(2) The mini-pill acts in such a way that during the first 4-5 months glandular secretory activity is strongly enhanced. After this period we find the glandular epithelium to be irregularly secretory.
(3) There is no true decidual transformation in the mini-pill endometrium but there is a moderate predecidual reaction.
(4) Under the lynestrenol treatment (Exlutona 0.5 mg/day) nucleolar channel system (NCS) formation is suppressed completely, even though we have a rate of over eighty percent of ovulatory cycles in our patients. This is particularly important because NCS formation is believed to be dependent on ovulation having occurred.

Q: As the WHO task force proved five years ago that retroprogesterone had no contraceptive action in women if given orally, why use retroprogesterone instead of norgestrel or lynestrenol?
A: The study reported today was completed a few years before. The findings of WHO were not known to us. However, oral administration of a steroid is not equal to its local release. Oral administration subjects the steroid to first-pass liver metabolism, which may inactivate the steroid. Progesterone, for instance, is very active on the endometrium when released locally but it is inactive when given by mouth because of the liver metabolism. Norgestrel or lynestrenol may be a better choice but, although requested, these steroids were not made available to us by the manufacturers.

Q: The Progestasert was associated with a high ectopic rate in the original figures published by the Alza Corporation; this was about four times more common than that expected with an IUD. Have other studies shown different figures? Were any of the pregnancies ectopic with the norgestrel device?
A: At the present we have experience from over 4000 woman-months of use of the levonorgestrel-releasing IUD. No intrauterine nor extrauterine pregnancies have yet occurred.

Q: What was the infection, mortality and morbidity rate?
A: The rates were: infection 1.15 and perforation 0.7. No deaths were recorded.

Q: What is your experience of intermenstrual bleeding in women using the norgestrel IUD?
A: See Figure 1 and Figure 2.

Q: Is there any effect on lactation?
A: I am not aware of any effect of intrauterine progesterone on lactation per se. Recently Spellacy et al. (1978) reported an increase in plasma prolactin in women wearing progesterone IUDs. However, in a more critical prospective study this could not be confirmed (Spellacy and Buhi 1979). In any case, even if prolactin levels were increased, this would

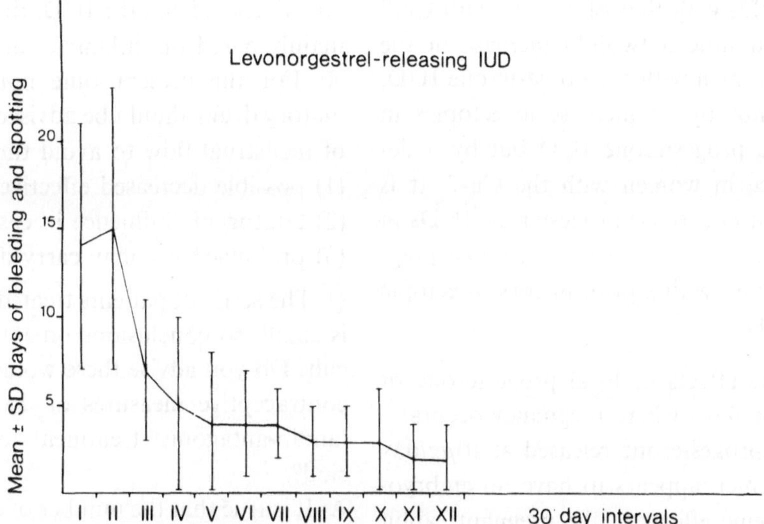

Figure 1. Means and standard deviations of total number of bleeding an spotting days during twelve postinsertional consecutive thirty day periods of thirteen volunteers using a levonorgestrel-releasing intrauterine device.

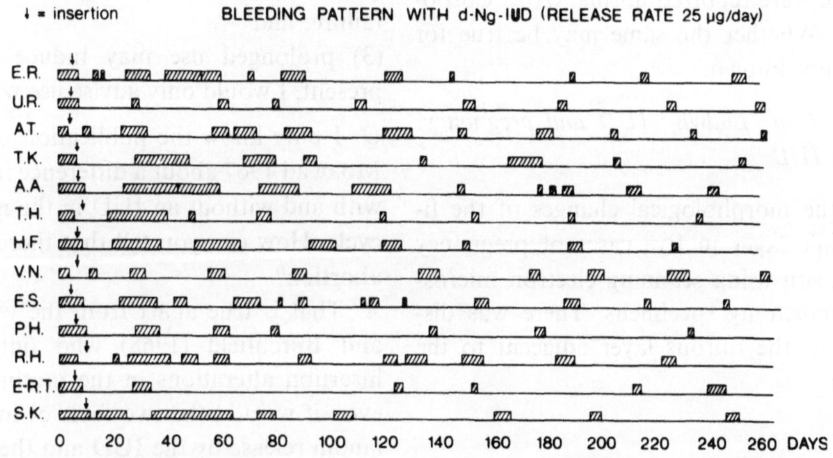

Figure 2. Bleeding pattern during the first 270 days after insertion of a levonorgestrel-releasing intrauterine device. The hatched rectangles denote bleeding, not distinguishing between bleeding and spotting.

not have a significant effect on established lactation. The amount of progesterone released by the IUD (60 μg per day) is too small to have any direct effect on the breast or on its milk production.

Q: No mention has been made of incidence of ectopic pregnancies with the progesterone IUD, but the reported high incidence of ectopic pregnancies has caused discontinuation of use of these devices in the United Kingdom. Could you comment please.

A: We have just completed a case control study relating to the risk of extrauterine pregnancies to various contraceptive techniques. The relative risk of ectopic pregnancy in women wearing a progesterone IUD was found to be 1.3. We can conclude that use of a progesterone IUD does not significantly affect the incidence of ectopic pregnancy. However, women wearing Cu-7 IUDs had a calculated relative risk of 0.6. If, therefore, we compare the ectopic pregnancy incidence of women with progesterone IUDs with that of women with Cu-7 IUDs, we would note a twofold increase in the ectopic rate of women with the progesterone IUD. This is caused not by an increase in ectopics in women with the progesterone IUD but by a decreased incidence in women with the Cu-7. It is therefore prudent not to use progesterone IUDs in women who have a higher risk for ectopic pregnancy, that is, those with a prior history of ectopic pregnancy or PID.

Q: What are the effects of local progesterone or norgestrel on the fetus where pregnancy occurs?
A: Intrauterine progesterone released at 10μg/day in the uterine lumen appears to have no embryotoxic or teratogenic effects in the pregnant rabbit nor is it detrimental to the general well-being of the developing embryo or neonate (Hudson et al. 1978). In humans, the physical examinations at 1-17 months of age of all infants known to have been exposed to an intrauterine progesterone contraceptive system were reported normal (Alza Corporation 1976). Whether the same may be true for norgestrel is not known.

Comment by Prof. Ludwig: IUD and pregnancy: dislocation of IUD

We studied the morphological changes of the fibrous chorionic layer in five cases of pregnancy with IUD in situ using scanning electron microscopy or hysterectomy specimens. There was disorganization of the fibrous layer adjacent to the device in situ.

IV. DEVICE PHYSIOLOGY

Dr. Abdalla, Aref, Hafez, Hall, Honmon, Kandil, van Kets, Lopez de la Osa, Ludwig, van Os, Sapire, Schijf, Thiery, Toppozada and Wolf

Q: As you showed the mode of action to be linked to prostaglandins, did you find in your study, using antiprostaglandins, that the pregnancy rate was raised?
A: The number was too small, and treatment was only given during menses so that the hazard of failure could be avoided.

Q: If you use anti-inflammatory treatment (indomethacin) against pain, do you not fear a lack of effectiveness from the IUD, the activity of which is mainly based on inflammation?
A: For the present time nonsteroid ant-inflammatory drugs should be advised only with the onset of menstrual flow to avoid three problems:
(1) possible decreased effectiveness,
(2) teratogenic influence in case of failure, and
(3) prolonged use may carry dry side effects.

Q: The series of patients treated with Indomethacin is small, so conclusions on IUD failures are difficult. Do you advise these women to use additional contraceptive measures or do you limit prostaglandin-antagonist treatment to the menstrual period?
A: It is true that the number of cases we treated was small. However, the treatment was only started with the onset of flow in order to avoid:
(1) possible decrease in contraceptive protection in case prostaglandins are involved in the mechanism of action,
(2) the hazard of a teratogenic influence in case of failure, and
(3) prolonged use may induce side effects. At present, I would only advise use with onset of flow.

Q: I only know the publication of Bengtsson and Moawad 1967 about a difference in uterine motility with and without an IUD in the normal ovulatory cycle. How can you tell that there will be an early abortion?
A: That is true apart from the work of Behrman and Burchfield (1968) who only showed post-insertion alterations in the uterine activity. However, if we add the two facts of increased prostaglandin release by the IUD and the known effect of prostaglandins on uterine activity one can reach such a conclusion. Also, recent evidence has shown that the recording systems may impose problems in interpretation and new systems may clarify existing controversies.

Q: (1) Will you please comment in short on the method used in the determination of prostaglandins produced by animal uteri?
(2) Do you suppose that there exist species-dependent variations, say between animals and humans, in the type or amount of prostaglandin release?
(3) What is the dosage dependency of the effect of anti-inflammatory drugs on prostaglandin release in animals or humans?

A: (1) Various methods have been used in animal studies; the most popular was radioimmunoassay. However, prostaglandin measurements is a complicated and difficult issue and false data can be easily achieved since tissue manipulation or even needle puncture of a vein can release a considerable amount of prostaglandins; our measurements simply reflect a tissue's ability to synthesize rather than actual levels of prostaglandins. It is a better policy to measure metabolites, especially by gas-mass methods.
(2) I certainly believe there is species variation, particularly in view of available data on other aspects such as luteolyis.
(3) This is difficult to answer since I know little about animal prostaglandin synthetase an sensitivity to anti-inflammatory drugs. I therefore do not know.

Q: What dosage regime of indomethacin was used?
A: The used dosage was 25-mg oral capsules with meals, 3-4 times a day. The majority received the higher dose level since a 75 mg dose may block prostaglandin synthesis incompletely.

Q: Do you think the hormonal changes you have shown could account for the clinical impression I have that the premenstrual syndrome is produced or increased in some women using IUDs? I have noted mood changes, particularly increased irritability, breast tenderness, bloating and weight gain premenstrually in patients who have not previously experienced these symptoms or have done so only mildly in the past. These symptoms have been the reason for requesting removal of a device; they improved after removal. The Lippes C, Saf-T-Coil, Gravigard and Orthogyroad-T were involved.
A: Premenstrual syndrome is directly related to hormonal changes in the non-IUD user. Correlation of psychological behaviour and hormonal levels was demonstrated recently by Abdalla et al. (1978a). We have no data on clinical or endocrine aspects of premenstrual syndrome in IUD users.

Q: Do you have any explanation for the higher testosterone level in IUD users? Did you assay prolactin?
A: This endocrine change may result from increase in prostaglandin secretion in IUD users. The effect of prostaglandin injection on the serum level of estradiol, progesterone, testosterone, FSH and LH was clearly demonstrated in both follicular and luteal phases by Abdalla et al. (1978b). The changes in testosterone levels in IUD users may be due to an alteration in the peripheral conversion of one circulating hormone into another. We did not assay prolactin.

Q: McRorie and his group have some preliminary data on the interfering effect of copper and zinc on the proacrosine process. Since you show a rise in copper levels could you comment on this possible anticapacitation effect?
A: I am sorry I do not have this at the present time.

Q: Does the indwelling intrauterine tip catheter work as a device itself?
A: It is possible, but the longest time the open-end catheter was in situ was four hours. We have never measured the prostaglandin levels. In obstetrics a known intrauterine catheter gives better contractions without oxytocin infusion.

Q: Is there any biochemical change in the cervical mucus which would explain the difference of motility with sperm mucus?
A: No.

Q: You have been inserting the ML without copper. Do you have data on the pregnancy rate with this device?
A: We have carried out fifty insertions and we stopped since we had some pregnancies.

V. CLINICAL PARAMETERS FOR THE USE OF INTRAUTER,INE DEVICES

Drs. Batar, Duncan, Hafez, Hamilton, Huber, van Os, Stryker and van Wering

Q: (1) To what were your patients addicted?
(2) Do you have data on alcoholic addicts?
A: Street heroin, poly-drugs and alcohol: usually all three. We have only a few patients who are using only on addictive drug. The pure alcoholics number about 3-5 percent.

Q: Is it correct what your last slide shows that the longer the use of an IUD, the less premature and immature delivery.
A: The frequency of immature and premature

deliveries was in inverse ratio to the duration of IUD use: the longer the wearing period, the lower the rate of immaturity and prematurity. The correlation was strongly negative, yet statistically significant, at the 0.05 level. Because this analysis evaluated the premature and immature deliveries together (gestational age was 29-37 weeks), I could not tell you how the premature deliveries changed separately parallel to IUD use within the group.

Q: Would it be reasonable to develop a list of patient characteristics (physical, medical, social) that could be used to select or reject individuals for (1) IUD use? (2) for use of a particular IUD if they meet the criteria for general IUD use? Do you feel a general consensus among physicians can be developed for support of these selection criteria?
A: No answer.

VI. CLINICAL TRIALS TO EVALUATE DEVICE PERFORMANCE

M. Thiery

The minimal requirements should be
1. To apply life-table analysis for calculating event rates (Tietze);
1. To provide a statistical background to allow interpretation of event rates (for example to add confidential limits at the 95-percent level, standard deviation or standard error);
3. To use a randomized setup when comparing the performance of various IUD models;
4. Because pertinent event rates are usually small, the volume of the material under study, both the number of IUD acceptors and the number of women months of experience, should be sufficiently great to allow valid conclusions to be drawn.

REFERENCES

Abdalla MI, Ibrahim II, Elwan O, Taher H, Taher Y: Serum progesterone in female patients with neurotic depression. Arab J Lab Med 4 : 244-251, 1978a.

Abdalla MI, Ibrahim II, Osman MI: Effect of prostaglandin-E_2 derivative (Sulprosterone) on the pituitary-ovarian function in nonpregnant females. Presented at the International Sulprosterone symposium, Vienna, 1978b.

Alza Corporation: The Progestasert: a monograph. Palo Alto, Alza Corporation, 1976.

Behrman SJ, Burehfield W: The intrauterine contraceptive device and myometrial activity. Am J Obstet Gynecol 100 : 194, 1968.

Bentsson LP, Moawad AH: The effect of the Lippes Loop on human myometrial activity. Am J Obstet Gynecol 98 : 951, 1967.

Hudson R: Contraception 17 : 489, 1978.

Population Reports: Intrauterine devices. Popul Rep [2] d, May 1979.

Ros Burine, Duval, Aviband: Contraccezione Fertilità Sessualità 1979.

Spellacy W: Contraception 17 ; 71, 1978.

Spellacy W, Buhi WC: Contraception 19 : 91, 1979.

INDEX*

* t = table, f = figure